The
Medical Device
R&D
Handbook

The Medical Device R&D Handbook

Theodore R. Kucklick

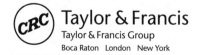
Taylor & Francis
Taylor & Francis Group
Boca Raton   London   New York

A CRC title, part of the Taylor & Francis imprint, a member of the
Taylor & Francis Group, the academic division of T&F Informa plc.

ST. PHILIP'S COLLEGE LIBRARY

None of the companies mentioned in this book have sponsored or otherwise paid for placement or mention in this book.

Published in 2006 by
CRC Press
Taylor & Francis Group
6000 Broken Sound Parkway NW, Suite 300
Boca Raton, FL 33487-2742

© 2006 by Taylor & Francis Group, LLC
CRC Press is an imprint of Taylor & Francis Group

No claim to original U.S. Government works
Printed in the United States of America on acid-free paper
10 9 8 7 6 5 4 3 2 1

International Standard Book Number-10: 0-8493-2717-2 (Hardcover)
International Standard Book Number-13: 978-0-8493-2717-9 (Hardcover)
Library of Congress Card Number 2005049422

This book contains information obtained from authentic and highly regarded sources. Reprinted material is quoted with permission, and sources are indicated. A wide variety of references are listed. Reasonable efforts have been made to publish reliable data and information, but the author and the publisher cannot assume responsibility for the validity of all materials or for the consequences of their use.

No part of this book may be reprinted, reproduced, transmitted, or utilized in any form by any electronic, mechanical, or other means, now known or hereafter invented, including photocopying, microfilming, and recording, or in any information storage or retrieval system, without written permission from the publishers.

For permission to photocopy or use material electronically from this work, please access www.copyright.com (http://www.copyright.com/) or contact the Copyright Clearance Center, Inc. (CCC) 222 Rosewood Drive, Danvers, MA 01923, 978-750-8400. CCC is a not-for-profit organization that provides licenses and registration for a variety of users. For organizations that have been granted a photocopy license by the CCC, a separate system of payment has been arranged.

Trademark Notice: Product or corporate names may be trademarks or registered trademarks, and are used only for identification and explanation without intent to infringe.

Library of Congress Cataloging-in-Publication Data

The medical device R & D handbook / edited by Theodore R. Kucklick.
    p. ; cm.
Includes bibliographical references and index.
ISBN 0-8493-2717-2
1. Medical instruments and apparatus--Design and construction--Handbooks, manuals, etc. I. Title: Medical device R and D handbook. II. Kucklick, Theodore R.
  [DNLM: 1. Biomedical Technology--Interview. 2. Entrepreneurship--Interview. 3. Equipment Design--methods--Interview. 4. Research--methods--Interview. W 82 M4883 2005]

R856.15.M43 2005
610'.28--dc22

2005049422

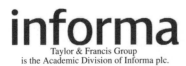

Taylor & Francis Group
is the Academic Division of Informa plc.

Visit the Taylor & Francis Web site at
http://www.taylorandfrancis.com

and the CRC Press Web site at
http://www.crcpress.com

ABOUT THIS BOOK

The Medical Device R&D (Research and Development) Handbook is the fruition of a personal desire to see some of the practical information on how to develop medical devices compiled in one place. I wanted to write a book that I wish had been available when I first started in medical device design.

This book contains three main threads. The first thread is practical. There are many excellent books that give in depth theory on specialized medical and technology subjects in medical device engineering, but not a general practical how-to manual. This part of the book seeks to serve that need.

There is a great deal of practical skill, developed by very intelligent and clever people, to be found in specialized areas of the medical device industry. Having worked for a succession of medical device start-up companies, each new area seemed to have its own fund of "tribal knowledge" that, for various reasons, did not seem to percolate much out of the tribe. Working for start-ups and developing products for different medical specialties was somewhat like joining a succession of guilds. There is also little cross-over between certain fields such as engineering and medical illustration. One of the goals of this book is to collect some of the knowledge of these practical skills, such as medical device prototyping, plastics selection, and catheter construction and make them more readily accessible to the hands-on designer. The skills may be well known to those who work in a specialized area, but not as well known to those outside that specialty. Some of this information is usually learned "on the job" if you happen to have that kind of a job. This book brings you this type of information. Having knowledge of these practical skills can allow the designer to combine and apply these specialized techniques in new and innovative ways, and save valuable time.

Another thread is entrepreneurial. This book contains interviews with some of the top leaders in the medical device industry. These are people who know by experience how to develop innovative new medical technology and how to start and grow successful companies. Each of them was unfailingly gracious and exceptionally generous with their time and insight, and they have my enduring gratitude for allowing me to interview them and pester them with my questions. Hearing them share their knowledge, experience, and wisdom has been one of the most enjoyable aspects of producing this book. The insights shared represent decades of distilled top-level experience. These are people that have helped build some of the most successful companies and key technologies in the medical device industry. They share what works, and what doesn't. These interviews are valuable resources that will reward the reader with fresh insights as they are read, and re-read. Where available, there are lists of additional material and resources on these individuals. This section will be of special interest to the designer with an idea for an innovative technology, the student, and the physician-entrepreneur.

Yet another thread in this book is historical. In my experience I am sometimes asked to design a product that is similar to or is inspired by a device already in use. Early on, I remember an incident, where one of our scientific advisors suggested that we look at a Veress needle for ideas on how to solve a design problem. Once that suggestion had been made, and he left, we looked at each other, and asked one another "what is a Veress needle?" Being new and green, I did not know, but the engineering managers in this medical device company did not know either. With apologies to Santayana, "Those who do not know history are condemned to reinvent the wheel." In the technical chapters I have made an effort to dig out the historical background of various technologies, and put them in a useful context. In the chapters on needles and catheters, for example, I have compiled glossaries with detailed historical footnotes. This will help the R&D engineer understand how certain devices developed and for what purpose.

In this thread you meet fascinating personalities — often people solving a problem just like you —who, through hands-on development, arrived at important solutions. People like Harvey, Veress, Luer, Forssmann, Sones, Tuohy, Dotter, Gruentzig, Fogarty, Foley, and numerous others who solved important clinical problems are recognized today for their groundbreaking contributions. It is important, as a medical device designer, to know these personalities, what they developed, and why, how they sometimes collaborated, and some of the technical challenges and institutional barriers they overcame to succeed.

Finally, the introductory chapter is on the subject of innovation and how it applies to medical device technology in particular and explores a useful framework for approaching the subject of creativity, invention, and innovation.

Taken together, this book helps give the working engineer, manager, technician, designer entrepreneur, or student some of the tools to more quickly and efficiently develop innovative medical devices, and to see their role in a larger business and societal context. This book covers a fair bit of ground; however, it is only a start. Examples of subjects not covered are patents, the role of industrial design in medical device development, adhesives, catheter tubing extrusion, operating room procedures and protocol, new company formation, and how and where to raise start-up capital among many other important topics. These areas are all as equally important to medical device design and development as the material already covered. These topics and several more are planned for future volumes. This book has also been designed with sufficiently wide margins to add your own notes, and to turn this into your own customized handbook.

The help, support, and encouragement of the many contributors, reviewers, and collaborators involved in this project are gratefully acknowledged, as well as those people those who have provided the opportunities and mentoring I needed to work in diverse areas of this endlessly fascinating medical device industry.

One resource especially useful in researching this book is the PubMed database of the National Institutes of Health (NIH), National Center for Biotechnology Information (NCBI), and the National Library of Medicine (http://www.ncbi.nlm.nih.gov/). Hundreds of medical journals and thousands of article abstracts are easily searchable with this resource, for free. PubMed has to be one of the better uses of taxpayer money and is an essential research tool for the medical device designer.

I would also like to acknowledge Taylor & Francis for its interest and support in publishing this title, as well as all of the work and support of the Taylor & Francis staff and editors.

This is the beginning of what is intended to be a work in progress and designed to be responsive to the needs and input of you, the reader. Your suggestions for future topics are welcome. Please email suggestions, feedback and questions to: editor@meddevbook.com

Ted Kucklick
Los Gatos, California

THE EDITOR

Ted Kucklick has extensive experience in the hands-on design and commercial development of medical devices, including radio frequency ablation devices, microwave catheters for minimally invasive therapy, in-home diagnostics devices, surgical closure devices, battery-powered devices, disposables, gene therapy manufacturing equipment, and general surgery tools. Ted has been involved in the early stages and development and productization of devices for companies such as Vidamed, Oratec, Neomend, Somnus, Curon, Starion Instruments, Sleep Solutions, RITA Medical, AfX (now Guidant), and Cannuflow. He is the former senior designer for RITA Medical Systems and Advanced Closure Systems (now Neomend). Ted is currently the cofounder, vice president of engineering, and CTO for Cannuflow, Inc., an arthroscopic instrument start-up company, and design director for TRKD Medical Device R&D, a medical device design and development company. Ted has a bachelor's degree in product design and is the inventor of several issued and pending patents; he is a member of the IEEE/Engineering in Medicine and Biology Society, the Industrial Designers Society of America, and the Association of Medical Illustrators. Ted is also a founding member of the Keiritsu Forum angel investment group of Silicon Valley; a graduate of the University of California, Berkeley Haas School of Business Bio-Entrepreneurship certificate program; and a member of the Eureka Medical advisory board.

CONTRIBUTORS

James Swick, D.V.M.
Lychron LLC
Mountain View, California

Thom Wehman, Ph.D.
Cupertino, California

CONTENTS

1 **Invention, Innovation, and Creativity** 1
  Ted Kucklick

2 **Introduction to Medical Plastics** 19
  Ted Kucklick

3 **Catheter-Forming Equipment and Operations** 51
  Ted Kucklick

4 **Basics of Catheter Assembly** 67
  Ted Kucklick

5 **Introduction to Needles and Cannulae** 89
  Ted Kucklick

6 **Rapid Prototyping for Medical Devices** 113
  Ted Kucklick

7 **Reverse Engineering in Medical Device Design** 161
  Ted Kucklick

8 **Using Medical Illustration in Medical Device R&D** 193
  Ted Kucklick

9 **Brief Introduction to Preclinical Research** 217
  James Swick

10 **Regulatory Affairs: Medical Devices** 223
   Thom Wehman

11 **Introduction to Biocompatibility Testing** 267

Interview with Thomas Fogarty, M.D. 295

Interview with Paul Yock, M.D. 305

Interview with Dane Miller, Ph.D. 313
Interview with Ingemar Lundquist 321
Interview with J. Casey McGlynn 325
Index 341

1

INVENTION, INNOVATION, AND CREATIVITY

Or How Thomas Edison Never Changed the World by Creating the Light Bulb

Ted Kucklick

CONTENTS

Science and Discovery 4
Art and Design 6
Finding the Need 9

Thomas Edison is perhaps the best-known inventor of all time. Edison also embodies many of the popular myths and misconceptions of invention and the invention process. If you ask the average person, "Did Edison change the world by creating the first light bulb?" he or she would probably agree, even though this statement is not correct. Examining this statement provides a convenient framework for discussing some of the misconceptions and challenges in understanding innovation, and how it relates to developing clinically useful medical device technology.

In medical device R&D what are we setting out to accomplish? We are seeking practical solutions to clinical problems — solutions with clinical utility. This seeking will involve several unsuccessful attempts before a solution is found. Once that solution is found, it then needs to be turned into a solution that is safe, effective, reliable, repeatable, scalable, and profitable.

From a business point of view it helps if the solution is unique and patentable, so that a company can charge enough for this solution to recoup the cost of finding it, developing it, testing it, and protecting it, and still have enough left to pay a return to the investors who put up the money to make it possible — and maybe a little left over for you, the innovator.

The purpose of this chapter is to give you a practical way to look at invention and innovation, and to try to remove some of the confusion over terms. If terms are defined, it becomes possible to think clearly and logically. If you can define and understand the innovation process better, this will help you to be a better innovator.

One source of misunderstanding comes from the common use of terms that are not quite accurate. Another comes from different compartmentalized specialties using similar terms to describe different things, or different terms for the same things.

> Vague and insignificant forms of speech, and abuse of language have so long passed for mysteries of science; and hard and misapplied words, with little or no meaning, have, by prescription, such a right to be mistaken for deep learning and height of speculation, that it will not be easy to persuade either those who speak or those who hear them, that they are but the covers of ignorance, and hindrance of true knowledge.
>
> **—John Locke,** ***English: An Essay Concerning Human Understanding*** **(1690)**

Let us start with a few dictionary definitions (from the *Oxford Universal Dictionary*, 1955 edition):

Invent: From the Latin *invenire*, to come upon, find, or discover. To find out in the way of original contrivance, to devise first a new method or instrument, to find out or produce by mental activity, to find out how to do something.

Innovate: From the Latin *innovare*, to make new. To change into something new, to alter, to renew, to introduce novelties, to make changes in something established, a new shoot at the end of a branch.

Create: From the Latin *creare*. To bring into being, cause to exist. To form out of nothing, to call into existence.

We see from these definitions that the emphasis of invention is discovery. The emphasis of innovation is change.

Here we have a basic conflict between the terms *invent* and *create*. To invent and innovate requires that you start with something to be able to put it into a new form. To create means you start with nothing. As

Thomas Edison once said, "To invent, you need good imagination and a pile of junk."

If Edison had not had his pile of junk to start with, he would not have been able to get anything done. Artists talk all the time about creating a work or being creative, yet we know this is not literally true. An artist, inventor, or innovator may be the first human being to put certain preexisting elements into a form that another human being has not done before, make a discovery that another human being has not made, or produce a solution to a problem, but this is very different from calling something into existence from nothing. God creates from nothing. People form and make from that which exists, whether physical objects and forces or from abstract mental processes.

> I invent nothing, I rediscover.
>
> —**Auguste Rodin**

> An inventor is a person who makes an ingenious arrangement of wheels, levers and springs, and believes it civilization.
>
> —**Ambrose Bierce,** *The Devil's Dictionary*

The more raw material we have to work with, the better methods we have, and the more focused energy we put into it, the more practical skill, the more times we can try new things, iterate and fail intelligently, the better our opportunity for success at invention.

In the heroic treatment, historical change is shown to have been generated by the genius of individuals, conveniently labeled "inventors." In such a treatment Edison invented the electric light, Bell the telephone, Gutenberg the printing press, Watt the steam engine, and so on. But no individual is responsible for producing an invention "*ex nihilo.*" The elevation of the single inventor to the position of sole creator at best exaggerates his influence over events, and at worst denies the involvement of those humbler members of society without whose work his task might have been impossible.[1]

---

[1] Burke, James, *The Day the Universe Changed*, Little, Brown & Co., Boston, 1985.

The other part of the Edison story most people know is how many thousands of unsuccessful attempts were made before a reliable light bulb was produced. The process of trying many different approaches in a systematic way with a clear goal in mind is an essential ingredient in producing innovation.

> Failure is the preamble to success.
>
> —**Thomas J. Fogarty, M.D.**

Design is a stepwise iterative process. Design starts with a need, and then applies technology until the need is solved in the best way possible given the time, resources, talents, and specifications available. This is the way medical device development usually occurs.

> An inventor is simply a person who doesn't take his education too seriously. You see, from the time a person is six years old until he graduates from college he has to take three or four examinations a year. If he flunks once, he is out. But an inventor is almost always failing. He tries and fails maybe a thousand times. If he succeeds once then he's in. These two things are diametrically opposite. We often say that the biggest job we have is to teach a newly hired employee how to fail intelligently. We have to train him to experiment over and over and to keep on trying and failing until he learns what will work.
>
> —*Charles F. Kettering*

SCIENCE AND DISCOVERY

Archimedes is known for having the original *Eureka!* moment. He discovered the principles of buoyancy and hydrostaics while contemplating a nondestructive way to test the golden crown of King Hiero of Syracuse. Archimedes observed these principles while stepping into his bathtub. Realizing that this was the answer to his problem, the story says he leapt from his tub, *au naturel,* and ran through the streets announcing his discovery to the citizens of Alexandria, shouting "Eureka!" (I have found it!). Whether the Alexandrians were more nonplussed at what he had discovered or that he was uncovered is not known.[2]

---

[2] *Eureka* is also the motto of the state of California. From this anecdote, it may apply to more than one situation.

Archimedes produced an innovation by matching a physical phenomenon to a problem he needed to solve. He uncovered this phenomenon through his keen powers of observation. Developing these powers of observation and the ability to apply these observations to problems is a key skill of the innovator.

> For what study is there more fitted to the mind of man than the physical sciences? And what is there more capable of giving him an insight into the actions of those laws, a knowledge of which gives interest to the most trifling phenomenon of nature, and makes the student find:
>
> Tongues in trees, books in the running brooks,
>
> Sermons in stones, and good in every thing?[3]
>
> **—Michael Faraday**

Scientists, especially those engaged in pure research, are often criticized for the lack of practical use for their discoveries. The U.S. produces an enormous quantity of publicly funded basic research, which by definition is directed toward the expansion of knowledge, not the production of useful inventions. Universities are becoming more skilled at cataloging these discoveries and offering them for use through their offices' technology licensing.

A fundamental tension in this process is the following: The incentive structure in universities and the sciences rewards basic discovery and publication of results. Commercial application relies on putting a discovery in the form of intellectual property, which requires a degree of secrecy prior to a discovery being published as a patent. The numerous and complex issues involved in moving basic research from the laboratory bench to the patient's bedside is the subject of intense interest. The National Institutes of Health (NIH) has a Translational Research Initiative (TRI) to help turn basic discoveries into applied therapies.[4]

> Michael Faraday's interest in knowledge for its own sake often baffled people of a more practical bent. British Prime Minister William Gladstone, observing Faraday performing a particularly unlikely experiment one day, pointedly asked him how useful

---

[3] *Harvard Classics*, Vol. 30, P.F. Collier and Son, New York, 1938, p. 85.
[4] http://ccr.cancer.gov/initiatives/TRI/default.asp, http://www.nih.gov/.

such a "discovery" could possibly be. "Why," Faraday smartly replied, "you will soon be able to tax it!"[5]

Donald E. Stokes' book *Pasteur's Quadrant* addresses the conflict between basic and applied science. Stokes draws a matrix with curiosity on the x-axis and practicality on the y-axis. The four quadrants are occupied by Niels Bohr in the upper left, Louis Pasteur in the upper right, Thomas Edison in the lower right, and accident in the lower left. Niels Bohr was entirely theoretical. If a discovery had a practical use, it was of little interest to him. Pasteur was a balance between pure and applied science. Pasteur was driven by an intense concern for the medical needs of people. Edison was by his own admission entirely practical. For Edison there was no "why," but only trial and error until a practical solution with commercial value emerged.[6]

ART AND DESIGN

Another pair of terms that are often used interchangeably are art and design. Again, some definitions:

Art: From *artem*, to fit. Skill as the result of knowledge or practice, human skill, technical or professional skill, perfection of workmanship, application of skill in the areas of taste, poetry, music, architecture, painting. The quality, production or expression according to aesthetic principles (*Old English Dictionary* (*OED*), *Webster's*). *Webster's* (1828) makes a distinction between the *polite,* or *liberal,* arts and the *useful,* or *mechanical,* arts or *trades.* One emphasizes mental skill, the other manual skill.

Design: From the Latin *de signo*, to seal or stamp (*Webster's*, 1828). To delineate by outline or sketch, to plan; the preliminary conception of an idea that is to be carried into effect by action (*OED*). Organization or structure of formal elements, composition, plan, blueprint (*Webster's Unabridged*, 1989).

Design helps to make a product logical, usable, and understandable to the end user. Good design is invaluable in making medical technology usable and even safer. It is part of providing complete utility and a satisfying and appealing experience for the user. Design is putting things

---

[5] Bolton, Sarah K. and Cline, Barbara L., *Famous Men of Science*, Crowell, New York, 1960.
[6] Stokes, Donald, *Pasteur's Quadrant*, Brookings Institution Press, Washington, DC, 1997.

together in a planned and purposeful way. It can be utilitarian mechanical design, aesthetic design, or a combination of the two. Design can range from the cool rationality of the Bauhaus to exuberant technological Rococo.

In art, the emphasis is on skill applied to aesthetics. Aesthetics is what appeals to the senses or feelings. Aesthetics is primarily subjective and emotional.

In design, the emphasis is on planning and organization. It is primarily a logical and objective activity. It is producing purpose and order.

In his work *The Two Cultures and the Scientific Revolution*, C.P. Snow describes the gulf between the scientific community and the literary intellectual communities. If anything, this gap has widened since Snow wrote his work in 1959.[7] On many levels the scientific and artistic communities view each other with a mixture of mutual suspicion and disdain. To the scientist, the arts lack rigor and purpose, and to the artist, science lacks feeling.

Why is the artist important to the scientific innovator? Because art communicates and also appeals to the emotions.

Art is a vital way to communicate scientific information. The medical illustration work of Vesalius, *De Humani Corporis Fabrica*, as well as the work of DaVinci, Albinus, Broedel, and, more recently, Dr. Frank Netter, have been essential to making the human body understandable to generations of clinicians.

Marketers know that buying decisions are primarily emotional. The effective marketer uses the tools of the artist to bring attention and desirability to a product. It turns technical specifications into an appealing emotional story that communicates value. Marketing communicates objective features and subjective benefits. Branding helps people recognize products. Marketing helps to communicate information in a direct and intuitive way. This can help a clinically useful innovation get to the person it is intended to help. People may need what you have invented, but they have to know what you have, want what you have, and like what you have. They have to "buy into" a product before they buy the product. Also, what you have has to ultimately be what people need. All the marketing in the world cannot "push a rope."

It has been said that sales is taking orders for water from thirsty people. Marketing is the art of making them thirsty. Advertising is getting people to crave things they do not yet know exist.

---

[7] Snow, C.P., *The Two Cultures and the Scientific Revolution*, Cambridge University Press, New York, 1998.

> In art, in taste, in life, in speech, you decide from feeling, and not from reason.... If we were obliged to enter into a theoretical deliberation on every occasion before we act, life would be at a stand, and Art would be impracticable.
>
> —**William Hazlitt**

People operate far more on intuition than logic than they may care to admit. The reason for this is that intuition takes less time. One way marketing persuades us to buy is to communicate the endorsement of a person or institution we trust. We assume that the "expert" has done his homework so that we do not have to.

One difficulty here is that the purists in the academic scientific community as well as the purists in the arts community look upon the process of practical commercialization with suspicion or even distaste. In some circles if someone "goes commercial" they have prostituted themselves beyond redemption. Again, the goal is not to be an academic purist, but to develop practical solutions for the real needs of real patients. This will in turn produce value for the workers, owners, and investors of a company and society, and generate capital for reinvestment and growth. Fields of activity, distilled and isolated, can be as dead as a body part cut off from the bloodstream. Art for art's sake and knowledge for knowledge's sake are no more defensible that profit for profit's sake.

The arts suffer from an internal conflict between pure and applied forms. In his 1891 essay "The Soul of Man under Socialism," Oscar Wilde wrote:

> Indeed, the moment that an artist takes notice of what other people want, and tries to supply the demand, he ceases to be an artist, and becomes a dull or an amusing craftsman, an honest or dishonest tradesman. He has no further claim to be considered as an artist.[8]

To the aesthete purist, the moment art serves a practical purpose it is no longer fine art. It becomes an inferior applied art. This passage also illuminates the political bent found in some of the fine arts. In the conservative classical view, which prevailed in Western art from Greek and Roman times through the late 19th century, the purpose of art is to evoke noble emotions and teach moral values.[9] In the modernist view,

---

[8] Wilde, Oscar, *The Soul of Man under Socialism*, Lowling, Linda, Ed., Penguin Books, USA, 2001.
[9] http://witcombe.shc.edu/modernism/artsake.html.

the ultimate goal of art to produce social change in the context of class struggle. The classical conservative definition has been virtually eradicated in academic circles. For example, the familiar term *avant-garde* applied to the innovative leading edge of modern art was originally the name for the shock troops of a revolutionary people's army. In this class-warfare model, art that does not annoy or infuriate the conservative middle class is considered a failure, mere illustration, or kitsch. There is a persistent argument over the definition of what is art. The fundamental dispute is actually not over what is art, but a noisy clash between the presentation of fundamentally irreconcilable world views. In the fine art world Norman Rockwell is recognized for his technical talent, but scorned for his idyllic portrayal of bourgeoisie values. Corporations contribute to and taxpayers are forced to pay for *épater les bourgeois* and *art brut* that is hostile to middle-class values and advocates the overthrow of free-market capitalism. The dissonance this produces in the arts-based industrial design field remains unresolved.

> During the Renaissance, ... little cleavage was felt between the sciences and the arts. Leonardo passed back and forth between fields ... that later became categorically distinct. Furthermore, even after that steady exchange had ceased, the term "art" continued to apply as much to technology and the crafts ... as to painting and sculpture. Only when the latter unequivocally renounced representation ... did the cleavage we now take for granted assume anything like its present depth.[10]

FINDING THE NEED

Necessity, who is the mother of invention

—**Plato, *The Republic***

Restlessness and discontent are the first necessities of progress.

—**Thomas A. Edison**

Medical innovation usually starts with a need, and then matches an appropriate technology to solve the problem. This is the way the vast majority of medical innovations occur. Some innovations are technology

---

[10] Kuhn, Thomas, *The Structure of Scientific Revolutions*, University of Chicago Press, Chicago, 1996, p. 161. This is an influential work that popularized the terms *paradigm* and *paradigm shift*.

driven. However, according to Beckie Robertson, cofounder of Versant Ventures, a major life science investment fund, these technology-driven products are by far in the minority.

The ability to find and understand important clinical needs is an essential skill of the medical device entrepreneur. One of the ways to find needs is from thought leaders in a field. This approach has been formalized by Eric von Hippel of MIT into the lead user method. These lead users are leaders and early adopters who anticipate where a technology may be going, translating this information into a product that one of these early adopters will use is one thing. Making a product that the early and late majorities will adopt is another. Between these early adopters and the majority market is a gap, the so-called valley of death that many technologies fail to cross.

Need finding is not as easy as it sounds. One would think that all you have to do is ask people what they want. Some of the most important needs are latent needs, where people do not know what they want and do not what they are missing. Market research is especially ill-suited to finding latent needs. How do you predict market share for an innovative product where no comparable product yet exists? Balloon angioplasty and magnetic resonance imaging are two breakthrough technologies initially thought to have no market. Doctors, for many reasons, will seldom admit that they have a need. To admit a need is to say that they are not providing the best standard of care. Gathering and interpreting clinical needs information is another art in itself. For example, Dr. Thomas Fogarty, in a talk on this subject, stated that "What a doctor wants, what they say they want, what they need, and what they will pay for are all different things."

Technology-driven products have a seductive appeal. These are products with intriguing technology, with a wide range of potential uses, but ill-defined clinical utility. The problem with the technology-driven approach is the panacea trap. Medical lasers had this problem. When laser technology became available for medical use, it was applied to a wide range of products. Few of these products were ultimately successful. The most successful medical device products and companies have compelling technology appropriately focused on a very specific clinical need, not solutions in search of a problem, and not science projects. Two responses to a new medical technology that you do not want to hear are "that's interesting" or "you have a great solution to a problem I don't have."

Innovation, by definition, is practical, applied, and meets the needs of people. Applied science, invention, applied art, and design work together to produce innovations, solutions to human problems that have commercial value. Peter Drucker writes the following:

> Above all, innovation is not invention. It is a term of economics rather than technology. Non-technological innovations — social or economic innovations — are at least as important as technological ones. Innovation can be defined as the task of endowing human and material resources with new and greater wealth-producing capacity. Managers must convert society's needs into opportunities for profitable businesses. This too, is a definition of innovation.[11]

Innovation is about finding and solving the real needs of real people, and generating economic wealth in the process. It is taking all of the skills and talents of the scientist, doctor, engineer, artist, businessperson, and technician to bear on solving the medical needs of patients and building a viable business.

> An idea in and of itself has no value. It's when you implement an idea, by means of an innovation, then you create value for society.[12]
>
> —Thomas J. Fogarty, M.D.

To really solve a medical problem, and get it to the people who need it, you cannot do it all alone. To produce a product of real value, it takes the combined, committed, and organized efforts of people with a range of skills and talents. To get these people to work together and organize their efforts takes skilled management, and this art of management requires very different skills than most innovators have. It takes meticulous science. It takes people with skill at negotiating an ever-changing regulatory landscape. To bring these people together takes capital, and if successful, produces more capital that can then be put to work solving other problems. Managing capital requires yet another set of specialized and very necessary skills.

Invention is a means to an end, not an end in itself. It does not matter how rapidly you are able to produce iterations of an idea, how cleverly you solve a problem, and how original you are at doing it; what matters in the end is the importance of the human clinical need you are solving and the effectiveness with which you solve it. One needs to get past having a technologically driven solution in search of a problem, or trying to market solutions to problems patients and doctors do not have. Medical

---

[11] Drucker, Peter F., *The Essential Drucker*, Harper Business, New York, 2003, pp. 22–23.
[12] From "Celebrating a Lifetime of Innovation" reception program at Stanford for Thomas J. Fogarty, 2000 Lemelson–MIT Award for Invention and Innovation.

innovation with real value is the matching of a well-executed solution with an important unmet clinical need.

Edison is known also for his prolific output of patentable ideas. He is credited with 1093 patents during his life. Edison was focused on patenting ideas with commercial value.

> Anything that won't sell, I don't want to invent. Its sale is proof of utility, and utility is success.
>
> —**Thomas A. Edison**

There is a common misconception that all one needs to have is a patent, and this alone will produce wealth. The truth is that few patents make enough money to cover the cost of filing them. A patent is a fence. You can build a fence around a swamp or a gold mine. A swamp with a fence around it is still a swamp.

The purpose of patents is not to make inventors rich. It is to preserve a record of technology for the benefit of society, and for other inventors to build on. The social contract between the inventor and society is a temporary monopoly on the sale of the patented product. This is the compensation given to the inventor in exchange for making the details of his invention public. It is up to the inventor to practice his patent or sell it to someone who generates wealth.

Another more subtle, yet vitally important issue arises when it comes to patents and intellectual property. This is the concept of freedom to operate. Just because you have a patent on a technology does not mean you can actually practice your invention. A common tactic, especially in crowded fields, is the filing of blocking patents. These are meant to fence off key areas of technology that may not be the product itself, but some of the essential means of practicing the invention. Establishing intellectual property protection as well as verifying freedom to operate are essential to successfully commercializing a medical device innovation.

So, did Edison create the light bulb? According to the literal definition, no. Did Edison invent the light bulb by himself? No. On the contrary, Edison organized a large team of skilled technicians and researchers that made his innovations possible. Employees of Edison Laboratories searched the ends of the earth for a material that would make a reliable light bulb filament. They invented means to insulate and bury reliable electrical cables. They worked on the myriad of challenges to make electric lighting and electrical generation and distribution a reality. In fact, according to James Burke, one of Edison's great innovations was the establishment and structure of Edison Laboratories, which became the prototype of the modern R&D organization. Edison states the structure of his method as follows:

Edison's Six Rules for Invention:

1. Define the need for innovation. If there is no market, don't start.
2. Set yourself a clear goal, and stick to it.
3. Analyze the major stages through which the invention must pass before it is complete.
4. Make available at all times data on the progress of the work.
5. Ensure that each member of the team has a clearly defined area of activity.
6. Record everything for later examination.[13]

Was Edison even the first to invent the light bulb? Again, the answer is no. The light bulb had been invented some 50 years before. Several inventors, including Sir Joseph Wilson Swan in England, had already developed working light bulbs. Edison even had to share credit with Swan when first marketing electric lighting in England, calling his English subsidiary the Ediswan Company. In fact, the bayonet lock light bulb base used in automobile taillight bulbs today was an invention of Sir Joseph's brother, Alfred Swan.

When discussing Edison, lighting, and electricity, another name that comes up is Nikolai Tesla. Tesla was a mirror image of Edison. Cultured, educated, and a brilliant if eccentric theoretician, he disdained the "empirical dragnet" approach of Edison. Tesla would construct an invention in his mind, and when it was fully formed, build a machine according to his vision, as opposed to the iterative stepwise approach of Edison.

Edison plays to an American saga of the rough, untutored, self-taught, practical natural genius. Tesla was the European educated, refined, theoretical visionary. Tesla was possibly more technically brilliant; however, commercial success and recognition eluded him at every turn. Tesla and Edison fought costly and acrimonious battles over the merits of Edison's direct current (DC) vs. Tesla's and Westinghouse's alternating current (AC).

In the medical device industry it is possible to be an innovator with little formal medical education, but it is an uphill battle. Persons entering the field owe it to themselves to get the best relevant education, to get a solid technical foundation as early as possible.

---

[13] Burke, James, *Connections*, Little, Brown & Company, Boston, 1978.

Tesla was further frustrated by Guglielmo Marconi's commercialization of radio. Marconi used inventions and discoveries pioneered and patented by Tesla to make his system work, such as the Tesla oscillator. Tesla thought that his invention of radio was safe because his basic radio patent predated Marconi by 3 years. The Patent Office, for reasons not entirely clear, invalidated Tesla's 1894 patent, and Marconi became the father of radio and was awarded the Nobel Prize in 1911.

Tesla loved basic research. One of the reasons he was unable to get financial backing for his projects was that he would accept investments (in one example from financier J.P. Morgan) to work on a project and then spend the money on what he felt like working on. This doomed Tesla to penury. Tesla was ridiculed in the press for producing brilliant but eccentric scientific novelties. Society recognizes and rewards those who produce solutions for their problems. Genius, unfortunately does not speak for itself. Tesla achieved as much success as he did through his association with George Westinghouse, who hired Tesla away from Edison, and recognized the practical potential of Tesla's "polyphase current" and focused his efforts.[14]

Tesla designed intuitively. It took the work of Charles P. Steinmetz to describe the mathematical basis of alternating current, which eventually allowed AC systems to be understood, designed, and controlled. Among Steinmetz's many accomplishments were the discovery of the law of hysteresis, symbolic calculation methods for predicting the performance of AC circuits, and the invention of three-phase power.[15]

So then, what did Edison do? Edison identified an important unmet market need and focused the resources of Edison Laboratories to solve it. Edison made a practical and reliable light bulb and the methods to produce them inexpensively, in quantity.[16] His research and development team, under his direction, also developed the generating equipment and the wiring infrastructure to deliver electricity to where the light bulbs were. It was not even the ultimate solution. Tesla's alternating current eventually replaced the direct current that originally flowed over Edison's

---

[14] http://www.pbs.org/tesla/index.html.
[15] http://chem.ch.huji.ac.il/~eugeniik/history/steinmetz.html. It is interesting to note that Steinmetz was instrumental to the growth and success of one of America's largest corporations, General Electric, a company virtually synonymous with capitalism, although he was a dedicated socialist. Steinmetz kept up a correspondence with V.I. Lenin, and in his office proudly displayed an autographed picture sent to him by the communist dictator (http://www.uh.edu/engines/epi276.htm).
[16] "In 1876 Maximilian Nitze modified Edison's light bulb invention and created the first optical endoscope with a built-in electrical light bulb as the source of illumination. Like the Lichtleiter from Bozzini, this instrument was only used for urologic procedures" (http://www.laparoscopy.com/shows/lapstry3.htm).

wires. Edison invented the simple and reliable screw-in fixture system that is still used in home lighting today. Edison developed a sales, marketing, and promotion structure. Solutions to problems such as how to generate electricity, how to manufacture the bulbs,[17] and how to insulate wires had to be invented. He formed a research organization that spawned other innovations such as the phonograph, moving pictures, and a superior way to manufacture Portland cement. Then, perhaps one of the more important parts of the system, and possibly the most overlooked invention in this whole structure, was the electric meter. This, too, was an Edison invention. Not only was a complete, integrated system devised that solved an especially important unmet need, but it also had economic life. Edison devised the linchpin of the whole system, a way to make money at it, which in turn generated the capital to produce many more breakthrough innovations and gave people lighting that was far superior in cost, performance, and safety to the gas lamps it displaced.[18]

It was the importance of the need, the effectiveness of the solution, and the sustainability of the system that made Edison a great innovator and earned him a place in history and in the popular imagination.

One significant difference must be noted between the environment Edison operated in and the one in which the medical device innovator operates. Edison did not operate in a highly regulated environment. In the U.S., for example, medical devices have been under the control of the federal Food and Drug Administration (FDA) since 1976 and drugs since 1906.[19] The purpose of the FDA is to protect the public from unsafe or adulterated medical products. Their charter is to ensure that medical devices and pharmaceuticals are safe and effective before they are cleared for sale. These regulations become increasingly strict as the potential risk

---

[17] Edison's bulbs were produced by the Corning Glass Company, pioneers in glass technology, including the glass/phenolic insulation originally used for high-temperature insulation for electric trains. It was the research into high-temperature insulators that led to the synthesis of silicone, a polymer of silicon and carbon, by a young Harvard-trained chemist, Dr. James Franklin Hyde, working for Corning, and the successful development of the methyl silicone polymer by Eugene Rochow in a joint venture between General Electric and Corning (http://www.chemcases.com/silicon/sil4cone.htm, Kennesaw State University). The synthesis of silicates into silicone rubber was a fiendishly difficult chemical engineering problem that eluded the best efforts of chemists for over 70 years. Silicone found its way into demanding wartime applications such as high-temperature seals for superchargers in the B-29, and in one of the most famous (or infamous) medical devices of all time, the silicone breast implant, litigation over which eventually forced the bankruptcy of the Dow-Corning Corporation.

[18] For more information on Edison, see Baldwin, Neil, *Edison Inventing the Century*, Hyperion Press, New York,1995.

[19] http://www.fda.gov/oc/history/default.htm.

to the patient goes up. One person I once worked with referred to the FDA out of frustration as "Forbidding Development in America." Wilson Greatbach, inventor of the cardiac pacemaker, said, "If I did today what I did twenty years ago, I would go to jail. Imagine making pacemakers in a barn, and taking them to a hospital and putting them into patients. We did it, and it worked."[20]

Even though the process may be expensive and slow, I recall the statement made to me by a longtime FDA regulator at a medical device materials conference when he was new at the agency. His supervisor told him: "Remember, doctors can only kill patients one at a time. With a bad decision, you can kill them by the thousands."

Another significant difference is that Edison sold his electricity and lights directly to his customer. As medical device innovators, our focus is the patient; however, we rarely, if ever, sell a device to the patient. By law, we sell only to medical professionals. Furthermore, the medical professional we market the device to is often not the one paying for it. Discontinuous economic factors such as insurance reimbursement and managed care must be understood and dealt with if the medical device innovator is to develop an economically viable product.

The goal of the medical device innovator is to save, lengthen, and improve the quality of life for people, and in doing so, generate economic value and value for society. The focus is the patient and his needs. At a Stanford Innovator's Workbench talk, John Simpson, M.D., pioneer in balloon angioplasty, stated the importance of doing right by the patient, and the rewards that can follow, and how it will catch up with you if you do not.[21]

We can help people live longer, feel better, and look better. We can help save lives and limbs. We can improve quality of life. We can give a child her grandmother back. It is hard, rewarding work, and it is an important and noble enterprise.

> Does a student know how to tackle a problem with no background in the subject? And does he or she know how to get

---

[20] Brown, Kenneth, *Inventors at Work*, Tempus Books/Microsoft Press, Redmond, WA, 1988, p. 24.

[21] "The whole concept that you do this for the money is absolutely flawed. If you do it for the patients and it works out really well for the patients, you'll make a ton of money. But if you do it for the money and you figure you've got something and it becomes a scam, then it is really going to be a frighteningly long road. It absolutely does not work" ("John Simpson: Reluctant Entrepreneur," interview by David Cassack, *In Vivo*, April 2003).

the knowledge needed? Accumulating methodology matters more than accumulating knowledge of subject matter.

—Herbert Kroemer, Nobel Laureate, on physics and education[22]

It takes a thousand men to invent a telegraph, or a steam engine, or a phonograph, or a photograph, or a telephone, or any other important thing — and the last man gets the credit and we forget the others. He added his little mite — that is all he did.

—Mark Twain[23]

I recognize that many physicists are smarter than I am — most of them theoretical physicists. A lot of smart people have gone into theoretical physics; therefore, the field is extremely competitive. I console myself with the thought that although they may be smarter and may be deeper thinkers than I am, I have broader interests than they have.

—Linus Pauling

A good scientist is a person with original ideas. A good engineer is a person who makes a design that works with as few original ideas as possible.[24]

—Freeman Dyson

---

[22] *IEEE Spectrum*, June 2002.
[23] Letter to Anne Macy. Reprinted in *Anne Sullivan Macy: The Story Behind Helen Keller* (Doubleday, Doran, and Co., Garden City, NY, 1933), p. 162. Twain was also a friend of both Edison and Tesla.
[24] For more information on Freeman Dyson, see http://www.sns.ias.edu/~dyson/.

2

INTRODUCTION TO MEDICAL PLASTICS

Ted Kucklick

CONTENTS

Biocompatibility 21
Biomaterials Availability 22
Materials Performance 23
Processablility 23
What Is a Polymer? 24
Basics: Thermoplastic and Thermosets 24
Cross-Linked Thermoplastics 25
What Is a Medical-Grade Plastic? 25
Finding Plastics 27
Plastics for Machining 30
Plastics for Processing by Machining 31
    Acrylonitrile–Butadine–Styrene (ABS) 31
    Acrylic 31
    Polyvinylchloride (PVC) 32
    Polycarbonate (PC) 32
    Polypropylene (PP) 33
    Polyethelene (PE) 33
    Acetal 34
    Nylon (Polyamide) 34
    Fluorinated Ethylene Propylene (FEP) 35
High-Performance Engineering Plastics for Machining 35
    Ultem® Polyetherimide 35
    PEEK™ (Polyetheretherketone) 36

PTFE (Teflon®)...36
Polysulfone and Polyphenylsulfone..37
Polyimide Rod and Sheet (Vespel®, Kapton®)...................................38
Injection Molded and Extruded Plastics...38
    Considerations...38
Commodity Plastics..39
    ABS..39
    PC/ABS...40
    Acrylic...40
    Polycarbonate 40
    Polyethelene..41
    Polyolefin 41
    Styrene..41
Elastomers...41
    Elastomeric Plastics 41
        Polyurethane (PU)..42
        Kraton®..42
        K-Resin®..42
        Monoprene®..43
        Pebax®...43
        Polyvinylchloride (PVC) 43
        Ethylene Vinyl Acetate (EVA)...44
Thermosets 44
    Santoprene® 44
    Silicone...44
    Polyisoprene 44
    Nitrile..45
    Latex...45
High-Performance Engineering Plastics for Molding 46
    Polyetherimide (PEI), Ultem®, PEEK®, Polysulfone............................46
Useful Specialty Plastic Material Forms 46
    Extruded PTFE (Zeus, Texloc)..46
    Expanded PTFE (EPTFE) 46
Sheet and Film and Foam Plastics...47
    Polyethylene Terephthalate (PET) and Polyethylene
       Terephthalate Glycol (PETG) 47
    Tyvek..47
    PVC and Polyethelene Film..47
    Polyester Film (Mylar®)...47
    Polyimide 48
    Styrene Butadiene Rubber (SBR) Foam and Elastic Fabric
       (Wetsuit Material)...48
    Foam Sheet Material...48

Resources..49
  Radiation Effects on Plastics...49
Acknowledgments..49

When working with medical plastics, there are some basic considerations: relative biocompatibility, performance, processability, bondability, cost, and availability. Using these basic characteristics as a starting point will help to sift through the myriad of available plastics to arrive at a short list of candidates that best suit your design criteria.

In addition to materials for devices, another category of medical plastics is those that are used in packaging. These plastics need to not react with whatever is contained in them, be resistant to degradation when sterilized, and be at the lowest possible cost.

For the sake of simplicity, this chapter will sort some of the common plastics according to the more common methods of processing, as not all plastics are readily available for all processes. In the R&D environment, rapid development, cost-effective materials, and short lead times are key considerations.

BIOCOMPATIBILITY

This is a subject that could fill several books, and does. This concept may be understood as relative biocompatibility, as the requirements for the medical devices are all different: for example, one that does not come into much contact with a patient, such as an instrumentation case, compared to one that comes into intermittent or continuous skin contact, compared to an invasive surgical device, compared to an implantable device. It is biocompatible relative to the application. If choosing a material for a medical device application, biocompatibility is the first and most important consideration. If the material is not biocompatible, it may not be used, no matter what the potential performance. The most basic indicator that a material might be used is if it carries a U.S. Pharmacoepia (USP) Class VI, or medical-grade designation, or is marketed by the manufacturer as suitable for medical use. It is the responsibility of the designer to determine if any particular material is suitable for its particular application.

The companion chapter in this book, "Assessing Biocompatibility" (Chapter 11) provides a very useful guide to understanding this topic.

Note: If a material is to be used for human use, it *must* have appropriate biocompatibility data on file *before* it is used clinically. Avoid using industrial-grade or "hardware store" materials and adhesives in *in vivo* or preclinical studies. It is good practice to use only medical-grade materials from the beginning. This way you can be more confident that you are building a device that remains usable as you move from bench tests to *in vivo* to clinicals.

The amount of biocompatibility testing required varies with the class of device, duration of contact with the patient, and amount of mucous membrane or blood contact. Discuss these testing requirements with your regulatory affairs person and your testing lab *before* you begin any human clinical study. Schedule and allow enough time to do these tests. It is also good practice to use materials that are medical grade, and you are confident will pass appropriate biocompatibility tests when doing preclinical work. Biocompatibility testing is done on the material in its *finished form*, as processed, as colored, and as it will be used in the device.

BIOMATERIALS AVAILABILITY

In response to a looming biomaterials crisis[1] precipitated by ruinous judgments against medical device manufacturers, and the associated liability exposure of suppliers of bulk raw materials, Congress passed the Biomaterials Access Assurance Act of 1998.[2] This gives a degree of protection to suppliers of materials that may become included in medical devices. A series of liability suits based on sometimes dubious science drove some major materials suppliers to exit from knowingly supplying materials for medical use, especially implants.[3] With the act, the situation is somewhat improved. In some cases (e.g., silicones), smaller companies have stepped into the breach to supply these essential biomaterials, although at substantially higher cost than their industrial-grade equivalents. Ultimately, it is the responsibility of the medical device manufacturer to

---

[1] Nadim, J. Hallab, Biomaterials crisis looms, *AAOS Bulletin*, Vol. 45, No. 1, January 1997.

[2] The text of this act may be found at http://www.biomaterials.org/community/comact.htm.

[3] The most well known of these cases are those involving Dow Corning and silicone breast implants. Despite scientific evidence to the contrary, Dow Corning was driven into bankruptcy, and billions of dollars paid out to plaintiffs and trial lawyers over alleged autoimmune disorders from silicone gel-filled implants. Other well-known cases involved the Dalkon Shield IUD made by A.H. Robins, several cases involving pacemaker leads, and suits against Vitek for its TMJ joint implant product. In the Vitek case, DuPont found itself spending millions of dollars to extricate itself from deep-pocket liability over the use of a few cents' worth of material by a small company. This case led DuPont to embargo the sale of its Teflon material for medical use. See Ratner et al., *Biomaterials Science*, 2nd ed., *Legal Aspects of Biomaterials*; Legal Analysis of Biomaterials Access Assurance Act of 1998, Public Law 105-230, http://www.advamed.org/publicdocs/legal021599.htm; and Limiting Liability of Medical Device Materials Suppliers, http://www.packaginglaw.com/index_mf.cfm?id=113.

ensure that a material used is suitable for medical use, is properly selected for use in a well-designed product, and meets applicable regulatory and biocompatibility requirements.

MATERIALS PERFORMANCE

Under this category are considerations such as the mechanical properties of the material, its stiffness or flexibility, and its heat resistance, chemical resistance, and dielectric properties.

For example, heat resistance becomes a consideration if a device is meant for autoclave sterilization. For these applications, a heat-resistant high-performance engineering plastic like Ultem™ PEI (polyetherimide) or PEEK™ (polyetheretherketone) might be considered. If high dielectric strength in a thin material is desired, a polyimide tube or sheet may be a good choice. If ease of molding and low cost are important, acrylonitrile–butadine–styrene (ABS) plastic may be a good choice. Determining the properties, performance, and processing of a plastic material for your application are important selection criteria.

PROCESSABLILITY

Once you have found a plastic that meets your performance and biocompatibility requirements, the issue of how the plastic will be processed into its final shape needs to be considered. If a device is a one-off or low-production prototype, it will most likely be machined from a stock shape. Numerous plastics that are suitable for medical use and are available in stock shapes are described in this chapter.

One thing to keep in mind is your strategy for scaling up production if a prototype design proves successful. Think design for manufacture from the beginning. Is the material from which you are machining the part available in an injection moldable form? Or, is a plastic that you want to injection mold available in a stock shape? Can the plastic be machined to a tolerance and surface finish acceptable for the application? Are you specifying a plastic that cannot be radiation sterilized or is not available in a form for injection molding? Planning ahead on these issues will save time, expense, and headaches down the road.

Another consideration when selecting a plastic for molding is how easy or difficult is the material to mold to get the parts you want without sinks, blushes, or blemishes. Is the part intricate with hard-to-fill thin areas? High-performance engineering plastics that are stronger and tougher, and have high heat resistance, are usually more difficult to mold and are more expensive per pound. It is important to specify the appropriate plastic for the application, and not overspecify. For example, a part that may be made in a more expensive polycarbonate, which runs hotter in the mold, may be made in an easier-to-mold and less expensive acrylic, at lower temperatures and cycle times, and perform just as well in the application.

WHAT IS A POLYMER?

Polymers are chain molecules. *Poly* means many and *mer* means an individual unit. Polymer means many units (mers) together, e.g., polyester. In chemistry there is also an oligimer. *Oligi* means a few (like an oligarchy). So, an oligimer is an arrangement of a few units; monomer, one unit; and polymer, many units. Examples of monomers are styrene, methyl, and carbonate.

BASICS: THERMOPLASTIC AND THERMOSETS

Another very basic distinction for plastics is whether a plastic material is a thermoplastic or a thermoset. A thermoplastic is one that can be melted. Think of thermoplastic polymer molecules like strands of spaghetti. Ones with lower molecular weight, like styrene, are shorter. Ones with high molecular weight, like ultra-high-molecular-weight polyethelene (UHMWPE), are longer. When you boil a pot of spaghetti, the noodles become soft and pliable. You can pour spaghetti into a bowl, and it takes the shape of the bowl. When it cools, it still keeps the shape of the bowl. The spaghetti can then be reheated and softened, and formed into another shape.

If you think of the length of the strands and then think of squeezing boiled spaghetti through a large funnel, you will see how plastics process differently. Spaghetti chopped up into small strands will go through easily. Noodles in long strands will be harder to squeeze through. Styrene, for example, is a short molecule that flows very easily when melted. This makes it a popular material for low-cost products that need to hold high detail, such as styrene car and aircraft models. It also easily remelts.

The other basic type of plastic is a thermoset. This is a material that is cross-linked. Unlike the spaghetti in the earlier analogy, where the strands are separate and can be made to flow again if heated, a cross-linked plastic is more like a fishnet. The strands are hooked together. It cannot be boiled and made to flow like the spaghetti. Therefore, thermoset plastics, once they are cross-linked in an irreversible chemical reaction and form this molecular network, cannot be made to flow or melt. Examples of thermosets are epoxy, cast urethanes, and silicones.

A common example of a type of thermosetting reaction is a hard-boiled egg, where heat causes the proteins in the egg to denature and cross-link from a liquid to a solid in an irreversible reaction.

Whether a plastic is a thermoplastic or a thermoset obviously makes a great deal of difference in how the material is processed and shaped. Thermoplastics can be melted and molded, as in injection molding. Thermosets are shaped by some form of casting. Thermoplastics assume their shape when they cool. Thermosets assume their shape when a chemical reaction causes the material to cross-link.

CROSS-LINKED THERMOPLASTICS

A special case found in some modified plastics used for medical devices is that of cross-linked thermoplastics. This is where a thermoplastic is irradiated with ionizing radiation to release free radicals and induce the formation of three-dimensional cross-linked structures in a thermoplastic. This modification can have a dramatic effect on the properties and performance of the plastic material. Common applications of this process in medical devices are irradiated polyester tubing for angioplasty balloons and irradiated UHMWPE for joint implants.[4]

Radiation cross-linking allows a material to be processed like a thermoplastic and then be given the properties of a thermoset. Modified Polymers Corporation (Sunnyvale, CA) offers these materials modification services to the medical device industry.

Note that radiation sterilization can cause unintentional cross-linking, stiffening, or embrittlement of some polymers. See the section in this chapter on sterilization effects on plastics for more information.

WHAT IS A MEDICAL-GRADE PLASTIC?

First, there is no such thing as an FDA-*approved* material. This is a misnomer, because the FDA does not approve materials. The FDA supplies regulations and guidance for material compliance for manufacturers to follow. There are U.S. Pharmacoepia (USP), International Organization of Standardization (ISO), and FDA-*compliant* materials.

---

[4] Irradiated Plastics: Applications and Perspectives for the Automotive and Electrotechnic Industries, Sophie Rouif, IONISOS S.A., France, http://www.radtech-europe.com/download/rouifpaperjuly.pdf; Sobieraj, M.C., Kurtz, S.M., and Rimnac, C.M., Notch strengthening and hardening behavior of conventional and highly crosslinked UHMWPE under applied tensile loading, *Biomaterials* 2004.

These are materials manufactured in compliance with particular regulations and standards.[5,6]

USP is responsible for establishing legally recognized product standards for drugs and other health-related articles in the U.S. In the 1960s, methodology and requirements were established for plastic materials used for pharmaceutical containers and closures, and were subsequently adopted by medical device manufacturers. USP tests measure biological reactivity of plastics in contact with mammalian cell cultures (*in vitro*) and via implantation and injection of extractables into laboratory animals (*in vivo*). Plastics are classified into one of six classes, each requiring different levels of testing. USP Class VI requires the most extensive testing. Not all plastics manufacturers wish to undertake the expense of testing their materials to this level; therefore, the number of materials meeting this classification for your application may be limited.

USP does not regulate compliance or certification of plastics tested according to its published methods. The FDA has adopted some the tests specified by USP for regulation of medical devices.

For further information on USP test methods, reference USP 23 — NF 18, Chapters 87 to 88 and contact USP at U.S. Pharmacopeia, 12601 Twinbrook Parkway, Rockville, MD 20852, by phone at 800-822-8772.[7]

Whenever a plastic is used in a medical device in human use, even if it is advertised as a USP Class VI material, it needs to be tested by the manufacturer according to the standards relevant to the amount of contact it has with the patient. This is because several factors, such as the addition of colorants, processing, and the use of the plastic in

---

[5] "The United States Pharmacopeia (USP) is a nongovernmental, standards-setting organization that advances public health by ensuring the quality and consistency of medicines, promoting the safe and proper use of medications, and verifying ingredients in dietary supplements. USP standards are developed by a unique process of public involvement and are accepted worldwide. In addition to standards development, USP's other public health programs focus on promoting optimal health care delivery and are listed below. USP is a nonprofit organization that achieves its goals through the contributions of volunteers representing pharmacy, medicine, and other health care professions, as well as science, academia, the U.S. government, the pharmaceutical industry, and consumer organizations. USP's Internet address is www.usp.org" (from the usp.org website).

[6] CFR Title 21, Food and Drugs 170–199, http://www.access.gpo.gov/nara/cfr/waisidx_99/21cfr177_99.html.

[7] Boedeker Plastics Regulatory Standards and Compliance Overview, http://www.boedeker.com/regcomp.htm#FDA. Good overview of several other standards, e.g., ASTM, Canadian, 3A Dairy, UL, etc.

combination with other materials and adhesives, can affect the biocompatibility characteristics of the material.[8]

These tests need to be done even if the same material is in use in another medical device. However, using a material that is already in use in another medical device that is known to have passed biocompatibility testing can help, as you can have some confidence that the material will pass testing in your application.

Additionally, if any part of the material changes, such as the addition of colorant or fillers to an injection molded part, testing will need to be done on that combination of materials even if the plastic has already been tested in its natural state, and even if the additives have been tested separately.

The biocompatibility test matrix in Table 2.1 and in Chapter 11, "Assessing Biocompatibility," gives a quick reference to the testing to be done for several categories of medical device applications. Again, it is the responsibility of the designer and manufacturer to determine if a particular material is suitable for its particular use.

FINDING PLASTICS

There are seemingly endless varieties of plastics under hundreds of trade names. A convenient way to sort through these materials is the "Polymer Trade Name" section of Matweb.com (http://www.matweb.com/search/SearchTradeName.asp). This can help locate the manufacturer of a material you are interested in, as well as the composition of a trade name

---

[8] "The best starting point for understanding biocompatibility requirements is ANSI/AAMI/ISO Standard 10993, *Biological Evaluation of Medical Devices*. Part 1 of the standard is the guidance on selection of tests, Part 2 covers animal welfare requirements, and Parts 3 through 17 are guidelines for specific test procedures or other testing-related issues. Testing strategies that comply with the ISO 10993-1 are acceptable in Europe and Asia. In 1995, the FDA issued a Blue Book Memorandum G95-1, which replaced the Tripartite Guidance (the previous biocompatibility testing standard). The FDA substantially adopted the ANSI/AAMI/ISO guideline, although in some areas FDA's testing requirements go beyond those of ISO. The specific test procedures spelled out in the ISO standard vary slightly from the USP procedures historically used for FDA submissions. The ISO procedures tend to be more stringent, so companies planning to register their product in Europe and the U.S. should follow ISO test methods. FDA requirements should be verified since additional testing may be needed. Japanese procedures for sample preparation and testing are slightly different from either USP or ISO tests. Northview highly recommends discussing your proposed biocompatibility testing plan with a FDA reviewer before initiating testing (*Assessing Biocompatibility: A Guide for Medical Device Manufacturers*, Northview Bioscience Laboratories, Chicago, IL and Hercules, CA.

Table 2.1 Biocompatibility Matrix

Device Categories		Examples
Surface device	Skin	Devices that contact intact skin surfaces only; examples include electrodes, external prostheses, fixation tapes, compression bandages, and monitors of various types
	Mucous membrane	Devices communicating with intact mucosal membranes; examples include contact lenses, urinary catheters, intravaginal and intraintestinal devices (stomach tubes, sigmoidoscopes, colonoscopes, gastroscopes), endotracheal tubes, bronchoscopes, dental prostheses, orthodontic devices, and IUDs
	Breached or compromised surfaces	Devices that contact breached or otherwise compromised external body surfaces; examples include ulcer, burn and granulation tissue dressings, or healing devices and occlusive patches
External communicating device	Blood path, indirect	Devices that contact the blood path at one point and serve as a conduit for entry into the vascular system; examples include solution administration sets, extension sets, transfer sets, and blood administration sets
	Tissue/bone/dentin communicating	Devices communicating with tissue, bone, and pulp/dentin system; examples include laparoscopes, arthroscopes, draining systems, dental cements, dental filling materials, and skin staples
		Devices that contact internal tissues (rather than blood contact devices); examples include many surgical instruments and accessories

	Circulating blood	Devices that contact circulating blood; examples include intravascular catheters, temporary pacemaker electrodes, oxygenators, extracorporeal oxygenator tubing and accessories, hemoadsorbents, and immunoadsorbents
Implant device	Tissue/bone	Devices principally contacting bone; examples include orthopedic pins, plates, replacement joints, bone prostheses, cements, and intraosseous devices
		Devices principally contacting tissue and tissues fluid; examples include pacemakers, drug supply devices, neuromuscular sensors and stimulators, replacement tendons, breast implants, artificial larynxes, subperiosteal implants, and ligation clips
	Blood	Devices principally contacting blood; examples include pacemaker electrodes, artificial arteriovenous fistulae, heart valves, vascular grafts and stents, internal drug delivery catheters, and ventricular assist devices

Courtesy of Northview Bioscience.

material. Plastics.com also has a listing of materials by trade name and composition (http://www.plastics.com/tradenames.php). Plastics distributors (Port Plastics, Westlake Plastics, Polymer Plastics Corporation, Boedeker Plastics) are also good sources of information when choosing and sourcing plastic materials.

PLASTICS FOR MACHINING

This category of plastics consists of materials that are readily available in shapes that are easily set up for machining. These plastics tend to have high costs relative to weight, as most of the material is lost as chip waste during machining.[9]

Listed are some of the more readily available materials suitable for machining that are sold in FDA-compliant grades. These are listed with plastics vendors as mechanical plastics. Check with your vendor to be sure that the material you are ordering is sufficiently FDA-compliant for your intended use.

Not all of the plastics listed here are available in USP Class VI grades. This, however, is not an issue if the application does not involve patient contact or passing of liquids intended for patient contact.

Also listed are a number of high-performance engineering plastics. These are intended for particular demanding applications. The cost of these plastics can be very high relative to commodity plastics.

Most plastics in stock shapes are available only in natural (often a cream color), transparent, black, or white. Colored plastics are normally not available off the shelf. The exceptions to this are PVC rod and acrylic sheet and some nylon shapes.

Polymer Plastics Corporation, Mountain View, CA (www.polymerplastics.com), has an online catalog with a quotation function for each of the standard shapes it carries. This can be a very useful tool when choosing a cost-effective material, and planning and budgeting a prototyping or short-run manufacturing project.

Boedeker Plastics, Shiner, TX, offers a broad range of information on plastics for medical and food processing use (http://www.boedeker.com/agency.htm).

---

[9] Some descriptions of plastics and their stock shapes. Courtesy of Polymer Plastics Corporation, Mountain View, CA.

PLASTICS FOR PROCESSING BY MACHINING
Acrylonitrile–Butadine–Styrene (ABS)

A terpolymer is made from SAN (styrene–acrylonitrile) and butadiene synthetic rubber. The SAN gives ABS its hardness and surface finish, and the butadiene gives it its toughness.

Commonly available plastic in sheets to 4 inches thick and rods up to 6 inches in diameter, it can easily be bonded and laminated to form thicker sheets and assemblies. Due to its reasonable cost and ease of machining, it is a popular material for computer numerical control (CNC)-fabricated prototypes.

Rod: 0.250 to 6.000 inches
Sheet: 0.062 to 0.250 inches
Plate: 0.250 to 4.000 inches
Standard color: Natural (cream), black

Acrylic

Acrylics were actually one of the first medical device plastics[10] and are still commonly used in molding of anaplastic prosthetics.[11] Acrylic is basically polymethyl methacrylate (PMMA). It is one of the most readily available plastics, found at signage and hobby shops. It is rigid, clear, very machinable, and bondable. One popular method of bonding acrylic is solvent bonding with methyl chloride. Acrylic is available in nearly unlimited varieties of rod, sheet, and plate shapes, and a variety of colors. Acrylics are especially suitable for light pipes and optical applications.

One project I worked on required a clear tube, 12 inches in diameter, for a hyperbaric chamber that needed to be clear for observation. I was able to locate this shape, preformed in acrylic, in an appropriate wall thickness, and had parts fabricated at reasonable cost at an acrylic fabrication shop.

---

[10] "PMMA was introduced to dentistry in 1937. During World War II shards of PMMA from shattered gun turrets unintentionally implanted in the eyes of aviators, suggested that some materials might evoke only a mild foreign body reaction" (Ratner, B.D. et al., *Biomaterials Science*, Academic Press, New York, 1996, p. 1). PMMA was developed and marketed in the 1930s by the Rohm and Haas company under the name Plexiglas®, and with lesser success by DuPont under the name Lucite®.

[11] For more information on anaplatological modeling, see McKinstry, Robert L., *Fundamentals of Facial Prosthetics*, ABI Professional Publications, Vandamere Press, Clearwater, FL, http://www.abipropub.com/fundfapro.htm. This book contains detailed how-to information on numerous medical modeling techniques.

Acrylics for signage and display may be used for bench testing and prototypes; however, care must be taken to identify a medical-grade version before using in any clinical trials. Commercial-grade acrylics may contain UV inhibitors for weatherability, flame retardants, impact modifiers, and other chemicals that render them unsuitable for clinical use.

Medical-grade acrylics are available from Cyro Corporation (Rockaway, NJ; www.cyro.com) For more information, see the entry on acrylics in the injection molding materials section of this chapter.

Polyvinylchloride (PVC)

PVC is available in both rigid and flexible forms, depending on whether plasticizers are added. PVC is commonly used for water pipes.

The major disadvantages of PVC are poor weatherability, relatively low impact strength, and fairly high weight for thermoplastic sheet (specific gravity of 1.35). It is easily scratched or marred, and possesses a relatively low heat distortion point (160_i).

Unplasticized PVC is produced in two major formulations: type I (corrosion resistant) and type II (high impact).

Type I PVC is the most commonly used PVC, but in applications where higher impact strength than that offered by type I is required, type II offers better impact properties, with a slight loss in corrosion resistance. In applications requiring a high temperature formulation, polyvinylidene fluoride for high-purity applications (PVDF) is usable to approximately 280°F.

Rod: 0.250 to 12.000 inches
Sheet: 0.032 to 2.000 inches
Hollow bar: From 0.562 inches inner diameter (I.D.) to 0.625 inches outer diameter (O.D.)
Hex bar: 0.432 to 2.000 inches
Standard color: Gray, white, clear

PVC rod is available from Gehr Plastics (http://www.gehrplastics.com/products/pvc/pvc.htm) in 10 different colors and up to 6 inches in diameter.

Note: PVC is one of the few mechanical plastics available in stock shapes in colors.

Polycarbonate (PC)

Polycarbonate is an extremely tough plastic, commonly sold under the trade name Lexan®. It is the toughest transparent plastic available. It is very useful for prototype medical devices, especially if UV cure bonding is to be used. It is available in rod, plate, and sheet. It bonds readily.

While more than a dozen performance characteristics of polycarbonate are utilized singly or in combinations, seven are most commonly relied on. These are high impact strength, water-clear transparency, good creep resistance, wide-use temperature range, dimensional stability, abrasion resistance, hardness, and rigidity despite its ductility.

PC tends to discolor with radiation sterilization. Radiation-stable grades are available.

Rod: 0.250 to 6.000 inches
Plate: 0.375 to 4.000 inches
Sheet: 0.030 to 0.500 inches
Film: 0.003 to 0.030 inches
Tubing: 0.250 inches I.D. to 4.000 inches O.D.
Standard colors: Optical clear, black, gray

Polypropylene (PP)

PP is a lightweight, inexpensive polyolefin plastic with a low melting temperature, making it popular for thermoforming and food packaging. PP is flammable; therefore, look for a flame retardant (FR) grade if fire resistance is required.

Rod: 0.250 to 14.000 inches
Sheet: 0.060 to 2.000 inches
Tubing: From 0.060 inches I.D. to 2.000 inches O.D.
Standard color: Opaque white, natural

Polyethelene (PE)

PE is a material commonly used in food packaging and processing. Ultra-high-molecular-weight PE (UHMWPE) has a high abrasion resistance, low coefficient of friction, self-lubrication, nonadherent surface, and excellent chemical fatigue resistance. It also retains high performance at extremely low temperatures (e.g., with liquid nitrogen, at $-259°C$). UHMWPE starts to soften and lose its abrasion resistance characteristics around 185°F.

Because UHMWPE has a relatively high expansion/contraction rate when subjected to temperature changes, it is not recommended for close tolerance applications in these environments.

Because of its high-surface-energy nonadherent surface, PE can be difficult to bond. Assemblies may most readily be put together with fasteners, interference, or snap fits. Loctite Corporation makes a cyanoacrylate adhesive (CYA) (Loctite Prism® surface-insensitive CYA and primer) to bond these types of plastics.

UHMWPE is also used in orthopedic implants with great success. It is the most common material used in acetabular cups in total hip arthroplasty, and in tibial plateau components in total knee replacements, bearing against highly polished cobalt–chrome.[12] Note that material suitable for orthopedic implant use is a specialty material, not the industrial-grade version. A medical-grade UHMWPE is marketed by Westlake Plastics (Lenni, PA) under the trade name Lennite®.

Acetal

Delrin® by DuPont is one of the best-known acetals, and most designers refer to this plastic by this name. Acetals are synthesized from formaldehyde. Acetal was originally developed in the early 1950s as a tough, heat-resistant nonferrous metal substitute.[13] It is a tough plastic with a low coefficient of friction and high strength.

Delrin and similar acetals are difficult to bond and are best assembled mechanically. Delrin is commonly used in machined medical device prototypes and close tolerance fixtures. It is highly machinable, making it popular for machined device prototypes that require strength, chemical resistance, and FDA-compliant material.

One drawback of Delrin is its sensitivity to radiation sterilization. This tends to make acetals brittle. Snap fits, plastic spring mechanisms, and thin sections under load may crack and break if radiation sterilized. If acetal parts are to be sterilized, consider using EtO, Steris, or autoclave, depending on whether the device contains any sensitive components such as electronics.

Acetals are sold by Westlake Plastics, BASF, and Celanese. DuPont markets an improved acetal, DelrinII® with improved properties. Westlake Plastics markets an FDA-compliant grade under the trade name Pomalux®.

Nylon (Polyamide)

Nylon[14] is available in 6/6 and 6/12 formulations. Nylon is tough and heat resistant. 6/6 and 6/12 refer to the number of carbon atoms in the polymer

---

[12] For detailed information on UHMWPE in orthopedic applications, see Kurtz, Steven, *The UHMWPE Handbook*, Elsevier Academic Press, New York, 2004. See also the related website at www.uhmwpe.org.

[13] See http://heritage.dupont.com for the history of Delrin®, Nylon, and many other DuPont plastics and their inventors.

[14] Nylon was a discovery of Dr. Wallace Carrothers, who also discovered neoprene. Nylon was not trademarked, with the hopes that it would become a generic term and popularize use of the fiber. Neoprene was likewise a name coined at DuPont, and allowed to go generic. Dupont has been the source of many of the most important materials used in medical devices, such as PTFE, polyimide, Mylar, Tyvek, nylon, and Delrin.

chain. 6/12 is a longer-chain nylon with higher heat resistance. Nylon is not as machinable as ABS or Delrin, as it tends to leave stringy swarf on the edges of a part that may require deburring.

Nylon 6, most commonly known as cast nylon, was first developed prior to WWII by DuPont. However, it was not until 1956, with the discovery of chemical compounds (cocatalysts and accelerators), that cast nylon became commercially viable. With this new technology, the speed of polymerization was greatly improved, as well as reducing the steps necessary to achieve polymerization.

Because there are fewer processing limitations, cast nylon 6 provides one of the largest arrays of sizes and custom shapes of any thermoplastic. Castings are available in rods, tubes, tubular bars, and sheets. They range in sizes from as small as 1 pound to as large as 400 pounds per part.

Hydlar® is a high-performance version of nylon 6/6 reinforced with Kevlar fiber for use in bearings and bushings. Note: Filled and fiber-reinforced plastics of this kind are generally *not* FDA compliant.

Rod: 2.00 to 20.000 inches
Plate: 0.250 to 4.000 inches
Tubular bar: From 2.00 to 20.000 inches O.D.; unlimited I.D.

Fluorinated Ethylene Propylene (FEP)

FEP has all the desirable properties of tetrafluoroethylene (TFE) (polytetrafluoroethylene (PTFE)), but with a lower survive temperature of 200°C (392°F). Unlike PTFE, FEP can be injection molded and extruded by conventional methods into rods, tubes, and special profiles. This becomes a design and processing advantage over TFE. Available in rods up to 4.5 inches and sheets up to 2 inches, FEP fares somewhat better than PTFE under radiation sterilization.

HIGH-PERFORMANCE ENGINEERING PLASTICS FOR MACHINING

Note: These high-performance engineering plastics may be more limited in availability (special order). Some can also be quite expensive.

Ultem® Polyetherimide

Ultem 1000 is a thermoplastic polyetherimide high-heat polymer designed by General Electric for injection molding processing. Through the development of new extrusion technology, manufacturers such as A.L. Hyde, Gehr, and Ensinger produce Ultem 1000 in a variety of stock shapes and sizes. Ultem 1000 combines excellent machinability and provides a cost savings benefit over PES, PEEK, and Kapton in high-heat applications (continuous use to 340°F). Ultem is resistant to autoclave sterilization.

PEEK™ (Polyetheretherketone)

PEEK, a trademark of Viktrex plc (U.K.), is a crystalline high-temperature thermoplastic that offers excellent thermal and chemical resistance properties and outstanding resistance to abrasion and dynamic fatigue. It is recommended for electrical components where a combination of high continuous service temperature (480°) with very low emission of smoke and toxic fumes on exposure to a flame is required.

PEEK meets Underwriters Laboratories (UL) 94 V-0 requirements at 0.080 inches. This product is extremely resistant to gamma radiation, even exceeding the resistance of polystyrene. The only common solvent that will attack PEEK is concentrated sulfuric acid. Hydrolysis resistance of PEEK is exceptional and it can operate in steam up to 500°F.

PEEK is also a very hard plastic. PEEK tubing can be sharpened to a point that can pierce tissue. It is an excellent insulator. It also has stiffness that approaches that of metal tubing. PEEK is highly biocompatible, being used in demanding applications such as orthopedic implants and heart valves.

Victrex plc supports medical device manufacturers closely through their Invibio subsidiary. It supplies medical device manufacturers with implantable-grade PEEK-OPTIMA® and medical-grade PEEK-CLASSIX™ polymers.

PTFE (Teflon®)

TFE or PTFE (polytetrafluoroethylene), more commonly known as Teflon, is one of the three fluorocarbon resins in the fluorocarbon class composed wholly of fluorine and carbon. The other resins in this group, also referred to as Teflon, are perfluoroalkoxy fluorocarbon (PFA) and fluorinatedethyle neopropylene (FEP).

The forces binding the fluorine and carbon together provide one of the strongest known chemical linkages in a compact symmetrical arrangement of atoms. The result of this bond strength plus the chain configuration is a relatively dense, chemically inert, thermally stable polymer.

TFE resists attack by heat and virtually all chemicals. It is insoluble in all organics with the exception of a few exotics. Its electrical properties are excellent. Although it has high impact strength, its resistance to wear, tensile strength, and creep resistance are low in comparison to other engineering-type thermoplastics.

TFE exhibits the lowest dielectric constant and lowest dissipation factors of all solid materials. Because of its strong chemical linkage, TFE shows very little attraction for dissimilar molecules. This results in a coefficient of friction as low as 0.05.

Though PTFE has a low coefficient of friction, it is *not* suitable for use in load-bearing orthopedic applications, due to low creep resistance and poor wear. This was discovered in a classic case by Sir John Charnley in the late 1950s in his pioneering work on total hip arthroplasty.[15]

Note: Fluoropolymers (TFE and PTFE) are very sensitive to radiation sterilization. PTFE is obviously very difficult to bond; however, chemical or plasma etching may be used to produce a bondable surface.

Polysulfone and Polyphenylsulfone

Polysulfone was originally developed by BP Amoco and is currently manufactured by Solvay Advanced Polymers, S.A. (Brussels, Belgium), under the trade name Udel®. Polyphenylsulfone is sold under the trade name Radel®.

Polysulfone is a tough, rigid, high-strength transparent (light amber) thermoplastic that maintains its properties over a wide temperature range from −150 to above 300°F. Designed for use in FDA-recognized devices, it also passed all tests of the U.S. Pharmacopeia Class VI (biological). It complies with the National Sanitation Foundation's potable water standard up to 180°F.

Polysulfone has very high dimensional stability. The changes in linear dimensions after exposure to boiling water or air at 300°F are generally 1/10 of 1% or less.

Polysulfone has very high resistance to mineral acids, alkali, and salt solutions; resistance to detergents and hydrocarbon oils is good, even at elevated temperatures under moderate stress levels. Polysulfone is not resistant to polar organic solvents such as ketones, chlorinated hydrocarbons, and aromatic hydrocarbons.

Radel is used in instrument trays that require high heat resistance and high impact strength for hospital autoclave tray applications.

Polysulfone engineering resins combine high strength with long-term resistance to repeated steam sterilization. These polymers have proven successful as alternatives to stainless steel and glass. Medical-grade polysulfones are biologically inert, display unique long life under sterilization procedures, can be transparent or opaque and are resistant to most common hospital chemicals.[16]

---

[15] Brown, S.A., Let's Not Repeat History: Good Examples of Bad Ideas, paper presented at Proceedings of the Materials and Processes for Medical Devices Conference, ASM International, 2003.

[16] *J. Biomater. Appl.*, 3, 605–634, 1989.

Polyimide Rod and Sheet (Vespel®, Kapton®)

Vespel is a graphite-filled polyimide material for extreme service bearings. It is *not* an FDA-compliant material.

Ryton (polyphenyl sulfide), unmodified or modified with glass fibers or other modifiers such as PTFE, molybdenum sulfide (MoS), or graphite, is used primarily in structural components. Characteristics are high stiffness, extremely high-use temperature (up to 600°F), excellent chemical resistance, and excellent electrical properties.

In both modified and unmodified forms, Ryton exhibits excellent machineability, with optical finishes possible by grinding and lapping.

Note: These types of filled and fiber-reinforced plastics are generally *not* FDA compliant.

Injection Molded and Extruded Plastics

Injection molded and extruded plastics are available in the widest array of materials and properties. They can be custom compounded in almost endless combinations. When choosing a material, a good rule is to use a plastic that is readily available with proven biocompatibility appropriate for its use, and that meets the mechanical design and assembly requirements. Most mechanical plastics available in shapes for machining that are thermoplastics are available in injection molding pellet form.

The injection molding process will accommodate virtually any thermoplastic. Extrusion for catheters is usually done from the more flexible plastics such as Pebax®, polyurethane, polyvinylchloride (PVC) nylon, thermoplastic elastomers (TPEs), and flourinated ethylene propylene (FEP). Extrusion from rigid plastics such as PEEK (polyetheretherketone) is available where more pushability and torqueability of a catheter is required. Flexibility in these stiffer plastics in extrusions is achieved by use of thinner wall sections.

Considerations

One of the issues with injection molded plastics is that plastics manufacturers tend to sell their material in large minimum quantities. For example, a minimum quantity order of Magnum® ABS from Dow is 760 kg (1600 lb). This can be difficult to manage in an R&D environment, especially if you are molding a relatively low quantity of small-shot-size parts. One way to manage this is to request 20- or 50-lb samples, which most manufacturers will provide. Another is to deal with an injection molding vendor that specializes in medical molding. They may keep on hand cartons of common stock materials that they can subdivide for customers with smaller material requirements.

When choosing a material for injection molding, it is important to have a material that meets the design requirements, but is not overengineered. Selecting a material with more properties than you need may result in higher material costs, longer cycle times, and possibly a less cosmetically pleasing part. This can drive up costs and erode margins, especially for single-use disposables. It is also important to choose a material carefully because different materials have different shrink factors and will produce slightly different size parts from the same mold if materials are changed.

A way to work with plastics available only in injection molding pellets is to have a custom extrusion made from the material that you want to use. A number of feet of extrusion can be made from a material sample. This allows the use of a material that may be machined into prototypes.

When evaluating candidates for a plastic material, be sure to look at the example applications of a manufacturer's material used in a medical application. Not only will this help determine if the material is suitable for your application, but you may find also innovative ways to use these materials that you had not considered before.

In the following section some of the more common medical plastics for molding are described.

COMMODITY PLASTICS

ABS

ABS (acrylonitrile–butadine–styrene) is the most common plastic for injection molding. ABS is a two-phase polymer blend. A continuous phase of styrene–acrylonitrile copolymer (SAN) gives the materials rigidity, hardness, and heat resistance. The toughness of ABS is the result of submicroscopically fine polybutadiene rubber particles uniformly distributed in the SAN matrix.[17]

ABS is a very versatile, less expensive plastic with a combination of high processability, excellent surface finish, and toughness. It resists the

---

[17] "Styrene acrylonitrile copolymers have been available since the 1940s, and while their increased toughness over styrene made them suitable for many applications, their limitations led to the introduction of a rubber (butadiene) as a third monomer and hence was born the range of materials popularly referred to as ABS plastics. These became available in the 1950's and the variability of these copolymers and ease of processing has led to ABS becoming the most popular of the engineering polymers" (http:// www.bpf.co.uk/bpfindustry/plastics_materials_Acrylonitrile_ Butadiene_Styrene_ABS.cfm and www.basf.com).

formation of blemishes from flow marks and knit lines, even with more difficult part geometries.

Medical-grade ABS is sold under the Magnum® name by Dow Chemical,[18] and Lustran® by Bayer Plastics,[19] and Cycolac® by GE.

PC/ABS

PC/ABS is a versatile blend of ABS and polycarbonate. It is especially suitable for molded housings and parts that require high impact strength. The ABS component makes the material more moldable, and the PC provides high toughness.

PC/ABS is more expensive than ABS, and while highly moldable, it is not as moldable as plain ABS. More care needs to be taken in part design to avoid flow and knit lines.

PC/ABS is available from Bayer Plastics in its Bayblend® material, from GE in its Cycoloy® blend, and from Dow as Emerge®.

Acrylic

Acrylic for injection molding is available in a wide range of properties, depending on the modifiers, copolymerization, and alloying of the base PMMA.

Acrylic can be an attractive and cost-effective alternative to polycarbonate in less demanding applications. It has lower heat deflection performance; however, this means that it also molds at lower temperatures, allowing better fill of thin walls and intricate parts. Acrylic is water clear and has excellent optical properties, as well as alcohol and lipid resistance. Unlike polycarbonate, which discolors yellow under gamma sterilization, acrylic takes on a blue-green tint.

Acrylic for injection molding of medical devices is marketed by the Cyro Corporation under the trade name Cyrolite® acrylic-based multipolymers and Cyrex® acrylic–polycarbonate alloys.

Polycarbonate

Polycarbonate is one of the workhorse materials in medical devices. It is clear, tough, and tolerates a variety of sterilization methods. Since it is clear, it is especially suited to assembly with UV cure adhesives. Polycarbonate is a popular material for molding smaller devices such as luer fittings and stopcock bodies.

---

[18] http://www.dow.com/engineeringplastics/bus/na/med/#magnum.
[19] http://www.bayerus.com/new/2000/01.21.00plas.html.

PC tends to yellow under radiation sterilization. Radiation-stable grades of PC are available for these applications.

PC is sold under the trade names of Markolon® and Apec® from Bayer, Dow Calibre®, Zelux® from Westlake, and GE Lexan®.

Polyethelene

PE is an easy-to-mold plastic with excellent surface lubricity and flexibility. high-density polyethylene (HDPE) and low-density polyethylene (LDPE) are used in fluid fittings, stopcock valves, and syringe bodies. It is excellent for snap fits, but does not bond easily.

Polyolefin

Polyolefin is a plastic commonly found in blow molding applications. It is very flexible under a wide range of temperatures. It is also a popular material for molding toys, especially rotationally molded (e.g., Little Tikes). It is a low-surface-energy plastic and can be difficult to bond.

Polyolefin is also used in a majority of heat shrink tubing used in the electronics industry. Texloc Corporation (Ft. Worth, TX) produces a medical-grade polyolefin heat shrink tubing.

Styrene

Styrene is an economical commodity plastic. It has low heat resistance and is readily attacked by many aromatic solvents. It is useful in items such as cups and trays and other low-cost applications. One common application of styrene is insulated foam beverage containers (styrofoam cups).

ELASTOMERS

Elastomeric Plastics

When specifying an elastomer, a balance of properties is needed. For example, in extruded catheters there is a balance between pushability, flexibility, torqueability, and lubriciousness. In general, the softer the plastic, the higher the surface tackiness will be, and the catheter will be softer and more flexible, but less lubricious and harder to push. Fillers such as barium, in addition to providing radiopacity, can improve the lubricity of an elastomeric catheter.

Thermoplastic elastomers are useful when molding rubber-like parts. Some TPEs have excellent properties, making them candidates for replacement of thermoset silicones in some applications. Below are some of the more common TPEs.

Polyurethane (PU)

Polyurethane is a material that may exist as either a thermoplastic or a thermoset. Polyurethane is a product of diisocyanates and diamines, and was invented by Otto Bayer and his associates in 1937. Thermoplastic PU is used in film applications such as heat seal bags, and is a common material for extrusion of soft catheters. PU is highly versatile, in molded and extruded solid plastic, as well as polyurethane foams, both open cell and self-skinning. Polyurethanes are some of the most commonly used plastics in catheter manufacturing.

Polyurethanes are common rigid casting materials for model-making applications, as well as two-part mixes for dip molding and casting prototype rubber parts.

An innovative use of PU is the Synbone® (Switzerland), an injection molded bone model for training orthopedic surgeons, made from Bayer Baydur 60®.

Medical thermoplastic PUs are sold under trade names such as Pellethane® (Dow Chemical); Baydur® (Bayer); Tecoflex®, Tecothane®, Tecophillic®, and Carbothane® (Noveon Thermedics, Wilmington, MA); and Chronoflex® (Cardiotech Inc.). PUs such as Pellethane are not plasticized to achieve their flexibility, making them suitable for uses where leaching of extractable plasticizers can cause biocompatibility problems.

Kraton®

Kraton is a styrenic block copolymer made by the Kraton Corporation of Houston, TX. Kraton is a very moldable TPE plastic in a very wide range of hardness and properties.

Kraton styrenic TPEs are compounded for medical and consumer applications by the GLS Corporation (McHenry, IL) under the Versaflex®, Versaloy®, and Dynaflex® trade names. These are a family of materials based on Kraton styrenic TPE, and are offered in a wide range of durometers and surface tackiness from 3 Shore A to 80 Shore A. These materials are especially suited to overmolding applications, with grades specified for many medical applications. GLS Kratons are particularly suited to overmolding to difficult-to-bond olefinic substrates.

K-Resin®

K-Resin is a family of styrene–butadiene rubber copolymers (SBCs) made by Chevron-Phillips Chemical. It is used in numerous disposable medical devices, toys, and food packaging applications.

Monoprene®

Monoprene is manufactured by the Teknor Apex Company, a privately held company founded in 1924 and headquartered in Pawtucket, RI. Monoprene TPEs are a versatile family of TPEs composed of saturated styrene block copolymer rubbers and thermoplastic olefin resins. Monoprene is available in softness from gel to 90 Shore A. Monoprene is used in applications such as resuscitator bags and other applications requiring a rubbery material that is FDA compliant.

Pebax®

Pebax is a highly versatile family of polyether block amides that are plasticizer-free thermoplastic elastomers. Pebax has been utilized in high-performance industrial articles, medical textiles, and sporting goods. It is manufactured by the Arkema Group (France).

It is one of the more common materials in catheter extrusion. It is easy to bond, is readily formed in secondary operations, such as flaring and tipping, and releases easily from glass molds that are pretreated with mold release.

Polyvinylchloride (PVC)[20]

PVC is used in rigid (nonplasticized) and flexible (plasticized) forms. It is a common commodity plastic for disposable medical devices, especially tubing. One common type of PVC tubing is Tygon®, made by Norton Performance Plastics, a subsidiary of Saint-Gobain (France). PVC was once found in nearly 60% of all disposable medical devices until concern over phthalate plasticizers[21] (diethylhexyl phthalate (DEHP)) was raised by the EU and activist groups. A concern over DEHP-plasticized PVC in medical use is its potential release of chlorine when incinerated, as well as alleged health issues. Another potential drawback of some PVCs is their corrosiveness to P-20 steel injection molds.

Saint-Gobain has removed DEHP from its PVC tubing, and other manufacturers have sought alternatives to PVC in their devices. However, PVC has a set of desirable properties, such as clarity, sterilizability, and economy. Vendors now offer DEHP-free PVCs for medical use.

---

[20] For more information on medical molding of PVCs, see http://www.thecannongroup.com/immaginigruppo/papers/MedicalMouldingPVC.pdf.

[21] Lichtman, Benjamin, Flexible PVC Faces Stiff Competition, http://www.devicelink.com/emdm/archive/00/03/special.html.

Non-DEHP-plasticized PVCs for molding are available from Colorite Polymers under the name Flexchem®. Solmed® and Solcare® are available from Solvay-Draka.

Ethylene Vinyl Acetate (EVA)

EVA is used as an alternative to PVC in film applications where plasticizers need to be avoided. EVA film is made by Solvay-Draka in its Solmed® film line.

THERMOSETS

Santoprene®

Santoprene is a thermoset rubber material that is processable by injection molding, and manufactured by Exxon-Mobil.[22] Santoprene is especially useful where abrasion resistance is important. It is known as a thermoplastic vulcanizate (TPV).

Santoprene and other vulcanized rubbers are often black. This is due to the addition of carbon black, a material that blocks UV and protects the rubber from degradation. Santoprene is commonly used in automotive interiors, grips, and rubber covers and bumpers.

Silicone

Silicone is a polymer of silicon and carbon first successfully commercialized in a joint venture between Corning and General Electric in the 1940s. It is very stable, very heat resistant, virtually inert, and well tolerated by the body (despite bad press from litigation over its use in certain cosmetic surgery applications). Silicone is cured with one of two catalyst systems, peroxide cure or platinum cure.

Silicone is used in tubing, seals, and prosthetics. In RTV (room temperature vulcanized) form, it is a popular material for producing rubber molds for short-run prototypes and production.

Silicone is provided to the medical industry mostly by smaller suppliers. NuSil (Carpenteria, CA) is a major supplier of silicones to the medical device industry.

Polyisoprene

Polyisoprene is a synthetic version of the natural rubber originally harvested by the Mayans and Aztecs from the hevea tree.[23] It is polymerized

---

[22] http://www.santoprene.com/home.html.

by the Ziegler–Natta vinyl polymerization reaction. Polyisoprene is used in balloons, syringe bulbs, and other dip-molded devices.

Nitrile

Nitrile is a popular substitute for latex in rubber gloves. It does not have the elongation of latex, but is free from potentially allergenic latex protein monomers. Nitrile is a terpolymer made up of acrylonitrile, butadiene, and carboxylic acid. It is processed as an emulsion, much like latex rubber. Nitrile has a superior resistance to oils and fats compared with latex or polyisoprene.[24]

Latex

Latex is a natural protein from the sap of the hevea tree grown in rainy, elevated areas of Southeast Asia. It is useful in thin-film applications such as surgical gloves, condoms, and other barrier devices. Concerns over latex allergies have led to the elimination of natural rubber latex in many medical devices, and many manufacturers will certify products containing elastomers as latex-free.

Latex is used as a film, usually in dip molding. This is how gloves and condoms are produced. Latex is often coated with cornstarch powder to prevent self-adhesion. When used, this powder becomes a further source of potential contaminants in surgical applications. Latex has exceptional tear resistance, elongation, and elastic recovery.[25]

Liquid latex is a water-based colloid of latex monomer micelles that polymerizes as it dries. Liquid latex is available in forms for glove-type mold making and dip molding from TAP Plastics and Douglas and Sturgess artists' and sculptors' supply house in San Francisco.[26]

Though problematic for use in medical devices, easily available natural latex is a very useful material for prototyping dip-molded membranes,

---

[23] http://www.psrc.usm.edu/macrog/isoprene.htm. This website at the University of Southern Mississippi, Department of Polymer Science, gives a very detailed and entertaining description of the Ziegler–Natta reaction.

[24] For more information on the barrier properties of nitrile, see Welker, Jeffrey L., Nitrile as a Synthetic Barrier, *Source to Surgery*, Vol. 6, Issue 2, December 1998, http://www.ansellhealthcare.com/america/latamer/source/dec98-4.htm.

[25] Latex has exceptional tear resistance and elongation to break in thin films. In fact, in a fraternity house trick, a latex rubber condom can be made to expand and hold nearly 1 gallon of water without breaking.

[26] Douglas and Sturgess, http://www.artstuf.com/, is a great resource for a wide range of hard-to-find sculpting, modeling, and casting materials.

balloons, and rubber tips and bumpers. The results obtained in testing should closely approximate what can be achieved with synthetic polyisoprene.

HIGH-PERFORMANCE ENGINEERING PLASTICS FOR MOLDING

Polyetherimide (PEI), Ultem®, PEEK®, Polysulfone

These materials are available in pellet form for injection molding when exceptional strength and heat resistance are required. The trade names, properties, and manufacturers of these materials are described earlier in the chapter.

Keep in mind that some engineering plastics can also be quite expensive per pound of material. When designing a cost-effective disposable device, it is important not to overspecify the plastic, and have a part that is more expensive than it needs to be, but also may be more difficult to mold.

If a product is to be reused and withstand high-temperature sterilization, or has other high-performance requirements, engineering plastics can be a very attractive alternative to formed or machined metal parts.

USEFUL SPECIALTY PLASTIC MATERIAL FORMS

Extruded PTFE (Zeus, Texloc)

Extrusion of PTFE is a specialty process, due to the high heat required and the difficult rheology of the fluoropolymer material. Teflon tubing is commonly available as a sheath for electronics wiring. Some vendors for medical-grade PTFE tubing are Zeus (Orange, NJ) and Texloc (Shiner, TX).

Expanded PTFE (EPTFE)

A special form of PTFE is a stretched or expanded PTFE. This material was originally developed by the W.L. Gore company. This produces a PTFE that is flexible, hemocompatible, and can act as a scaffold for ingrowth of intimal tissue.[27] EPTFE is available from W.L. Gore (Newark, DE), Zeus (Orange, NJ), Impra, a division of C.R. Bard (Phoenix, AZ), and International Polymer Engineering (Tempe, AZ). EPTFE is used as highly lubricious liners for catheters, lubricious and flexible heat-resistant liners for thermal ablation devices, seals and gaskets, low-friction catheter liners, and vascular graft material, which allows for ingrowth of endothe-

---

[27] For more information on EPTFE and medical textiles, see Gupta, Bhupender S., Medical Textile Structures: An Overview, *Medical Plastics and Biomaterials*, January 1998. Full text available at http://www.devicelink.com/mpb/archive/98/01/001.html.

lium, and cycles with the pulsatile expansion and contraction of blood flow. EPTFE is highly heat resistant. EPTFE was invented by the W.L. Gore company and sold under the trade name Gore-Tex. EPTFE for vascular grafts is available from Impra and Atrium (divisions of C.R. Bard) and W.L. Gore. Other EPTFE shapes are available from Zeus Corporation and International Polymer Engineering.

SHEET AND FILM AND FOAM PLASTICS

Polyethylene Terephthalate (PET) and Polyethylene Terephthalate Glycol (PETG)

PET and PETG are popular film and sheet material for vacuum-formed medical blister packs and trays that are closed with heat-sealed Tyvek® lids. PETG film is often treated with a silicone coating to prevent sticking while tray parts are nested together during shipment.

PETG film is sold under the Klöckner Pentaplast name and BP Chemical Barex®.

Tyvek

Tyvek is a nonwoven olefin fiber fabric developed by DuPont. It is especially useful in medical packaging, as the mesh of the material is breathable and allows the passage of gas molecules, such as ethylene oxide sterilizing gas, but is a barrier against larger-size microbes. Tyvek is thin, waterproof, and very tear resistant.[28]

PVC and Polyethelene Film

Polyvinyl and polyethelene films are widely used in bagging and packaging applications, especially heat-sealed bags and enclosures.

Polyester Film (Mylar®)

Polyester film was the material used on the first successful high-pressure angioplasty balloons. Polyester has the property of being extrudable into very thin tubing and being noncompliant, meaning it did not stretch

---

[28] "Tyvek® is a classic case of a slow starter. It grew out of a research into nonwoven fabrics begun by William Hale Charch in 1944, took 15 years to develop, and required another 15 years to become profitable. Today Tyvek® building wrap can be seen in nearly every housing development, and it has gained a firm foothold in the envelope market. Tyvek® is also popular as a sterile packaging and protective clothing in the medical field" (http://heritage.dupont.com/).

into a sphere, as would a latex balloon, for example. This allowed a device that would expand to slightly larger than a blood vessel, and no more, while holding high pressure to remold arterial plaque and restore blood flow by dilitation. Thin polyester tubing is used to blow a wide variety of medical balloons. It may also be irradiated to modify its properties.

Mylar was originally developed by DuPont. Polyester tubing is also very useful in medical devices, as very thin wall shrink tube as well as balloon stock tubing is manufactured by Advanced Polymers (Salem, NH).

Polyimide

Polyimide is a unique thermoset material that is both an exceptional insulator and very heat resistant. It is also resistant to attack from most chemicals. It is most commonly available in tubing form, which can be made in exceptionally thin walls. It can also be made into extremely small diameter tubing. Polyimide in thin films is very flexible and fatigue resistant. It is commonly used in flex circuit applications, and very thin and strong catheter tubing. Polyimide tube is supplied by the Microlumen Company (Tampa, FL), and in custom coextrusions from Putnam Plastics (Dayville, CT).

Styrene Butadiene Rubber (SBR) Foam and Elastic Fabric (Wetsuit Material)

A common material in braces and wraps is wetsuit material, which is a layer of rubber or TPE foam with an outer layer of Spandex® nylon stretch fabric. This foam comes in two basic forms, one a neoprene thermoset rubber foam material for UV-resistant durable wetsuits, and the other an SBR blend for lower-cost consumable and disposable applications, as well as padded bags and covers. One useful form of SBR foam material has a stretch nylon fabric side and a hook-compatible plush side. This allows the construction of bands and wraps closable with hooked Velcro® tabs.

Foam Sheet Material

Another type of plastic foam material is polyolefin foam. This is a popular material in the construction of backings for conductive hydrogel on several types of electrical conducting pads, such as adhesive electrode pads for radio frequency (RF) electrosurgery, EKG, and defibrillator pads.

RESOURCES

Radiation Effects on Plastics

A very important consideration with medical plastics is their tolerance of sterilization, especially by ionizing radiation such as electron beam or gamma radiation.

> Sterigenics Corporation has a detailed pdf article and chart on this subject online. It is available to download and print at http://www.sterigenics.com/SiteFiles/Library/Material%20Considerations%20-%20Irradiation%20Processing.pdf.
>
> *Biomaterials Science*, 2nd edition, edited by B.D. Ratner et al., Elsevier Academic Press, New York, 2004. This is completely updated and revised from the first edition. A comprehensive and definitive source of information on the subject. Highly recommended.
>
> *Handbook of Materials for Medical Devices*, edited by J.R. Davis, ASM International Press, Materials Park, OH, 2003. This book covers both plastics and metals, with an emphasis on orthopedic and dental applications.
>
> *Handbook of Materials for Product Design*, edited by Charles A. Harper, McGraw-Hill, New York, 2001. A comprehensive overview of industrial materials used in product design.
>
> *The UHMWPE Handbook*, Steven Kurtz, Elsivier Academic Press, New York, 2004. Covers the use of ultra-high-molecular-weight polyethylene in orthopedic applications.

ACKNOWLEDGMENTS

The assistance of Larry Stock of Polymer Plastics Corporation (Mountain View, CA) is gratefully acknowledged in the preparation of this chapter.

3

CATHETER-FORMING EQUIPMENT AND OPERATIONS

Ted Kucklick

CONTENTS

Basic Forming Operations 52
The Hot-Air Station.. 53
Hot-Air Station Setup... 54
Types of Compressors.. 54
Particle Filters.. 54
Moisture Filters.. 54
Safety 55
Features and User Controls 55
    Temperature Gauge... 55
    Airflow Control and Airflow Gauge 55
    Thermal Nozzle 56
    Cooling Air Nozzle... 56
Basic Forming Operations 56
    Mandrels... 56
    Glass Molds.. 57
    Balloon Blowing... 57
A History of the Development of Glass Catheter Molds 59
Hole Punching 61
Slug Ejection... 61
Automated Hole Punching.. 62
Balloon Dip Molds 63

Conclusion 65
Resources 65
Acknowledgments 65

BASIC FORMING OPERATIONS

Charles Dotter, considered the father of catheter-based interventional radiology, once said: "My favorite conceptual trademark is a sketch that I did years ago of a crossed pipe and wrench. It's a gross oversimplification, of course, but what it means to me is that if a plumber can do it to pipes, we can do it to blood vessels."[1]

Some of the basic forming operations to catheter tubing will be familiar to anyone who has worked with malleable copper water pipe. Necking, flaring, joining, etc. — much of catheter tubing is very similar to small plumbing parts, with tubes, tees, valves, and stopcocks. The difference is that you are working with plastic tubing, and the tube usually goes into a human blood vessel, a duct, or a hollow organ.

The basic forming operations for catheter tubing are tipping, bonding and laminating, necking, expanding, flaring, and forming. Tipping is to form a shape, usually cone or bullet, on the end of a catheter. Bonding is the process of thermally welding two compatible plastic materials under finely controlled heat without melting and distorting the plastic catheter tube. Necking is to reduce the outer diameter of a tube, by pulling the tube through a heated-reducing die. Flaring is to form a flange on the end of a tube with a cone-shaped heated die, or to mold the material into a clamshell mold. This flange is usually to produce a mechanical anchor when assembling the tube into a fitting. Expanding is using a heated tapered die to expand the end of a tube. Forming is the process of expanding a tube, usually under air pressure. Two types of forming are free blowing, or heating a tube while applying controlled pressure into the tube, and clamping one end with a hemostat, similar to glass blowing. This free-blowing process takes a fair bit of skill and practice. Tubing may also be blown into a mold, where the balloon takes the shape of the tool. Examples of these molds are shown later in the chapter. Shrinking and laminating using a shrink tube is also a basic operation. Laminating is where a fluoropolymer shrink tube is used as a tool to laminate a sandwich of an inner tubing, a reinforcing braid, and an outer layer. The shrink tube is used to squeeze this assembly together while it is heated, causing the plastic tubes to fuse together and flow around the

---

[1] Payne, Misty M., Charles Theodore Dotter: The Father of Intervention, http://www.pubmedcentral.nih.gov/articlerender.fcgi?tool=pubmed&pubmedid=11330737.

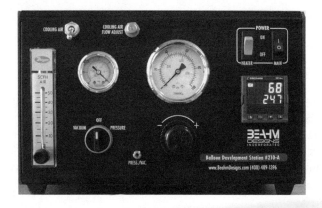

Figure 3.1   Control panel of prototype development hot-air station. (Courtesy of Beahm Designs.)

braid, capturing it in the middle layer of the finished tubing. A shrink tube is also used to bond joints between different sections of catheter tubing, such as a higher-durometer shaft and a softer-durometer distal tip. This is handled in more detail in Chapter 4. The basic tool for performing these thermal forming operations is the hot-air station.

Once catheter tubing has been formed, a common secondary operation is making holes in the tubing for aspiration, for a balloon inflation port, to inject medications or any other function a fenestration may have. Typically these holes are made with a small tube where the edge has been honed to a razor-sharp edge. Hole punches are not limited to round holes. Oval-shaped punches are also available to punch slots.

THE HOT-AIR STATION

A hot-air box is a basic piece of equipment for manufacturing catheters. It is used to perform forming and joining operations to extruded plastic catheter material. It is essentially a clean hot-air supply with fine air pressure and temperature control. The purpose is to bring the thermoplastic catheter material to its transition temperature, so that it may be formed into a desired shape, or melted and joined with another piece of catheter material. Another function of the hot-air box is balloon forming, where tubing is heated and compressed air is blown into the tube lumen. The balloon may be free blown, or blown into an exact shape into a heated glass mold. A hot-air box may also be used to form a conical tip on the end of a catheter, or to form a flare for mechanical assembly or a fluid fitting. Some of these operations require the use of nonsticking mandrels, which will be described in detail later in the chapter. Hot-air station forming is an evolution of the torch-forming methods used in early plastic catheter production.

HOT-AIR STATION SETUP

The first requirement in setting up the hot-air box is a supply of clean, dry compressed air. The requirements for the air supply are:

- Clean and dry, free from water, particulates, and oil
- Minimum 1.2 cubic feet per minute (CFM) per hot-air station at 15 PSI

An important consideration is to ensure that the air supply is free of contaminants. The three basic sources of these are dust, water, and oil from the compressor. The levels of compressed-air quality are commonly called shop air or plant air, which is basic unfiltered compressed air; instrument air for spray painting and laboratory use; and process air for food and pharmaceutical processing. ISO 8573 gives more detailed specifications for the quality of compressed air.

TYPES OF COMPRESSORS

Most compressors that meet the basic air output requirements may be used. An oilless compressor will eliminate the need to filter out oil. Some compressors are made to produce an oil mist to lubricate pneumatic air tools and should be avoided when supplying a hot-air station. Compressors and systems to supply automotive finishing spray guns can be used, as they are designed to supply clean, dry air free of oil and particulates.

PARTICLE FILTERS

To filter out particulates, the use of a small mesh filter is recommended. The size of the filter should trap particles down to the size appropriate to the manufacturing environment where you are working. For example, if you are operating the hot-air station in a class 100,000 clean room, the mesh filter should trap particles of 100,000 microns and larger. Use the largest-particle-size filter for your application. This will avoid line pressure drop and allow the compressor to operate most efficiently.

MOISTURE FILTERS

When air is compressed and decompressed, the water vapor in the atmosphere condenses, resulting in water in the compressed-air system.

Removal of this water and water vapor is required. Most compressor systems have a basic in-line water trap. An in-line trap is *not* adequate for water removal in a hot-air station setup. To ensure dry air to the hot-air station, a point-of-use (at the hot-air station) dessicator is required. A common point-of-use dessicator is a pellet cartridge. A point-of-use filter will ensure that the air used by the hot-air station is clean and dry. Consult your compressor dealer for information on filtering accessories.

SAFETY

Compressors generate noise and heat. Any compressed-air service must be handled carefully. Be sure that compressors are installed with proper ventilation, and in a location that does not produce excessive environmental noise. Be sure to install the compressor according to local building and electrical codes and applicable Occupational Safety and Health Organization (OSHA) regulations. Lines and tanks should be properly labeled. Keep the user's manuals readily accessible, and carefully follow the manufacturer's instructions for operation, safety, and regular maintenance.

FEATURES AND USER CONTROLS

Temperature Gauge

The temperature gauge is the most basic readout on the hot-air station. The temperature readout shows the air temperature at the thermal nozzle. (See Figure 3.1.)

The temperature should be set to the glass transition temperature of the plastic, or where the plastic begins to melt and becomes formable and weldable. There are several factors that can affect this temperature, such as ambient room temperature, the size of the thermal nozzle, and the nature of the material you are working with. Consult the material data sheet for the melt temperature of the plastic you are forming for the temperature at which to set the hot-air box. Try a few test pieces of your material to fine-tune to the optimum setting for your process. Remember that the melt temperature of your plastic in the data sheet is an average under laboratory conditions. You will need to find the setting that works best for your material under your conditions.

Airflow Control and Airflow Gauge

The airflow control knob regulates the velocity of airflow to the thermal nozzle. The airflow gauge shows the volume of airflow in cubic feet per minute (CFM). (See Figure 3.1.)

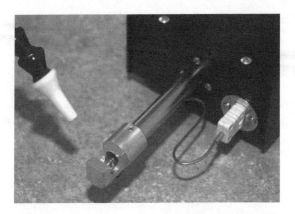

Figure 3.2 Temperature-controlled thermal nozzle and cooling air nozzle. (Courtesy of Beahm Designs.)

Airflow for welding and tipping operations should be set to 1.2 CFM. Airflow for other operations or balloon blowing should be set according to the material used and desired results.

Thermal Nozzle

Thermal nozzles are where the tubing material is heated. These nozzles come in several sizes according to your particular application. (See Figure 3.2.)

Cooling Air Nozzle

The cooling air nozzle is to cool off and set the plastic after melting and forming. The cooling air nozzle is typically foot pedal controlled.

BASIC FORMING OPERATIONS

Mandrels

A basic accessory in forming catheter tubing is mandrels. These are metal wires or fluoropolymer rods that keep tubing lumens open while forming and joining tubing.

Metal wire mandrels are made of either 304 stainless or nickel–titanium alloy (superelastic nitinol.) These mandrels are coated with polytetrafluoroethylene (PTFE, Teflon) to keep them from sticking to the melted catheter tube plastic. Mandrels may also be coated with paralyne polymer. Consult your mandrel vendor to determine which release material will best serve your needs.

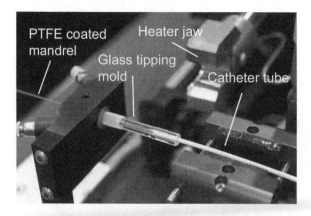

Figure 3.3 Parts of an automated tip-forming machine. Note how a mandrel is used to keep the guidewire lumen open. (Courtesy of Beahm Designs.)

While prototyping for bench testing, common piano wire may be used as a mandrel if a manufactured mandrel is not available. The wire may be polished, then sprayed with a PTFE mold release to keep it from sticking to the melted tubing plastic. Note: Never use such a mandrel for a device intended for human use. Always use materials that conform to Food and Drug Administration (FDA) good manufacturing practice (GMP) guidelines for devices intended for human use.

Glass Molds

Glass molds are another important and versatile accessory for forming catheter tubing. Glass molds are used for blowing small balloons and tipping catheters, and glass tubes for performing joining operations. (See Figure 3.4 and Figure 3.5.)

Balloon Blowing

In this operation a piece of thin-walled tubing is used, typically polyseter. One end of the tube is clamped with a hemostat. A glass mold that has the shape of the balloon inside is slipped over the tubing. The glass mold section is heated to the transition temperature of the plastic, and air pressure is blown into the open end of the tube. The result is that a balloon is blown into the shape of the inside of the glass mold. If you have never done this before, it may take some practice to get the desired results. Equipment is available from a number of vendors (e.g., Farlow's, Beahm Designs), including the hot-air station maker and glass mold maker to automate the process of balloon blowing. Also, a number of stock

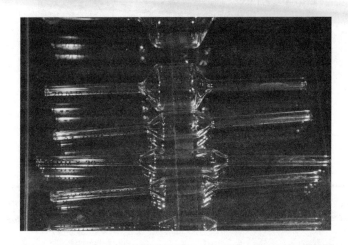

Figure 3.4 Assorted glass balloon blowing molds. (Courtesy of FSG, Inc.)

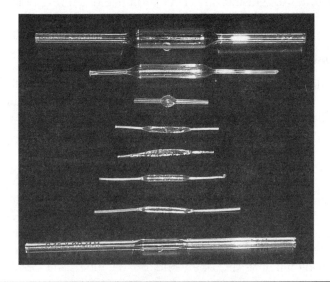

Figure 3.5 Balloon molds and blown plastic balloons. (Courtesy of FSG, Inc.)

balloon sizes and shapes may be ordered from Advanced Polymer Corporation in Salem, NH, if you do not want to blow your own balloons.

A HISTORY OF THE DEVELOPMENT OF GLASS CATHETER MOLDS[2]

Farlow's Scientific Glassblowing, Inc. (FSG), was established in 1980. The first shop was in a garage in Los Gatos, CA. In 1982, engineers from Advanced Cardiovascular Systems, Inc. (ACS) approached the company to develop the Glass Balloon Mold.

These molds were developed to form the plastic balloon catheters for the angioplasty industry. ACS at that time was forming their balloon in metal molds or by free blowing the plastic. The engineers discovered that using glass to form the balloons had some advantages. The glass allowed the engineer to see the balloon form and made the process of developing a program to blow the balloon much easier. When forming the plastic in the glass mold you could see how far to stretch the plastic. If the plastic separated or deformed, the engineer could quickly reprogram the machine to correct the problem. Another advantage of glass is that the inner surface is very smooth and would give the finished balloon a smooth surface with no flaws. Glass molds were able to hold very tight tolerances, ±.0002 on the inside dimensions of the glass molds.

As the Northern California medical device industry developed, engineers and doctors saw an opportunity to create their own niche and began leaving ACS to create new startup companies. These ACS engineers continued their development using the glass balloon technology with Farlow's. The engineers would bring glass mold technology and implement them into their new company's processes.

Along with the balloon molds Farlow's produces a part called capture tubes. This was needed for the attachment of the catheter to the balloons and dissimilar materials together.

---

[2] This history of glass catheter molds is adapted from a history of Farlow's Scientific Glassblowing, courtesy of Gary Farlow and FSG, Inc., Grass Valley, CA, www.farlowsci.com.

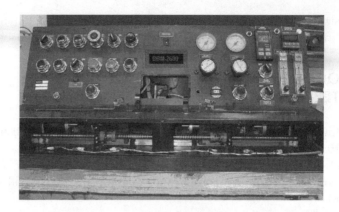

Figure 3.6 The original BMM-2600. (Courtesy FSG, Inc.)

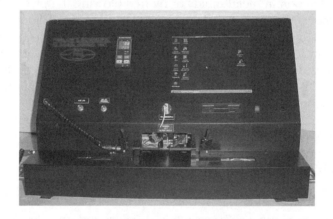

Figure 3.7 BBM-5100. (Courtesy FSG, Inc.)

Farlow's Glass and a medical company, Danforth Biomedical in Santa Clara, CA, entered into a joint venture in the medical mold business. They developed the BMM, a machine that uses glass molds to form catheter balloons for the medical industry.

Farlow's is currently producing and marketing a fourth generation of balloon blowing machines, the BBM-5100.

Farlow's now has many styles of molds, standard molds, and split molds; it has developed and is in the final stages of testing a clamshell mold.

Catheter-Forming Equipment and Operations ■ 61

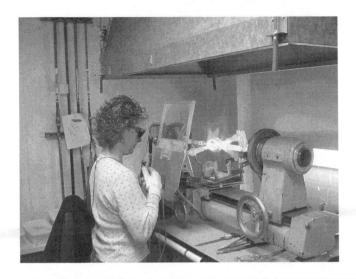

Figure 3.8 Producing a mold on a glass lathe. (Courtesy FSG, Inc.)

HOLE PUNCHING

As mentioned previously, holes are usually punched in catheter tubing with tubular cutting dies called catheter hole punches. A major supplier of these punches is Technical Innovations (Brazoria, TX). Types of hole forming are punching, where the hole punch tool is driven in perpendicular to the centerline of the tube, and skiving, where the tool cuts across the tube. Skived holes may also be made by making a notch with a sharp razor blade. Holes may be punched, where the die is held stationary and pressed into the catheter tube, or drilled, where the die is spun and driven into the tubing. Obviously, a round punch may be used in either punching or drilling, and an oval hole punch must be used as a nonrotating punch tool.

When punching holes, the durometer of the material has an effect on how easily and cleanly the hole can be punched. A thin, high-durometer tube will be more difficult to punch than a thicker, softer material.

SLUG EJECTION

When using a hole punch it is important to clear the slugs or chads from the tool. If slugs build up in the tool, the cutter will have no clearance, and the tool will stop cutting. This can be done in a rudimentary way by pushing a gauge pin into the cutter, when doing a few prototypes by hand. Technical Innovations sells a pin vise with a spring-loaded ejection mechanism for low-volume hole punching by hand.

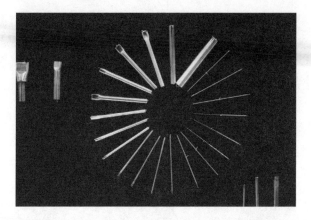

Figure 3.9 Assorted round and oval catheter hole punches. (Courtesy of Technical Innovations, Inc.)

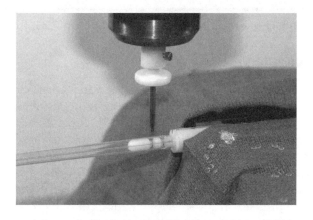

Figure 3.10 Hole-punching fixture with indexing and slug ejection mechanism.

Figure 3.10 shows a hole-drilling and manual-indexing mandrel fixture. This punch holder fixture was sized to fit into a collet in a Bridgeport-style mill. The free-spinning disc allows the chads to be ejected without stopping the mill. One thing to note is the slow speed at which the punch rotates. Higher speeds tend to cause excessive friction and melt the plastic, making a rough hole. In this setup the mill was run at about 850 to 1000 rpm to achieve good results.

AUTOMATED HOLE PUNCHING

Automated drilling and skiving setups are shown in Figure 3.11 to Figure 3.13. Catheter tubing is held in a collet and rotated using programmable

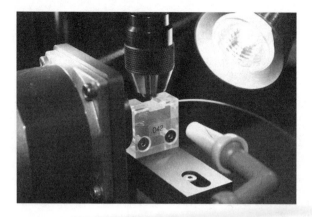

Figure 3.11 Small-hole (0.042-inch) automated hole drilling setup. (Courtesy of Technical Innovations, Inc.)

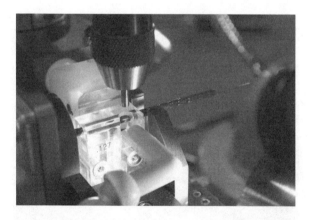

Figure 3.12 Automated skiving setup. Note skiving support block. (Courtesy of Technical Innovations, Inc.)

rotary and linear motion control. This allows the precise and repeatable punching of catheter tubes, even ones of very small diameter and hole size, as shown.

BALLOON DIP MOLDS

Another way to form balloons and shapes is with dip molds. Bullet-shaped forms are quite simple to achieve with dip molds. One of the limitations for dip molding a double-necked balloon is the stretch factor of the material. For example, if the material has a 300% stretch factor, or elongation to break, then the balloon cannot be more than 300% larger than

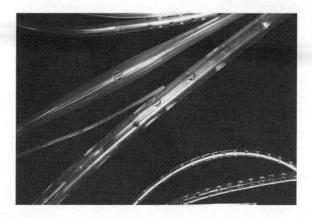

Figure 3.13 Examples of punched catheter tubes. (Courtesy of Technical Innovations, Inc.)

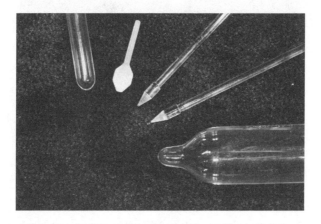

Figure 3.14 Assorted glass dip molds. (Courtesy Farlow's Glassblowing.)

the balloon necks. This can be overcome by building the balloon in two sections, then bonding the halves together.

Dip molds are also simple to make from polished brass, aluminum, or stainless steel on a lathe. When making a dip mold, make sure there are no gaps in the mold, such as testing the mold made from a bulb-shaped part by inserting a rod. The seam where the rod goes into the bulb is a place for air bubbles to form. It is better to machine the mold of one piece of material. Dip molding materials are latex, polyisoprene, nitrile, urethanes, silicones, and plastisol materials. Dip molds are useful for producing sheaths, condoms, gloves, balloons, bumpers, and numerous other elastomeric parts.

CONCLUSION

Catheter-making tools and equipment offer versatile capabilities to the medical device designer. Some of these pieces of equipment have only been widely available for a little over 10 years. Not that long ago, these types of capabilities had to be developed in-house from scratch, at significant expense, and some were closely guarded trade secrets. There is more capability and technology for developing innovative medical devices available off the shelf now than ever before. Processes that were once hand operations, and highly operator dependent, are being automated with programmable logic control, improving throughput, yield, and consistency. The tools and capabilities available to the imaginative engineer and designer to develop innovative medical devices have never been better.

RESOURCES

Hot-air stations and automated catheter manufacturing equipment:

Beahm Designs
568 Division St.
Campbell, CA 95008
Phone: 408-871-2351
Fax: 408-871-8295
www.beahmdesigns.com

Farlow's Scientific Glassblowing
200 Litton Dr. #234
Grass Valley, CA 95945
Phone: 800-474-5513
www.farlowsci.com

Technical Innovations
20714 Highway 36
Brazoria, TX 77422
Phone: 979-798-9426
Fax: 979-798-9428
www.catheterholes.com

ACKNOWLEDGMENTS

The assistance of Brian and Anita Beahm (Beahm Designs); Gary Farlow, Ralph Joiner, and Bobbie O'Brien (FSG); and Gail Brinson and Scott Thompson (Technical Innovations) in the preparation of this chapter is gratefully acknowledged.

4

BASICS OF CATHETER ASSEMBLY

Ted Kucklick

CONTENTS

How This Catheter Is Built 68
Forming the Distal Tip Assembly 71
Other Ways to Tip a Catheter 71
Joining the Distal Tip Assembly and the Proximal Shaft 73
Punching the Air Hole for Balloon Inflation 73
Attaching the Proximal Luer Fitting 74
Attaching the Balloon to the Catheter Shaft Assembly 76
Assembling the Proximal Steering Hub 77
Glossary of Catheter Terms 79
Resources 86
    Participating Vendors in the Relay Catheter 86
    Other Resources 86
Acknowledgments 87

Catheters are one of the more common medical devices. A catheter is a flexible tubular device inserted into a vessel, duct, body cavity, or hollow organ. This device is used in the introduction or withdrawal of fluids, delivery of energy, placement of a balloon, or placement of a device or biologic to the body. The device may be steerable to navigate through curved or branching structures. The catheter may also contain electronic sensors.

At a recent industry conference, an executive R&D manager of a major medical device company outlined the company's vision for delivery therapies via the "vascular highway." He stated that nearly every structure in the body is accessible by this route. This means that there are significant future opportunities available for innovative catheter design in less invasive therapy.

Catheters have been at the foundation of the revolution in minimally invasive and less invasive therapy. Advances in plastics, metals, electronics, sensors, and innovative construction techniques have produced catheters of unprecedented capability. Some of the largest medical device companies (e.g., Boston Scientific and Guidant) were founded on catheter products.

This chapter will present an example study of building a generic deflectable balloon catheter. In this example, you will see some of the basic parts of a balloon catheter, manufacturing methods of the components, and basic assembly techniques and equipment. One of the most basic pieces of equipment is the hot-air station, which is described in Chapter 3. Common adhesive bonding materials will be described. The end of the chapter will have a glossary of common catheter types.

The example for this will be a basic steerable catheter, the relay catheter, which was a demonstration piece for the annual Beahm Designs medical device technology open house, held in Santa Clara, CA. The reason for the name is that the device was built at the show, in relay fashion from one vendor's booth to the other, while onlookers watched. *The Medical Device R&D Handbook* gratefully acknowledges the support of Venture Manufacturing, Santa Clara, CA, and all of the vendors who participated in the relay catheter for their assistance with this chapter.

This demonstration catheter serves as a valuable introduction to a number of catheter-building concepts. In this demo, there are examples of heat bonding of different durometer catheter shafts, tipping, and anchoring of a pull wire at the distal tip, and some basic principles of building a steerable catheter. Tools such as the hot-air box and tipping dies are demonstrated. Another important method in catheter building is also demonstrated: the use of shrink tubing to form heat-bonded joints.

Another feature of this demonstration piece is that many of the items to build this device are readily available, and some are even off-the-shelf components. Knowing what can be acquired quickly and inexpensively is a key skill of the R&D technician, as this will allow the rapid iteration of prototypes while consuming the least amount of scarce and expensive capital money, and while quickly converging on a usable solution.

HOW THIS CATHETER IS BUILT

This catheter demonstrates some of the inner workings of a simple deflectable catheter that would not be obvious to one who has not seen

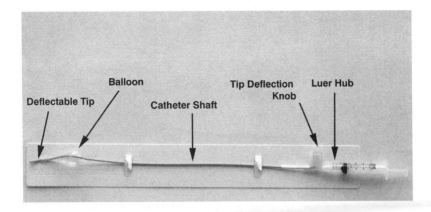

Figure 4.1 Parts of the relay catheter.

one put together before. The distal catheter shaft is a soft 30 Shore D Pebax material, and the proximal shaft is a stiffer 72D Pebax (Figure 4.1).

One of the things about catheter building, especially when seeing it for the first time, is how much touch and art are involved. Some of the features of the device are rather small and tricky to get right the first time. In an R&D environment, it can be very helpful to have the assistance of an experienced medical device assembler. This technician can be a valuable resource and partner with the designer to build the device for assembly from the beginning. It is one thing to hand-build a one-off device; however, it is another matter to build five or ten devices that are reliable and consistent, and yet another to scale up to make devices in the hundreds or thousands. Getting the input of a skilled and knowledgeable assembler will help the engineer design devices that are of higher quality, reliable, and consistent, with good yields and without unnecessary labor content. They often know efficient ways to put a device together that the engineer may not know.

This catheter consists of a proximal luer fitting for inflating the balloon and an integrated screw mechanism for actuating a pull wire to deflect the tip section. In this demo unit this feature is insert molded to the catheter shaft, meaning that the catheter shaft is placed into an injection mold, and the hub is injection molded around it. This allows the hub to be fused to the catheter shaft without adhesives. This is a useful method for higher production numbers; however, an off-the-shelf proximal hub may just as easily be bonded to the catheter shaft by either thermal bonding, cyanoacrylate, or UV cure adhesive.

Note that the joint between the luer hub and the catheter shaft is covered with heat shrink tubing. This is to provide a strain relief between the hub and the shaft, to prevent the shaft from kinking.

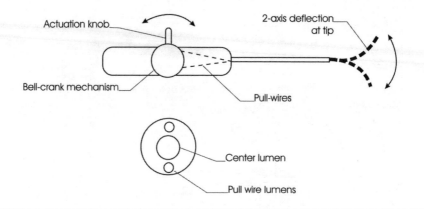

Figure 4.2 Two-axis steerable catheter and handle.

This deflectable catheter operates by having a proximal shaft that is relatively stiff, and a softer distal tip. A small-gauge stainless steel pull wire runs the length of the shaft to provide pulling force to the tip and deflect the catheter. The catheter shafts are a standard two-lumen design, with a small lumen for the pull wire and a larger lumen to pass air to inflate the balloon. Both the softer and stiffer shafts have the same extrusion profile. The catheter diameter is 8F (2.7 mm, or 0.105 inches).

The method shown in the example makes a catheter tip that deflects in one direction. Other ways to make a steerable catheter are as follows. If the catheter is to steer in two or more axes, the extrusion profile will have two wire lumens 180° apart, with the larger lumen in the center. These wires are anchored in the tip, and to get bidirectional steering, the wires are connected to a bell-crank mechanism in the handle (Figure 4.2). A lever bends the tip in its two directions of deflection. This may be expanded to allow four axes of deflection if wires are placed at the 12:00, 3:00, 6:00, and 9:00 positions in the catheter shaft, and connected to two bell-crank actuators at 90° to one another. Gastroscopes and sigmoidoscopes have this type of four-way steering. This type of mechanism makes the catheter more versatile; however, it also makes it larger, and more complex and expensive to build. This may be justified for a reusable endoscope costing thousands of dollars, but is difficult to justify in a single-use device. It is often just as simple to torque a device to turn the catheter tip as to make a more complex four-way steering device.

Another way to make a flexible tip on a catheter is by means of a vertebrated section. As the name implies, a tube of metal or plastic is notched to produce a series of rings, leaving a spine of material. This vertebrated tube is then covered with a flexible elastomeric sheath. The spine may be made of the remaining material in the tube, or it may be a piece of flat metal or wire spot welded to a series of rings.

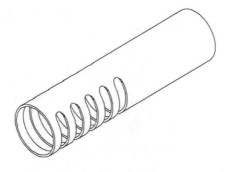

Figure 4.3 A vertebrated tube for flexibility.

FORMING THE DISTAL TIP ASSEMBLY

The distal tip assembly is formed with a bullet-shaped glass mold. These molds are described in detail in Chapter 3 on the use of the hot-air station and glass molds.

First, a wire is cut to the length of the catheter. A piece of small-diameter polyethylene (PET) tube liner, cut to the length of the distal shaft plus about a 1/2 inch, is then slipped over the wire. This liner will allow the wire to operate freely, and provide a bridge piece between the soft distal shaft and the stiffer proximal shaft when they are heat bonded together.

To form the anchor for the pull wire, the wire is bent back 180° in a hook, about 1/8 of an inch. This is then pulled back until the wire hooks into the large lumen of the extruded tubing. This assembly is then pushed into a heated mold, heated to the melt temperature of the plastic. This forms a bullet tip on the end of the distal end of the catheter and melts the plastic around the wire, anchoring it in place. Fine stainless steel wire is available from Small Parts, Inc., Miami Lakes, FL.

OTHER WAYS TO TIP A CATHETER

In this example, a custom-made glass mold is used to form the tip. Since many of these devices were to be built, this was the best solution. However, you may find yourself at the workbench late some afternoon or evening and need to put a tip on a catheter for an *in vitro* prototype. What do you do then?

One way to make a tipping die is to fabricate one out of brass or aluminum on a lathe. Drill out a metal rod to the diameter of the catheter tube with a plus tolerance for clearance. Grind a drill bit (hopefully an old dull one) to the shape of the tip you need, and grind a cutting edge on this tool. You can do this with the shank end of the drill if you cannot afford to destroy the drill. Use this as a form tool to carefully bore out

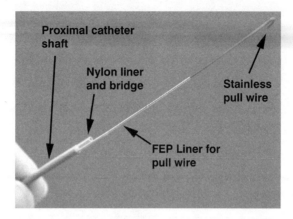

Figure 4.4 Pull wire and liver tubes of the catheter.

the tip shape in the metal rod. Machine the metal rod so that the wall thickness is about 1/8 inch for better heat transfer. Prime the tool with mold release, heat it to the transition temperature, push the catheter tube in until you feel that a tip has formed, cool the mold, and pull out your (hopefully) acceptably formed tip. One disadvantage over a glass mold is that you do not see the tip forming and need to do it more by feel. If you are really short on tools (you do not have a temperature-controlled hot-air station), an adjustable heat gun can work. With some trial and error and a barbeque thermometer that reads up to 500°F, you can calibrate your heat gun and get acceptable R&D or proof of concept level results. Another way to form a tip is with a plastic tip die. A Teflon rod can make a tipping die; however, it can be difficult to heat.

A tip can also be formed with a piece of thick silicone tubing that is just large enough to stretch over your catheter tube. Heat the tip of the tube. The silicone will not melt; however, the plastic inside the tube will soften and melt. Work the catheter tubing until the silicone tube squeezes down and melts the end of the tube closed. No mold release is needed, as the catheter plastic will not stick to the silicone. The plastic will flow more as you heat the distal end of the tube, and the temperature gradient from the tip back will produce a taper. If you need to keep an open lumen, use a piece of clean piano wire coated with mold release as a mandrel. (Pam™ no-stick cooking spray works in a pinch, again for *in vitro* prototype or bench testing only.) With some practice and the right size silicone tube, you can form an acceptable tapered tip with this method. One last way to form a rudimentary tip is to heat the plastic and (carefully, without burning your fingers) roll it between your thumb and forefinger until you get an acceptable tip.

JOINING THE DISTAL TIP ASSEMBLY AND THE PROXIMAL SHAFT

Once the pull wire and liner have been installed to the distal tip, and the tip has been formed, the distal tip assembly is ready to be joined to the catheter shaft. The way this is done is with fluorinated ethylene propylene (FEP) shrink tubing. FEP tubing, being a fluoropolymer, is far more heat resistant than Pebax, and the melted catheter shaft material does not stick to it.

An FEP shrink tube is purchased that when shrunk, recovers down to the diameter of the catheter shaft. The FEP shrink tube acts as a mold, allowing a butt weld between the distal and proximal catheter shafts, and pulls the shafts together as the tube shrinks lengthwise. As the FEP shrinks it squeezes the melted Pebax ends together to form a joint. Since the shrink tube recovers to the diameter of the catheter shaft, the joint is smooth and clean. Here you see why the liner tubes are important. Without the liner tubes, the plastic would melt and close off the catheter lumens, and the catheter would not function. The FEP liner for the pull wire and the nylon liner and bridge are essential parts to make this device work. Once the joint is formed, the FEP tubing is carefully cut off.

Using the nylon liner is actually a shortcut in constructing this particular catheter. It is a way to perform this joining operation without special tooling. Normally, catheter lumens are held open during joining operations with wire mandrels, ground to size, and coated with nonsticking polytetrafluoroethylene (PTFE) or paralene. These wires are removed after the joining operation, leaving a clean open lumen at the joint. The mandrel acts as a mold core. Another way to form a butt joint is with a tubular glass mold instead of the FEP shrink. With the glass mold method, a closely fitted mold is heated, and the catheter shafts are pressed together inside to form the joint. One of the advantages to the FEP shrink tube method is that the tube clamps down evenly on the tube while welding, and forms a very smooth and consistent joint. (See Figure 4.5 and Figure 4.6.)

PUNCHING THE AIR HOLE FOR BALLOON INFLATION

Typically, holes are punched in catheter tubes with a sharpened tubular punch. These punches are available from Technical Innovations (Brazoria, TX). Another simple way to make a hole in catheter tubing is to skive a small notch into the tube with a sharp razor blade. (Drilling is punching a hole perpendicular to the tube; skiving is slicing off a notch at a 90° angle across the tube.) This is a simple way to get a hole in a catheter tube when prototyping.

However, neither of these methods was used to make the small air hole in the catheter to inflate the balloon. In this case the hole was made

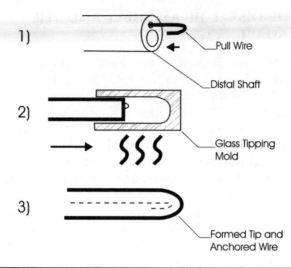

Figure 4.5 Steps in forming the wire anchor and tip.

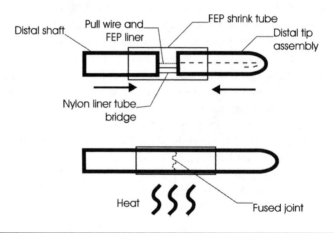

Figure 4.6 Fusing the proximal and distal shafts with FEP shrink.

with a clean, pointed, hot soldering iron tip. This method is a convenient way to make a small, clean hole in catheter tubing, quickly and consistently, without tooling.

ATTACHING THE PROXIMAL LUER FITTING

In this example, a custom luer fitting was insert molded to the proximal end of the catheter. Typically, an off-the-shelf Y connector or some other fitting is glued to the catheter shaft. Standard luer fittings are available from a number of vendors, such as Quosina, Merit, Value Plastics, Brevet, B Braun, and several others. Quosina (www.quosina.com) is a handy resource for all types of medical fittings. It carries a wide variety of fittings and accessories from several manufacturers, and has very reasonable minimum order requirements. Many times when building prototypes, a luer fitting with the exact diameter needed is not available off the shelf. In this case these standard fittings are often drilled out or modified to meet the need at the moment.

Another trick to fit a larger tube to a smaller hole is this: Say you have a slightly oversize tube and a fitting that you cannot or do not want to drill out. If possible, heat the catheter tube until is slightly soft, and pull carefully, like taffy. This will stretch the tube, reducing the cross-sectional diameter. If you pull the tubing until it stretches and breaks, you now have a tapered tube; you can slice it off with a razor blade at the desired diameter. This may not work all the time, but it is a useful trick in a pinch.

Usually the adhesive of choice for this application is a UV cure adhesive (made by Loctite, Inc., or Dymax, Inc.) Other adhesives like cyanoacrylates and epoxy can be used, but in this application UV cure is the most versatile.

To use UV cure adhesive, the fitting must be clear to allow the passage of UV light, and you must have a UV light source. These light sources can be expensive (around $1000 for a low-end model). These are a very useful accessory to have if you are doing a lot of catheter prototyping and assembly. Newer LED-based curing wands from Loctite may offer an economical alternative to lamp-based spot-curing wand systems. Another economical alternative is a used UV light source originally designed for curing dental composites.

UV adhesives are versatile and ubiquitous in medical device manufacturing. They are used for everything from gluing together oxygen masks to gluing hypodermic needles to luer hubs. UV cure adhesives are also used widely in the electronics industry. There are numerous types and grades of UV adhesives to bond nearly any material, where at least one is transparent to allow the passage of UV light. UV cure adhesives have excellent gap filling and solidify as soon as they are exposed to UV. The Dymax and Loctite websites have excellent information on how to choose the right adhesive for bonding your combination of materials.

It is important to design a part to be UV bonded so that UV light completely illuminates the adhesive. If any adhesive is in a shaded area, it will not cure. Also, just because a material is transparent to visible light does not mean it is transparent to UV. Most clear materials are, such as acrylic, styrene, and polycarbonate. A notable exception is polyimide tubing. It is amber colored and transparent to visible light, but opaque to UV. A glue joint that is under a polyimide tube will not cure under UV light.

It is important to use proper eye protection with UV cure systems. Use the eye protection provided by the manufacturer. *Exposure to high-intensity UV can cause permanent eye damage.*

Once the luer fitting is bonded to the catheter shaft, the joint is then covered with a length of standard polyolefin heat shrink tube. This is to provide a strain relief between the catheter shaft and the luer fitting.

ATTACHING THE BALLOON TO THE CATHETER SHAFT ASSEMBLY

The catheter is now ready for the attachment of the balloon. The balloon in this example is an off-the-shelf item available from Advanced Polymers (Salem, NH). The balloon for this example is a polyurethane balloon that is heat bonded to the Pebax catheter shaft.

To accomplish the heat bonding of the balloon neck to the tube as shown in Figure 4.7, a close-fitting PET heat shrink tube from Advanced Polymers is used. It is slipped over the balloon neck, and the assembly is heated. The shrink tube clamps down on the balloon neck, and the balloon neck fuses to the catheter shaft. When the balloon bonding is complete, the PET tubing is carefully cut away, as it does not bond to the materials used. A custom clamshell mold of this kind as pictured in Figure 4.8 is not a necessity; however, if a hot-air box heater jaw is to be used, the operation must be done very carefully to prevent damage to the catheter assembly.

In this example, a special clamshell mold is used to localize the heat and prevent damage to the thin balloon material.

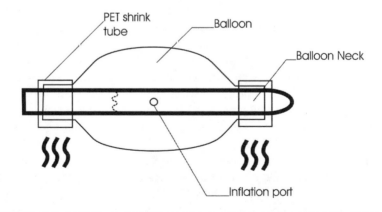

Figure 4.7 Balloon bonding with shrink tube schematic.

Basics of Catheter Assembly ■ 77

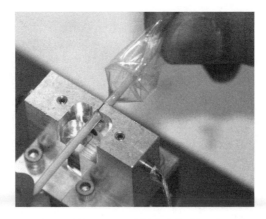

Figure 4.8 Balloon bonding using a custom-heated clamshell mold. (Courtesy of Venture Manufacturing, Santa Clara, CA.)

ASSEMBLING THE PROXIMAL STEERING HUB

In this example, a very compact, simple, and effective steering mechanism is used. The steering mechanism is a lead screw that when unscrewed pulls on the stainless steel wire and bends the distal catheter tip. The actuation anchor on the wire is a small steel bearing, drilled with a hole, soldered to the pull wire with silver solder. This bead sits in a coneshaped pocket at the top of the screw mechanism. Figures 4.9–4.12 show the construction and assembly of the steering hub.

This is an example of a generic catheter with rudimentary tip steering and balloon capabilities. For the designer, several approaches to make the catheter easy to build are apparent.

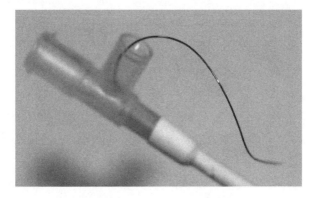

Figure 4.9 Pull wire and luer hub.

78 ■ The Medical Device R&D Handbook

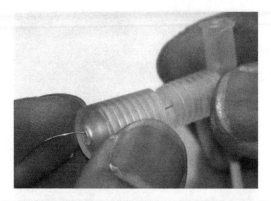

Figure 4.10 Assembling lead screw pull mechanism.

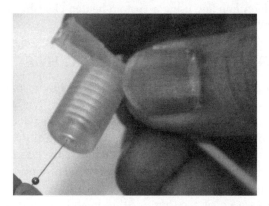

Figure 4.11 Fitting bearing bead to wire.

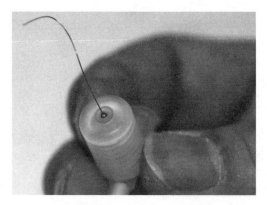

Figure 4.12 Soldering wire to bearing bead. Wire is trimmed, and cap glued over bearing.

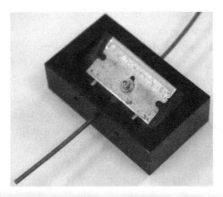

Figure 4.13 Fixture for slicing shrink tube from a catheter assembly. (Courtesy of Venture Manufacturing.)

This example shows how much may be done with simple tools and off-the-shelf components. The extrusions, both for the catheter shaft and for the liners and shrink tubes for assembly, must be custom ordered. For any particular catheter of this type, the sizes of the tubing must be carefully matched in order to produce a useable device.

Figure 4.13 shows is a fixture for trimming the shrink tube from the catheter when done.

GLOSSARY OF CATHETER TERMS

Acorn tip catheter: A catheter with a cone-shaped knob at the distal end to occlude the urethra when delivering contrast.

Amplatz catheter: A type of J-shaped guiding catheter to direct a cardiac catheter through the aortic arch and into a coronary artery. Also used in urology and other applications. Named for Kurt Amplatz, pioneer in radioliogy and development of guidewires.

Angiography catheter: A cardiac catheter for injecting contrast dye into the heart for an angiogram, a radiologic study of the blood flow in the heart that looks for blockages.

Atherectomy catheter: A device that cuts atherosclerotic plaque from the arteries, as opposed to squeezing it out of the way as with an angioplasty catheter.

Balloon catheter: A catheter with an expandable device affixed to a catheter for the purpose of either anchoring a catheter in place (Foley catheter), expanding and dilating a vessel (e.g., angioplasty catheter), occluding a vessel, or pulling out a thrombus (Fogarty catheter).

Bonding (heat): The method of assembling catheter parts together by welding or fusing, as opposed to bonding with adhesives.

Bougie tip: A soft, flexible tip at the end of a stiffer catheter to facilitate the passage of a catheter into a tubular structure. Usually cylindrical or conical. From the French word for a wax candle. Often used for dilating strictures. Specialized types are the Hurst and Maloney bougies. A wax bougie is used to detect calcific stones in the urethra, which scratch the surface of this bougie. A flexible bougie tip can help a device find the path through a passage without dissection, such as passing a stiff catheter tube into the esophagus.

Bozeman–Fritsch: A curved two-channel urinary catheter with fenestrations at the tip.

Braasch catheter: A bulb-tipped catheter for dilation.

Braid: A woven material thermally bonded to the surface of a catheter to increase its resistance to kinking and collapsing. A reinforcement structure to produce a composite structure with a plastic catheter. Braid is typically a woven tube of stainless steel wire.

Brush catheter: A catheter with a stiff bristled brush at the distal tip for collecting cell or biopsy samples.

Catheter: A tubular instrument. From Greek *katheter*, *kathemi*, to send down.

Catheter drill, punch: A sharpened tube for punching holes in catheter material.

Central venous catheter: A catheter inserted into a peripheral vein and placed into the thoracic vena cava.

Compliance: The tendency or resistance of a balloon to expand into a sphere. A compliant balloon is elastic and, when inflated, will eventually blow up into a sphere. A noncompliant balloon is not elastic and will inflate to a predetermined shape. An example of a compliant balloon is a latex Foley balloon. An example of a noncompliant balloon is an angioplasty balloon that is sized to expand only to the size of the vessel to be dilated, and no more, to prevent dissection of the vessel. Radiation cross-linking of balloon plastics is often used to produce a noncompliant balloon.

Coude: A bend in a catheter. A bi-coudate catheter has two bends, or elbows.

Cyanoacrylate adhesive: A versatile fast-setting acrylic-based adhesive commonly used in medical device assembly. A.k.a. crazy glue.

dePezzer: A self-retaining catheter with a bulb on the end.

Dotter, Charles: Dotter is considered the father of interventional radiology. Brilliant, energetic, and unconventional, he was nicknamed Crazy Charlie by colleagues. He is credited with such far-reaching and fundamental innovations as the use of x-ray roll film for angiography, the first percutaneous transluminal angioplasty (nicknamed Dottering), where stenoses were dilated with catheters. Dotter also developed the double-lumen balloon catheter, the safety guidewire, and the J-tipped guidewire. He was the first to experiment with self-expanding nitinol coiled stents. One of his students was Melvin P. Judkins, developer of the Judkins guiding catheters. He worked with Andreas Gruentzig and was instrumental in his success in developing balloon angioplasty. He also worked with Bill Cook to develop innovative new catheter designs.[1]

Drainage catheter: A tube for draining fluid from a body cavity.

Drew–Smythe catheter: A device for puncturing the amniotic sac for the purpose of inducing labor.

EP catheter: Electophysiology catheter. A device for delivering radio frequency energy to the heart for thermal ablation to interrupt aberrant cardiac heartbeat electrical signals.

Extrusion: A method of producing catheter tubing by squeezing melted plastic through a shaped die. Virtually any cross section and configuration of lumens are possible.

Fenestrations: Holes or openings. From Latin for "a window."

FEP: Fluorinated ethylene propylene, a fluoropolymer used in a type of heat shrink tubing, especially useful in catheter construction.

Flaring: Forming a flange on the end of a catheter tube with a heated cone-shaped die.

Fogarty catheter: The eponymously named embolectomy balloon catheter, which is advanced past a clot and inflated, then withdrawn to remove the clot. Invented by innovator, vascular surgeon, and noted medical device industry entrepreneur, Thomas J. Fogarty, M.D.[2,3]

---

[1] Misty M. Payne of the Oregon Health Sciences University, Portland, OR, has written an excellent biography of Dotter: Charles Theodore Dotter: The Father of Intervention, *Tex. Heart Inst. J.*, 28, 28–38, 2001. This article gives a picture of this remarkable innovator, his visionary contributions, and the institutional inertia he had to overcome. This full text of this article is available free from PubMed at http://www.pubmedcentral.nih.gov/articlerender.fcgi?tool=pubmed&pubmedid=11330737.

[2] "Before earning his MD in 1960 from the University of Cincinnati Medical School, Fogarty had designed his most significant invention. The Fogarty Balloon Embolectomy Catheter is, like many revolutionary inventions, simple in concept. It is a catheter (hollow tube) about the width of a pencil, with a small balloon at its tip: the catheter is inserted through an incision into a blood vessel, and pressed through an embolus (blood clot); then the balloon is inflated, so that when the catheter is extracted, the balloon drags the clot out with it. Fogarty built the prototype in his attic, attaching the fingertip of a latex surgical glove to a catheter using fly-tying techniques familiar to him from boyhood fishing expeditions." Dr. Fogarty was winner of the year 2000 Lemelson Prize for Innovation and is an inductee into the Inventor's Hall of Fame. From a Lemelson–MIT Program article on Thomas Fogarty. Fogarty was also a resident at the University of Oregon.

[3] See Interview with Thomas Fogarty, page 295.

Foley catheter: A urinary catheter with a balloon at the distal tip to provide retention in the bladder.[4]

Forssmann, Werner: The first person to demonstrate cardiac catheterization in Eberswald, Germany, in 1929. Because the procedure was considered especially risky, he performed it on himself, injecting contrast into his own heart through a catheter inserted into his arm, while an assistant operated a fluoroscope. Despite his repeated demonstrations of the safety and usefulness of the method, Forssmann was scorned as an eccentric. He switched specialties to urology and became a country doctor. The importance of his work was at last recognized in a shared Nobel Prize in 1956.

French (catheter scale): Catheters are most often measured according to the French catheter scale. A French is a unit of linear measure: 1 French is equal to 1/3 of a millimeter. French size measures the circumference, not the diameter, of a catheter, e.g., 3 Fr = 3 mm circumference and approximately 1 mm diameter. The French size, for example, is not the diameter of a catheter with an oval cross section at its widest point. The name and the symbol Ch refer to the Charrière gauge scale, which is often called the French scale.[5] This makes the French scale useful for measuring catheters that are not round. French size is abbreviated Fr. French is usually used when describing the diameter of flexible catheters, or larger tubes. On medical packaging French is often abbreviated F (e.g., 10F).

Gouley's catheter: A curved instrument with a groove on the lesser curvature to slide over a guidewire. Inserted into a urethra to dilate strictures.

---

[4] "Ninety-five years ago, Charles Russell Bard began research for the treatment of urinary discomfort. This led to the development of the first balloon catheter in cooperation with Dr. Frederick E.B. Foley." The first Foley catheters were sold in 1934. From C.R. Bard, Inc., www.crbard.com.

[5] "Joseph-Frederic-Benoit Charriere, a 19th century Parisian maker of surgical instruments, has by virtue of his ingenuity and advanced thinking, continued to have his presence felt in medicine throughout the 20th century. His most significant accomplishment was the development of a uniform, standard gauge specifically designed for use in medical equipment such as catheters and probes. Unlike the gauge system adopted by the British for measurement of needles and intravenous catheters, Charriere's system has uniform increments between gauge sizes (1/3 of a millimeter), is easily calculated in terms of its metric equivalent, and has no arbitrary upper end point. Today, in the United States, this system is commonly referred to as French (Fr) sizing. In addition to the development of the French gauge, Charriere made significant advances in ether administration, urologic and other surgical instruments, and the development of the modern syringe." Iserson, K.V., J. F. B. Charriere: the man behind the French scale, *J. Emerg. Med.*, 5, 545–548, 1987.

Gruentzig, Andreas: Pioneering figure in balloon angioplasty. Born in Dresden, Germany, he worked at the University Hospital in Zurich, Switzerland. After learning of the work of Charles Dotter, he set out to expand on Charles's work by adding a balloon to a dilating catheter. He built many early prototypes in his own kitchen, building the first balloon catheter device in 1975.[6] Gruentzig performed the first coronary balloon angioplasty on a patient in 1976. His meticulous work and superior presentation skills helped to shepherd this new technology through the intense scrutiny and skepticism of practicing cardiologists. The technology of balloon angioplasty spawned a revolution in minimally invasive alternatives to open surgery, and a major Silicon Valley success story, Advanced Cardiovascular Systems (ACS, now a division of Guidant). Andreas Gruentzig died in a plane crash in 1985.

Guidewire: A flexible wire, usually of stainless steel. This wire often has a lubricious coating of PTFE fluoropolymer and an atraumatic soft-coiled wire tip. The guidewire is placed into a blood vessel; a catheter slides over this wire to the target location. This is called the over-the-wire technique, and was pioneered by John Simpson, M.D.

Guiding catheter: A stiffer catheter tube that guides another, more flexible catheter into place. Examples of these are Judkins catheters and the Amplatz catheter.

Hemostasis valve: A type of valve that allows the passage of a guidewire through an elastomeric bushing. A screw mechanism squeezes the bushing against the guidewire, forming a blood-tight seal, while allowing advancement of the guidewire. A type of Tuhoy–Borst valve.

Hub: Generally, the round proximal end of a catheter.

Hydrophillic: A coating or material that absorbs water.

Hydrophobic: A coating or material that repels water.

---

[6] All of the pioneers of minimally invasive vascular interventions mentioned in this chapter, Fogarty, Sones, Judkins, and Dotter, were all skilled hands-on product developers: "And he [Andreas Gruentzig] showed me where he made his catheters in his kitchen, and I took one look at how he was making his catheters and you had to marvel at it, because he took single lumen tubing and in order to get two lumens into the catheter, he would put a sheath over the outside. The first lumen was on the inner tube and the second lumen was in that space in-between. The problem had been, if he applied suction, it would tend to collapse the outer sheath. In order to prevent that sheath from collapsing, he took a razor blade and went all the way down the catheter twice making a 'V' groove. Which is, if you've ever tried that, trickier to do than brain surgery, to say the least." From an interview with John Abele, cofounder of Boston Scientific, on his memories of Andreas Gruentzig, http://www.ptca.org/archive/interviews/970315int.html.

Indwelling catheter: A catheter left in place for a long period. It is specially designed to prevent infection and irritation. An old term for an indwelling urinary catheter is *catheter à demeure*.

Introducer: A shorter sheath that allows the easier entry of a longer catheter. A catheter that forms an entry port in tissue.

Judkins catheter: A preformed guiding catheter for accessing the coronary arteries. Named for Melvin P. Judkins, who developed the femoral artery access method of cardiac catheterization.[7]

Luer fitting: A 6° taper fluid fitting originally developed by Otto Luer. Later Farliegh Dickinson added a lead screw sleeve, inventing the Luer-Lok™ fitting.

Manifold: A rack of stopcock valves to control a plurality of fluid sources.

Olive tipped: A catheter with a bulbous end in the form of a prolate spheroid (olive).

Pacing catheter: A cardiac catheter with electrical leads at the tip to provide a pacing signal to the heart.

Pebax: Polyether block amide. A versatile plastic common in catheter construction.

Pushability: The ability of a catheter to be pushed into a long vessel without excessive frictional resistance, or without collapsing. Pushability is enhanced by the columnar strength of the catheter shaft and its lubricity, or slipperiness.

Seldinger technique: Named for Sven-Ivar Seldinger, Swedish radiologist, this is a method for percutaneous puncture and catheterization of the arterial system. This method involves puncturing the femoral artery with a needle and stylet set, and verifying location in the vessel from spurting blood. A guidewire is inserted through the needle, the needle is withdrawn, and a catheter is advanced over the guidewire. This method made possible quick and simple transfemoral arterial access, without the invasive cut-down techniques used previously.

---

[7] Equipped with a plastic-impregnated human heart, a roll of wire, a wire-cutter, and pliers, Dr. Judkins began creating shaping wires. When not scrubbed in his cath lab, he concentrated on bending shaping wires, using various pipes and faucets at the scrub sink to mold the wires," writes Mrs. Judkins. "He would scrutinize the shape, place the wire over a chest radiograph on the view box, contemplate, and make changes. If a shape seemed workable, he would thread a catheter over the shaping wire, immerse it in boiling water to set the shape, and experiment on the heart specimen." It is interesting to note that Judkins did not enter the cardiology specialty as a resident until he was almost 40, after a stint as a solo family physician. He went to the University of Oregon, the only program willing to take him, where he worked with Charles Dotter. The Society for Cardiovascular Angiography and Interventions (SCA&I), http://www.scai.org/drlt1.aspx?PAGE_ID=3734.

This is the access method used for nearly all vascular catheter interventions.

Simpson, John: Cardiologist, learned of balloon angioplasty from Andreas Gruentzig. Developed the over-the-wire angioplasty system. Helped to commercialize, develop, and improve the technology as a founder of Advanced Cardiovascular Systems (now Guidant).

Sones, Mason: Performed the first selective coronary angiography at the Cleveland Clinic, Cleveland, OH. Conventional wisdom taught that the insertion of a catheter into a coronary artery would result in immediate and fatal cardiac arrest. Sones accidentally slipped a catheter into a coronary artery, injected contrast, and was able to image the artery, without ill-effect to the patient. Sones then developed and perfected this technique. Selective angiography is now a routine and vital diagnostic procedure.

Steerable catheter: A catheter with a pull wire deflectable tip.

Stent: A metal mesh tube expanded to prop open a blood vessel or duct. Julio Palmaz and Richard Schatz are credited with the first modern, approved coronary stent. Drug-eluting stents (e.g., Boston Scientific Taxus™) have achieved blockbuster status.

Stent delivery catheter: A balloon catheter specially designed to place and expand a stent.

Stopcock: A small valve for the control of fluids or gasses. Available in either reusable metal or disposable plastic versions. For medical use, the ports are configured with male or female luer fittings.

Swan–Ganz: H.J.C. Swan and William Ganz invented the balloon-tipped, flow-directed pulmonary artery catheter in 1970. The Swan–Ganz catheter made possible simplified right-heart catheterization.

Tipping: To form a tip on a plastic catheter tube by means of heat and glass-, metal-, or heat-resistant plastic mold.

Thermodilution catheter: A catheter device that measures cardiac output by means of either injecting cold saline into the right ventricle or heating a volume of blood and recording the volume of heated or cooled liquid at the pulmonary artery.

Torqueability: An important performance characteristic of a catheter. Torqueability is the ability of a catheter to transmit twisting forces without kinking or absorbing the torsion in the catheter. Torqueability is enhanced by braid reinforcement of the catheter shaft.

Trackability: The ability of a catheter to be pushed through tortuous vasculature. A way to test for the pushability, torqueability, and trackability of a catheter is with an anatomical glass tube bench model.

Tuhoy–Borst valve: A valve device developed in part by Edward Tuhoy. This valve has an elastomer grommet with a central lumen in a screw compression setup. As the grommet is squeezed it closes the center lumen. This valve is often used to pass guidewires. *See* hemostasis valve.

UV cure adhesive: A versatile cure-on-demand adhesive commonly used in medical device assembly. Significant advantages are the adhesives' lack of volatile solvents, fast curing times, and ability to join dissimilar materials.[8]

Vertebrated catheter: A flexible catheter consisting of a notched tube with a remaining spine of material, or a series of rings joined by a strip or wire spine, and covered with an elastomeric sheath.

RESOURCES

One useful website chronicling the past, present, and future of angioplasty and interventional radiology is www.ptca.org. It is sponsored by Boston Scientific, originally underwritten by John Abele, and supported by Richard Myler, M.D. It is edited by Burt Cohen and is chock-full of historic information and catheter industry news.

Participating Vendors in the Relay Catheter

Advanced Polymers, Salem, NH — Shrink tube and balloon
Beahm Designs, Campbell, CA — Hot-air station
Centerline Precision, San Jose, CA — Steering hub insert molding
Extrusioneering, Inc., Temecula, CA — Catheter tubing
Farlow's Glassblowing, Grass Valley, CA — Tip mold
Peridot, Pleasanton, CA — Wire mount

Other Resources

- Small-gauge wire for pull wires
  Small Parts, Inc.
  13980 NW 58th Court
  P.O. Box 4650
  Miami Lakes, FL 33014-0650
  Phone: 800-220-4242
    Every R&D engineer should have a copy of the Small Parts, Inc., catalog.
- Adhesives
  Dymax, Inc.
  www.dymax.com

---

[8] For a general white paper on the use of UV light curing systems, see EXFO Corporation application notes 089, http://documents.exfo.com/appnotes/anotc089-ang.pdf.

Loctite, Inc.
www.loctite.com
> Both companies make a wide range of UV cure and cyanoacryate adhesives. Both offer extensive design guides and compatibility charts to help find the right adhesive for your combination of materials.

- Luer fittings

Quosina
www.quosina.com
> Every R&D engineer working on catheters should have a Quosina catalog. Nearly every plastic fitting you might need is available from them, as well as Tyvek sterilization pouches and many other component supplies.

Merit Medical
Merit Medical Systems, Inc.
1600 West Merit Parkway
South Jordan, UT 84095
Phone: 801-253-1600
> Merit manufactures and carries a wide range of off-the-shelf accessories specific to angioplasty, cardiology, and radiology.

ACKNOWLEDGMENTS

The kind assistance of Eric Lowe, Karl Im and Marlone Legaspi of Venture Manufacturing, Santa Clara, CA is gratefully acknowledged.

5

INTRODUCTION TO NEEDLES AND CANNULAE

Ted Kucklick

CONTENTS

Needle Gauges and Sizes 90
    Gauge Size 91
    French Catheter Size 92
Metric and English 92
Working with Hypodermic Tube 92
Common Hypodermic Tubing Materials 94
R&D Needle Grinding 95
Simple Compound Needle Grinding Fixture 95
Suture Needles 98
Basic Types of Suture Needle Tips 99
    Conventional Cutting 99
    Reverse Cutting 99
    Side Cutting 99
    Taper Point 99
    Blunt Point 99
Suture Attachment Methods 101
    Swaging Sutures to Needles 101
    Drill 101
    Channel 101
    Nonswaged, Closed Eye, French Eye, Slit, Spring 101
Suture Sizes 101
Suture Types 102
    Natural Absorbable 102

    Natural Nonabsorbable 102
    Synthetic Absorbable 103
    Synthetic Nonabsorbable 103
Trocars and Dilators 103
    Trocars 103
    Blunt Dilators 103
    Plastic Sharps and Trocars for Disposables 104
Glossary of Needles and Related Terms 105
Resources 110
    Hypodermic Tube, Needle, and Sharps Vendors 110
    Sharps, Disposal of, by Mail Order 112
Acknowledgments 112

One of the most common materials used in medical devices is small-diameter (hypodermic) stainless steel tubing. One of the most common medical devices is the hypodermic needle. Another is the suturing needle, and others are trocars and cannulae. Needles have been used in medicine since the dawn of recorded history. Needles are used for a wide variety of functions, such as injection, suturing, biopsy, gaining access to a surgical space, delivery of radio frequency (RF) energy for tissue ablation, delivery of electrical impulses for evoked potential tests, holding thermocouples for temperature measurement, guiding other devices such as guidewires and catheters, and numerous other uses.

    A typical needle works by piercing tissue with its sharp point, then smoothly slicing through tissue with its sharpened edges. The needle is usually designed to penetrate tissue with the least amount of resistance, thus causing minimum disruption to tissue. The sharpness of the needle as well as the polish of the tubing and freedom from burrs and roughness contribute to the effectiveness of the needle to penetrate tissue with the least resistance, and cause a minimum of tissue damage and discomfort.

    Needles and cannulae have been used since ancient times. The ancient Egyptians used metal tubes to gain access to the bladder and other structures.

NEEDLE GAUGES AND SIZES

There are several (confusing and mutually incompatible) ways to measure hypodermic needle diameter. The first is needle gauge. This is based on the Stubs wire gauge. Others are the French catheter gauge, and metric sizes in millimeters, or decimal or fractional English units.

Gauge Size

Hypodermic tubing is commonly sized according to the English Birmingham or *Stubs iron wire gauge*.[1] Note that this is *not* the same as the Brown and Sharpe, nor the W&M music wire gauge.

In the Stubs wire gauge world, as the gauge number goes up, the size goes down. This is because the gauge number was originally based on a 19th-century standard of approximately how many times the wire was drawn to get smaller sizes. The more draws, the smaller the wire and the higher the gauge number. This means that there is no number that adds up to a gauge. In most cases, the gauge became based on a geometric constant, and each manufacturer had its own. In the Stubs iron wire system, which is used to measure hypodermic tubing, a 10-gauge is 0.134 inch, and a 20-gauge is 0.035 inch. The Stubs gauge was originally developed in the late 1800s[2] and continues to be used as a matter of convenience and convention.

Obtaining a reference chart of gauge and decimal needle sizes from your tubing vendor is very helpful.

Certain gauge sizes have become commonly used in medicine, e.g., the 22-gauge needle for venipuncture. It has become a convenient way for practitioners to remember needle sizes as opposed to a fractional or decimal measurement, but otherwise quite counterintuitive.

The other thing to remember about gauge size is that this measurement refers to *outside diameter* (OD). Inner diameter (ID) is measured in English or metric diameter.

---

[1] The gauge system for sizing medical catheters and equipment is used widely around the world. Yet both its origins and its interpretation, in terms of conventional measurements, have long been obscure. The gauge, formally known as the Stubs Iron Wire Gauge, was developed in early 19th century England. Developed initially for use in wire manufacture, each gauge size arbitrarily correlates to multiples of .0010 inches. This sizing system was the first wire gauge recognized as a standard by any country (Great Britain, 1884). It was first used to measure needle sizes in the early 20th century. Today it is used in medicine to measure not only needles, but also catheters and suture wires. However, owing to the potential confusion inherent in using a gauge system, the iron wire gauge is rarely used in manufacture of nonmedical equipment." From Iserson, K.V., The origins of the gauge system for medical equipment, *J. Emerg. Med.*, 5, 45–48, 1987. See also Poll, J.S., The story of the gauge, *Anaesthesia*, 54, 575–581, 1999.

[2] For further reference, see http://www.sizes.com/materls/wire.htm. It is interesting to note that the Morse drill bit gauge system used today was copied from the Lancashire wire gauge system (yet another system), since this is the wire the Morse company apparently imported from England to manufacture its twist drills.

French Catheter Size

A French is a unit of linear measure; 1 French is equal to 1/3 of a millimeter (making it somewhat incompatible with the base 10 metric system). French size measures the circumference, not the diameter, of a catheter; 3 Fr = 3 mm circumference and approximately 1 mm diameter. The French size, for example, is not the diameter of a catheter with an oval cross section at its widest point. The name and the symbol Ch refer to the Charrière gauge scale, which is often called the French scale.[3]

This makes the French scale useful for measuring catheters that are not round. Think of it as the way you measure around your waist to get your pant size. Since most catheters are round, the French size in diameter is fairly consistent, even though this is not really what is being measured.

French size is abbreviated Fr. French is usually used when describing the diameter of flexible catheters, or larger tubes. On medical packaging French is often abbreviated F (e.g., 10F).

METRIC AND ENGLISH

In Europe and Asia, needle sizes and catheter sizes tend to be described in metric units, according to the diameter, either OD or ID. Engineers tend to describe diameters in either decimal English or metric units, according to their preference, and then translate these sizes into the units used by the medical professionals they are dealing with.

WORKING WITH HYPODERMIC TUBE

When working with hypodermic medical tubing it is especially important to know how the tubing is made, especially if an assembly is being designed where an obturator, stylet, catheter, wire, tube, or rod is being designed to fit into the inner diameter (ID) of the tube.

---

[3] "Joseph-Frederic-Benoit Charriere, a 19th century Parisian maker of surgical instruments, has by virtue of his ingenuity and advanced thinking, continued to have his presence felt in medicine throughout the 20th century. His most significant accomplishment was the development of a uniform, standard gauge specifically designed for use in medical equipment such as catheters and probes. Unlike the gauge system adopted by the British for measurement of needles and intravenous catheters, Charriere's system has uniform increments between gauge sizes (1/3 of a millimeter), is easily calculated in terms of its metric equivalent, and has no arbitrary upper end point. Today, in the United States, this system is commonly referred to as French (Fr) sizing. In addition to the development of the French gauge, Charriere made significant advances in ether administration, urologic, and other surgical instruments, and the development of the modern syringe." Iserson, K.V., J.-F.-B. Charriere: the man behind the French scale, *J. Emerg. Med.*, 5, 545–548, 1987.

Table 5.1 Units Conversion Chart

Gauge Number	Metric (mm)	French Catheter (Fr.) (mm × 3)	Stubs Gauge	American (A.W.G.) or Brown and Sharpe (inch)
6	5.16	15.5	0.203	0.1620
7	4.57	13.7	0.180	0.1442
8	4.19	12.6	0.165	0.1284
9	3.76	11.3	0.148	0.1144
10	3.40	10.2	0.134	0.1018
11	3.05	9.2	0.120	0.0907
12	2.77	8.3	0.109	0.0808
13	2.41	7.2	0.095	0.0719
14	2.11	6.3	0.083	0.0640
15	1.83	5.5	0.072	0.0570
16	1.65	5	0.065	0.0508
17	1.47	4.4	0.058	0.0452
18	1.27	3.8	0.049	0.0403
19	1.07	3.2	0.042	0.0358
20	0.91	2.7	0.035	0.0319
21	0.82	2.4	0.032	0.0284
22	0.72	2.2	0.028	0.0253
23	0.64	1.9	0.025	0.0225
24	0.57	1.7	0.022	0.0201
25	0.51	1.5	0.020	0.0179
26	0.46	1.3	0.018	0.0159
27	0.41	1.2	0.016	0.0141
28	0.36	1	0.014	0.0126
29	0.34	—	0.013	0.0112
30	0.31	—	0.012	0.0100
31	0.26	—	0.010	0.0089
32	0.23	—	0.009	0.0079

The first consideration is this: tubing is made by reducing the OD of the tube through a die. What this means is that the OD is controllable. The ID of the tube then becomes a function of the OD minus the nominal wall thickness of the tube after forming. This means that the ID is not absolutely controlled. The ID is a theoretical number. This can be seen in the accompanying illustration. This must be taken into account when calculating tolerances between the ID of the tube and whatever you are designing to slide into the tube. (See Figure 5.1.)

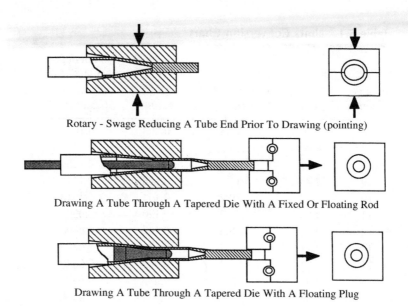

Figure 5.1 Typical metal tube drawing methods. (Courtesy of Microgroup, Inc.)

It is possible to draw tubing over a mandrel of a precise size, or hone the inner diameter; however, this is more expensive than using readily available standard-size hypotube.

Also, when designing a part to fit in to the inner lumen of a hypotube, remember that tubes are never perfectly round, nor perfectly straight, nor perfectly smooth on the inside. All of these factors will affect how much tolerance to allow in order to fit a part into the hypotube lumen.

If you are planning to insert a long part into a long hypotube, remember to allow enough tolerance. Even if a part fits easily into a short section of tube, frictions and tolerance stack-ups rapidly accumulate, where a part may fit initially, but becomes jammed as the part is advanced through the full length of the tube.

When measuring tubing with a pin gauge, be sure that the end of the tube is free from burrs. Deburring the end of the tube with a 60° cone burr held in a pin vise is a convenient way to clean up a tube before measuring. Also, remember that a gauge pin the exact diameter of the tube will not fit in the tube. For example, a 0.125-inch pin will not fit in a 0.125-inch lumen.

COMMON HYPODERMIC TUBING MATERIALS

The most common is 300 series stainless; 400 series stainless is required for heat treating. Nickel–titanium tubing is also now readily available from

Introduction to Needles and Cannulae ■ 95

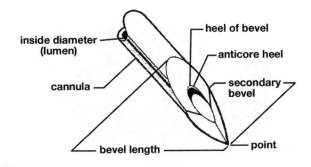

Figure 5.2 Typical hypodermic needle features. (Illustration courtesy of Popper and Sons, Inc.)

vendors such as Memry Corporation (Bethel, CT) and Nitinol Devices Corporation (NDC) (Fremont, CA). Tubing of other alloys such as titanium are available for use in magnetic resonance imaging (MRI) radiology applications.

If you look at a hypodermic needle, you will notice that the end is not ground to a simple bevel. Hypodermic needles are usually ground with a compound bevel, typically called a lancet point, and the angles of these bevels give the needle its characteristics. (See Figure 5.2.) Some needles are designed to pierce veins and arteries, others to penetrate into muscle, and yet others to penetrate tough fascia and joint capsule tissue.

R&D NEEDLE GRINDING

Glendo Corporation (Emporia, KS) makes a versatile grinder that works very well for grinding prototype sharps. It is a low-heat slow-rpm diamond grinder originally designed to sharpen carbide tools. (See Figure 5.3.)

SIMPLE COMPOUND NEEDLE GRINDING FIXTURE

A simple fixture can be made for grinding prototype lancet sharps. Here are the general specifications:

> Take a block of Delrin or other abrasion-resistant plastic and mill two surfaces as shown. These establish the angle of the first main bevel and the secondary bevels. Next, drill two holes through the block perpendicular to these planes. Note: The length of these holes needs to be equal so that when the second bevels are ground, they form a point and do not obliterate the first bevel. The grinds need to

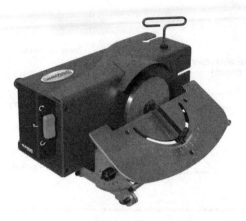

Figure 5.3 Glendo Accu-Finish® grinder. (Glendo, Inc.)

meet at the point. The angle of the secondary bevel must be steeper than the first bevel to form a lancet point.

Next, drill holes for the index pin. It will be at the 12:00 position, as shown in Figure 5.4, for the primary bevel, and at approximately the 11:00 and 1:00 positions for the secondary bevels, depending on the desired angle of rotation for the secondary bevels. Next make an index pin holding collar and mount it to a pin vise. Insert an index pin as shown in Figure 5.4. When the hypotube is held in the pin vise, this will index the angles of rotation for the bevels.

To grind a needle, place the pin vise in the index hole for the first bevel, and slide the hypotube through the pin vise and the fixture block for the first bevel. With just enough tube sticking out to grind the bevel, tighten the pin vise and grind the first bevel. The Glendo™ grinder works well for this application. Next, move the tube to the secondary bevel grinding position. The tip of the first bevel should sit right at the edge of the hole for the second bevel, with a slight overlap to ensure a complete sharp-tip grind. Insert the index pin into the 11:00 position and grind the first secondary bevel; then move the pin to the 1:00 position and grind the next secondary bevel. The heel of the needle should then be dulled with a small fine-grained grindstone if tissue coring is to be prevented.

With this fixture setup it is simple to make a set of blocks for a variety of combinations of first bevel angle, second bevel angle, and angle of rotation for the secondary bevels. Once proof of concept is achieved, one of the vendors listed in the "Resources" section can produce your needles in volume under good manufacturing practice (GMP) guidelines, or supply an off-the-shelf version.

Introduction to Needles and Cannulae ■ 97

Table 5.2 Basic Types of Needles and Typical Applications

Bevel Type	Gauge Range	Bevel Angle (approximate degrees)	Mean Bevel Angle (degrees)	Typical Use
Regular	7–12	15–17	12	Subcutaneous and intramuscular injection
	13–16	13–14		
	17–21	12		
	22–27	12		
	28–33	13–14		
Intravenous	15–18	12–14	13	Disposable IVs
Medium	13–16	16–17	15	Subcutaneous IV and intramuscular injection
	17–21	15		
	22–27	13–15		
Short	10–12	23–25	19	Nerve block, IV intra-arterial
	13–16	19–22		
	17–21	18–19		
	22–27	15–18		
Arterial	15–17	21–22	20	Intra-arterial injection
	18–20	18–19		
Spinal	7–12	26–31	22	Spinal anesthesia
	13–16	23–25		
	17–21	18–22		
	22–30	15–17		
Intradermal	26	23.5	23.5	Intradermal
Regular Quincke	—	22	—	—
Short Quincke	—	30	—	—
Pitkin	—	45	—	—

Data courtesy of Popper and Sons, Inc., New Hyde Park, NY.

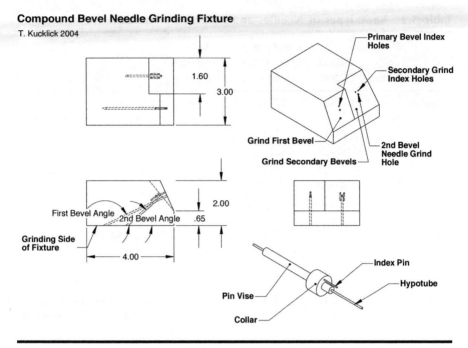

Figure 5.4 Prototype needle grinding fixture.

SUTURE NEEDLES[4]

Curved suture needles, very similar to needles used today, were used in ancient India.[5] Other shapes of needles are straight needles, which are less commonly used for suturing, the common curved needle, the half-curved ski needle, and the compound curved needle for specialty applications, such as microvascular surgery.

The most important feature of a suture needle is that it passes through tissue, causing the least amount of trauma. It is also important that the needle pass through smoothly. Some needles are coated with silicone or other lubricious coating. The needle must be of a material that will hold its shape while being passed through tissue, hold a sharp point or edge, and not be so hard that the needle becomes brittle and prone to breakage. Suture needles are driven through tissue with needle holders. Some needle

---

[4] For a complete introductory article on sutures and needles, see http://www.emedicine.com/ent/topic38.htm by Steven Lai, M.D., and Daniel Becker, M.D. This is an excellent and detailed overview of the subject of needles and sutures, describing many of the important parameters in needle and suture selection.

[5] Lyons, Albert S. and Petruccelli, R.J., *Medicine: An Illustrated History*, Abradale Press, New York, p. 115.

holders have special carbide inserts in the jaws to provide extra grip on the needle while driving the needle through tough tissue.[6]

BASIC TYPES OF SUTURE NEEDLE TIPS

Conventional Cutting

In this configuration, there are three cutting edges with a cutting edge facing the inside of the needle arc. This is known as a surface-seeking needle.

Reverse Cutting

Reverse-cutting needles cut on two sides and have the third cutting edge on the outside of the needle arc. This is known as a depth-seeking needle.

Side Cutting

Side-cutting needles, or spatula needles, have two cutting edges perpendicular to the arc of the needle. These are used for ophthalmic procedures.

Taper Point

A taper point is similar to a regular sewing needle. The sharpness is determined by taper ratio and tip angle. The needle is sharper if it has a higher taper ratio and lower tip angle. The taper-point needle is used for easily penetrated tissues, such as abdominal viscera and subcutaneous tissue, and minimizes potential tearing of tissue.

Blunt Point

Blunt needles dissect, rather than cut, tissue. Blunt needles are used to suture friable tissue such as liver.

---

[6] "During the last two decades, major advances in surgical needle and needle holder technology have markedly improved surgical wound repair. These advances include quantitative tests for surgical needle and needle holders performance, high nickel stainless steels, compound curved needles, needle sharpening methods, laser-drilled holes for swages, needle:suture ratios of 1:1, and the atraumatic needle holder." From Edlich, R.F., Thacker, J.G., McGregor, W., and Rodeheaver, G.T., Past, present, and future for surgical needles and needle holders, *Am. J. Surg.*, 166, 522–532, 1993.

Table 5.3 Suture Needle Identification Chart

Needle Type	Description	Point Shape(s)
Regular Trocar Point	A Round Bodied Needle With Triangle Cutting Edges	
Regular Taper Point	A Round Tapered Point Needle	
Regular Taper Cutting	A Round-Tapered Point Needle With Short Cutting Edges	
Regular Reverse Cutting Edge	A Triangle Cutting Edge Needle	
Regular Diamond Point	A Side Cutting Needle	
Regular Conventional Cutting Edge	An Inside Apex Triangle Cutting Edge Needle	
Regular Blunt Taper Point	A Blunt Tapered Point Needle	
Regular Ball Point	A Blunt Point Needle	
Premium Lancet Point	A Hand Honed Side Cutting Needle	
Premium Diamond Point	A Hand Honed Side Cutting Needle	
Premium Cutting Edge	A Hand Honed Triangle Cutting Edge Needle	
Cardiovascular (CV)	A Round-Tapered Point, Square Bodied Needle	

Courtesy of BG Sulzle, Inc., N. Syracuse, NY.

SUTURE ATTACHMENT METHODS

Swaging Sutures to Needles

Suture is usually permanently swaged to the needle. Needles with sewing needle-style eyelets require two strands of suture, which causes more tissue damage as the double strand is passed through tissue.

Drill

Here the proximal end of the needle is drilled with a hole, and the needle is swaged to retain the suture. This makes the proximal end smaller than the needle body.

Channel

In this method the end of the needle is formed into a channel, and the needle is crimped to retain the suture. In this case, the proximal end becomes larger than the needle body.

Nonswaged, Closed Eye, French Eye, Slit, Spring

These are various methods of retaining the suture. These have the disadvantage of pulling a double strand of suture through the tissue.

SUTURE SIZES

Sutures are sized in the U.S. according to a system from the U.S. Pharmacopoeia (USP). Sutures are gauged not only by diameter, but tensile strength and knot security. Sutures sizes are measured on two scales:

1. A whole number system for larger sutures, from 5 (largest) to 0 (smallest).
2. A composite number system for smaller sutures (smaller than 0), from 1-0 (largest) to 12-0 (smallest). These are the "aught" sizes, e.g., 12-0 is pronounced 12-aught or 12-oh.

Following is a chart of suture sizes with the largest on the left and the smallest microsurgery sizes on the right:

Larger																Smaller
5	4	3	2	1	0	1-0	2-0	3-0	4-0	5-0	6-0	7-0	8-0	9-0	10-0	11-0	12-0

Various types and sizes of suture needles are illustrated in Figure 5.5.

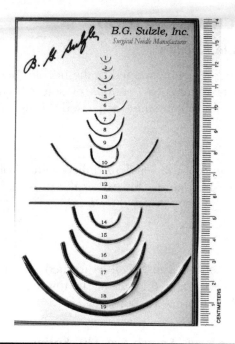

Figure 5.5 Assorted suture needles. (Courtesy of B.G. Sulzle, Inc.) For a complete chart of sizes, see http://www.bgsulzle.com/products/.

European suture is measured in diameter; however, two sutures of the same size can be very different in tensile strength. The USP system tries to rank suture gauge where two sutures of the same gauge will have similar tensile strength.

SUTURE TYPES

There are two basic categories of suture material, natural and synthetic. There are two basic types of performance characteristics, absorbable and nonabsorbable. Suture is constructed in either braided or monofilament forms.

Natural Absorbable

Gut (made from sheep or beef intestine) fast and slow absorbing types. Chromic gut is treated with chromium salts to slow absorption.

Natural Nonabsorbable

Surgical silk, surgical stainless steel (for suturing bone, e.g., a sternotomy), and cotton. Note: Surgical steel wire is specified according to the Brown and Sharpe wire gauge, *not* the Stubs needle gauge.

Synthetic Absorbable

Examples: Polygalactin 910 (Vicryl™), poliglecaprone 25 (Monocryl™), polydioxanone (PDS II™), polytrimethylene carbonate (Maxon™).

Synthetic Nonabsorbable

Nylon (Ethilon™, Dermilaon™, monofilament Nurlon™, Surgilon™ braided), polybutester (Novofil™), polyester fiber (Mersilene™/Dacron (uncoated) and Ethibond™/Ti-cron™ (coated)), polypropylene (Prolene™).[7]

TROCARS AND DILATORS

Trocars

Trocars are usually larger-diameter devices used to make a surgical entry into the body. Trocars are common features of laparoscopic and arthroscopic surgical ports.

Blunt Dilators

A blunt dilator is used to dissect rather than cut tissue. A blunt dilator is used to minimize a tissue defect from cutting, or to protect sensitive tissues distal to the axis of penetration, e.g., bowel in laparoscopy or articular cartilage in arthroscopy.

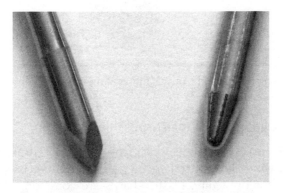

Figure 5.6 Metal trocar and blunt dilator.

---

[7] For detailed engineering information on sutures, see C.C. Chu, J.A. von Fraunhofer, and H. Greisler. *Wound Closure Biomaterials and Devices*, CRC Press, Boca Raton, FL, 1997.

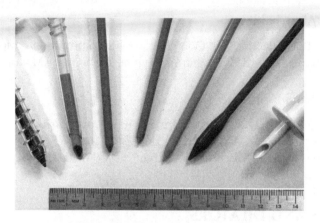

Figure 5.7 Assorted plastic sharp and blunt devices.

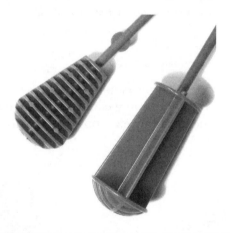

Figure 5.8 Plastic dilator and trocar handles showing coring out of thick sections.

Plastic Sharps and Trocars for Disposables

Plastic sharps, as well as dilators, are commonly used in single-use disposable medical devices. When properly designed, plastic parts have sufficient penetration acuity. Plastic sharps are common in disposable IV bag spikes. There are numerous designs for laparoscopic trocars that incorporate a combination of plastic and metal components.

An important design consideration in plastics is to minimize thick sections of material. Excessively thick sections make for long molding cycle times as well as potential voids and molded in stress.

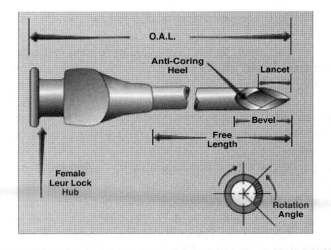

Figure 5.9 Needle terminology. (Illustration courtesy of Connecticut Hypodermic.)

GLOSSARY OF NEEDLES AND RELATED TERMS

Abrams' needle: A biopsy needle designed to reduce the danger of introducing air into tissues, used in pleural biopsy.

Acuity: The sharpness of a surgical needle.[8]

Agar cutting needle: A needle with a sharpened punch end and an obturator to pick up and transfer a sample of agar media.

Aneurysm needle: One with a handle, used in ligating blood vessels.

Angle of rotation: The amount of rotation performed on secondary grinds (lancets) of a cannula. This is an important variable for needle-point sharpness.

---

[8] The acuity (sharpness) of surgical needle points was assessed by measuring the force required for repeat needle penetrations through a medium-gauge latex sheet glued to a perforated Plexiglas frame. The data on the variation in the applied force with repeat penetrations showed that needles obeyed the general relation: $P = A + B \cdot n$; where P is the applied penetration force in grams, n is the number of penetrations, and A and B are constants. Constant A characterized the needle-point acuity and B the maintenance of acuity. This relationship indicated both needle acuity and acuity maintenance with repeated passes through a reproducible target material. Determining the microhardness of needles provided data on their strength, which helped to account for differences in the acuity of apparently similar needles. The tensile strength of the union between suture and needle was determined to evaluate the security of suture attachment." From von Fraunhofer, J.A., Storey, R.J., and Masterson, B.J., Characterization of surgical needles, *Biomaterials*, 9, 281–284, 1988. See also Frick, T.B., Marucci, D.D., Cartmill, J.A., Martin, C.J., and Walsh, W.R., Resistance forces acting on suture needles, *J. Biomech.*, 34, 1335–1340, 2001.

Anneal: A heat-treating process is performed on metal to make it more malleable. This can aid many small-diameter stainless steel tube components that are bent, flared, or swaged to prevent cracking or splitting.

Anticoring heel blast: The heel of a bevel is blasted with media to dull it in order to reduce coring. It is the heel of a needle that tends to produce coring. (See Figure 5.8 for location of needle heel.)

Aspirating needle: A long, hollow needle for removing fluid from a cavity.

ASTM A 967-96: Chemical passivation standard for treating stainless steel parts. Replaces QQP-35C.

Back bevels: Bevels that are ground on the side of a flat bevel. This provides a greater cutting edge on a short-bevel needle.

Bevel: Ground surface of a cannula or needle point. There are many styles, including but not limited to A-bevel, B-bevel, C-bevel, bias, Chiba, Crawford, deflected tip, Francine, Hustead, Huber, trocar, Tuohy, etc.

Bevel length: Length measured from tip of needle point to furthest distance of heel.

Bias: Angle grind.

Blunt end: Tube with square-cut (90°) end.

Brockenbrough needle: A curved steel transseptal needle within a Brockenbrough transseptal catheter; used to puncture the interatrial septum.

Burr: Deflection of the point. Usually considered unacceptable when perceptible to feel or greater than 0.001.

Cannula: A hollow tube meant to be inserted into a body cavity, sometimes with the assistance of an inner sharp trocar or blunt obturator.

Cataract needle: One used in removing a cataract.

Chiba needle: A common type of thin, flexible biopsy needle with a small-diameter needle and a stylet in the needle lumen.

Cope's needle: A blunt-ended hook-like needle with a concealed cutting edge and snare, used in biopsy of the pleura, pericardium, peritoneum, and synovium.

Deschamps' needle: One with the eye near the point, and a long handle attached; used in ligating deep-seated arteries.

Discission needle: A special form of cataract needle.

Echotip: Creates an enhanced visualization of the needle tip when used with ultrasonic imaging equipment. This is where the tip is roughened or knurled or coated with an acoustic reflectice material to increase echogenicity.

Emulsifying needle: A small tube with luer fittings at each end for mixing a liquid and an emulsifying agent by pushing the liquids through the tubing into opposing syringes. A simple type of static mixer.

Flared end: End of tube is spread out, increasing the diameter. Typically, flare diameter can be a maximum of 1.3 × tube diameter.

Free length: On a needle assembly free length is the length from the end of the part to where it protrudes from the hub.

Gauge: Stub gauge number referring to hypodermic tube size. For hypodermic tubing, the gauge number increases as the tube diameter gets smaller.

GG-N-196: U.S. government specifications for hypodermic needles dating back to 1947.

Grit blast: Refers to roughened surface added to components by means of pressure blasting with media. This may provide a better bonding surface for hypodermic needles or tubing or wire components.

Hagedorn's needles: Surgical needles that are flat from side to side and have a straight cutting edge near the point and a large eye.

Hasson cannula: A cannula made for laparoscopy with a blunt dialating obturator and an anchoring balloon at the distal end.

Hasson trocar: A blunt trocar inserted into the peritoneal cavity after a celiotomy. Used for insufflation and introduction of a laparoscope.

Hook burr: Burr on needle point that exceeds 0.002 inch.

Hub: Fitting at the end of a needle that can connect to a syringe or other component.

ID: Inside diameter of tubing, usually measured with pin gauges to determine proper size.

ISO 9626: International standard for stainless steel needle tubing for the manufacture of medical devices.

Knife needle: A slender knife with a needle-like point, used in discission of a cataract and other ophthalmic operations, as in goniotomy and goniopuncture.

Lancets: These are the two secondary bevels on a triple-ground point. Other common terms for lancets are side grinds and diamond points.

Ligature needle: A slender steel needle with a long handle and an eye in its curved end, used for passing a ligature underneath an artery.

Luer: Male or female taper on end of hub or syringe to connect a needle to a syringe or other Luer fitting. Hubs can be Luer Slip or Luer Lock, conforming to ISO 594-2.

Eponym for Otto Luer, who, in the 1880s, in Germany came up with the idea of a 6% taper as a way of putting a stopper in a bottle, keeping it there, and then getting it out again. Many years later, Luer's taper was used by hospital equipment manufacturers to ensure that one piece of IV set tubing would fit into another.[9]

---

[9] http://biotech.law.lsu.edu/cases/devices/hanson_v_baxter_app.htm. British Standards Institution, *Conical Fittings with 6% (Luer) Taper for Syringes, Needles, and Certain Other Medical Equipment: Lock Fittings*, BSI, London, 1997.

In 1925 Fairleigh S. Dickinson, cofounder of Beckton-Dickinson, patented what became known as the the Luer-Lok™ fitting, which added to the Luer's tapered fluid fitting a locking sleeve by incorporating a lead screw that prevented a hypodermic syringe from slipping off of a hypodermic syringe. [10] This made a hypodermic safer to use when dispensing viscous fluids, which tended to force the needle hub off of the luer slip fit. The luer lock fitting described in Dickinson's 1930 patent[11] is virtually identical to locking luer fittings in use today.

After plastic medical disposable devices were introduced in the 1950s, the Luer-Lok fitting and variations of it were incorporated into a wide range of plastic medical fluid fittings.

Lumen: This is the open space inside a tube.

Magnetic permeability: The property of stainless steel tubing that determines its relative influence in a magnetic field. Work hardening of 300 series stainless can affect the magnetic permeability.

Malleable: Easily bendable without breaking or cracking. Small-diameter stainless steel tubing can be drawn to less than full hard conditions to make more malleable. Another method is to have the hypodermic tube size parts bright annealed through heat treating.

Menghini needle: A needle that does not require rotation to cut loose the tissue specimen in a biopsy of the liver. This represented a significant advance in the previously slow and hazardous methods of liver biopsy. "Menghini introduced modern liver biopsy in 1958. He used a new, very thin suction needle. His original article was entitled 'One-Second Needle Biopsy of the Liver' in the journal *Gastroenterology*."[12]

Obturator: A blunt rod that fills the inner lumen of a cannula. A removable plug of a tubular instrument. From Latim *obturo*, "to close up."

Overall length (OAL): Entire length measured from one end to opposite end.

Passivate: Treat stainless steel with acid to prevent corrosion per ASTM A 967-96.

Pencil point: Tubing is swaged to conical point.

Pitkin bevel: A 45° bevel without a secondary lancet bevel.

Proximal end: Hub end of a needle, the end closest to you.

Quincke bevel: A type of needle grind named for Heinrich Irenaeus Quincke (1842–1922), German, who pioneered the lumbar puncture technique for aspirating cerebral spinal fluid (CSF) to diagnose neu-

---

[10] http://www.bd.com/aboutbd/history/timeline.asp.
[11] Patent nos. 1,742,497 and 1,793,068.
[12] http://www.vh.org/adult/patient/internalmedicine/aba30/2001/liverbiopsy.html.

rological disorders. A regular Quincke bevel is 22° and a short Quincke bevel is 30°.

Reverdin's needle: A surgical needle having an eye that can be opened and closed by means of a slide.

Seldinger needle: A needle with a blunt, tapered external cannula with a sharp obturator; used for the initial percutaneous insertion characteristic of the Seldinger technique for arterial or venous access. The Seldinger technique is the common method for placing a guidewire into a vessel (e.g., into the femoral artery for cardiovascular access), to allow the placement of catheters over the guidewire. Named for Sven-Ivar Seldinger (1921–1999), radiologist, born in Mora, Sweden. Dr. Seldinger published the description of a percutaneous-entry technique in the journal *Acta Radiologica*.[13]

Side port: Opening on the side of a tube. It can be a slot or hole.

Silverman needle: An instrument for taking tissue specimens, consisting of an outer cannula, an obturator, and an inner split needle with longitudinal grooves in which the tissue is retained when the needle and cannula are withdrawn.

Stop needle: A needle with a shoulder that prevents it from being inserted beyond a certain distance.

Stylet: A rod that fills the inner lumen of a hypodermic needle or trocar and is ground to match the sharp end of the needle or trocar.

Swaged needle: One permanently attached to the suture material. Curved needles for suturing tissue normally have the suture swaged to the proximal end of the needle.

Swaging: Forming process to reduce tube OD and shape to die configuration. Also a method to crimp together.

Transseptal needle: A needle used to puncture the interatrial septum in transseptal catheterization.

Trephine: A saw-type end on a needle or cylindrical tube that allows cutting of tissue as the needle or cannula is rotated, similar to a hole saw. Often used to cut a disc-shaped piece of bone or other firm tissue.

Triple grind: Typical three-sided grind of hypodermic needle.

Trocar: A cannula with a three-pointed obturator stylet. Sometimes refers to the sharp obturator alone. From Latin *trois* (three) and *carre* (the edge of a sword).

Trocar point: Three-sided point ground on stylet. Each grind is approximately 120° apart, usually to the center of the diameter.

Tuohy needle: One in which the opening at the end is angled so that a catheter exits at an angle. The end of the Tuhoy needle provides controlled penetration during the administering of spinal anesthesia

---

[13] http://www.cookgroup.com/history/seldinger.html.

and placement of an epidural spinal catheter. Named after Edward B. Tuohy, American anesthesiologist. Sometimes called the Huber needle, as it was designed jointly by Tuohy and Ralph Huber.[14] A pioneering development that made continuous epidural anesthesia in obstetrics possible.

Veress needle: Named for Janos Veress, a German doctor. A spring-loaded needle originally used to drain ascites and evacuate fluid and air from the chest. Was later adapted to use in laparoscopy. A hollow needle consisting of a sharp trocar with a slanted end surrounding an inner cylinder with a blunt end. After the trocar is introduced into a body cavity, the blunt cylinder is advanced outward so that internal organs are not injured by the sharp edge. Used for insufflation of a body cavity, such as for pneumoperitoneum in minimally invasive surgery.

RESOURCES

Hypodermic Tube, Needle, and Sharps Vendors

Avid Medical
9000 Westmont Dr.
Stonehouse Commerce Park
Toano, VA 23168
Phone: 800-886-0584
Fax: 757-566-8707

BG Sulzle
1 Needle Lane
N. Syracuse, NY 13212
Phone: 315-454-3221
Largest independent manufacturer of drilled end-suture needles.

Connecticut Hypodermics
519 Main St.
Yalesville, CT 06492
Phone: 203-265-4881
Fax: 203-284-1520

Disposable Instrument Company
P.O. Box 14248

---

[14] *Reg. Anesth. Pain Med.*, 27, 520–523, 2002.

Shawnee Mission, KS 66285-4248
Phone: 913-492-6492
Fax: 913-888-1762

Eagle Stainless
10 Discovery Way
Franklin, MA 02038
Phone: 800-528-8650
Fax: 800-520-1954

Electron Microscopy Services
P.O. Box 550
1560 Industry Rd.
Hatfield, PA 19440
Phone: 215-412-8400
Fax: 215-412-8450
EMS supplies microminiature needles and sharps.

K-Tube
13400 Kirkham Way
Poway, CA 92064
Phone: 858-513-9229
Fax: 800-705-8823

Medical Sterile Products
P.O. Box 338
Rincon, PR 00743
Phone: 800-292-2887
Fax: 787-823-8665
Manufactures sharps of all kinds.

Microgroup
7 Industrial Park Rd.
Medway, MA 02053
Phone: 800-255-8823
Fax: 508-533-5691

Point Technologies
6859 N. Foothills Hwy.
Boulder, CO 80302
Phone: 303-415-9865
Fax: 303-415-9866
Point Technologies provides electrochemical sharpening of microwires.

Popper and Sons
300 Denton Ave.
New Hyde Park, NY 11040
Phone: 516-248-0300
Fax: 516-747-1188

Vita Needle Company
919 Great Plain Ave.
Needham, MA 02492
Phone: 909-699-8790
Fax: 909-699-7490
Specialize in small minimum lot manufacturing.

Phlebotomy is the art of drawing blood with a needle. For more information see R.E. McCall and C.M. Tankersley, *Phlebotomy Essentials*, 3rd ed., Lippincott, Williams & Willkins, Baltimore, 2002.

Sharps, Disposal of, by Mail Order

GRP & Associates, Inc.
P.O. Box 94
Clear Lake, IA 50428
Phone: 888-346-6037

ACKNOWLEDGMENTS

The assistance of Bob Lamson of Microgroup, Zev Asch of Popper and Sons, Connecticut Hypodermics, and BG Sulzle, Inc., is gratefully acknowledged.

6

RAPID PROTOTYPING FOR MEDICAL DEVICES

Ted Kucklick

CONTENTS

Overview	114
Rapid Prototype Technology	116
In-House RP vs. Service Bureaus	119
RP Service Bureaus	120
Office-Based RP Machines	120
Types of Available RP Technologies	121
3D Systems: SLA®	121
Stereolithography Materials	122
Sony SCS™	123
3D Systems: SLS™	123
Stratasys: FDM	124
Resolution and Surface Finish	125
Solidscape	127
LOM™	127
Z Corp.: Three-Dimensional Printing	128
Polyjet Objet™ Printer	129
DLP: Envisiontec® Perfactory™	130
Sintering and Direct Metal	131
RP Applications in Product Design	131
CNC	133
Full-Size VMC CNC Machines	135
Machinable Prototype Materials	136
Rapid Tooling and Molding	137
Which Technology Is Best?	138
File Preparation	138

Other File Formats 139
RP Cost-Saving Tips 140
Secondary Processes to RP Parts 141
    Painting 141
    Electroplating 141
    Machining 141
    Threaded Inserts 141
        Installing the Inserts 141
UV Cure Sealing of Foam Parts 142
RP Casting Patterns 142
Reverse Engineering 143
Innovative Applications of RP 143
    RP and Surgical Planning 143
    RP and Training Models 144
        Molecular Modeling 144
    RP-Produced Medical Products 145
        Investment Cast Orthopedic Implants 145
    RP and RE Combined into a Product and Service 146
        Crowns in One Visit 146
    RP and Tissue Engineering 148
        The Envisiontec Bioplotter 150
    RP and Pharmeceuticals 152
    RP and Analysis 152
        Programmable RP Molding 153
        Printed Food and Inkjet Proteins 154
        Direct Manufacturing Freedom of Creation 154
        Direct Manufacturing: The Center for Bits and Atoms 155
Conclusion 156
Resources 156
    In-Print and Online Resources 156
    Professional Societies and Resources 157
Universities and Organizations 158
Acknowledgments 159

OVERVIEW

The past decade has seen an explosion of rapid prototyping (RP), rapid tooling, and reverse engineering (reverse modeling) technologies. All of these technologies have become more readily available, less expensive, and more flexible and capable each year. RP has only been widely available for less than 20 years. These technologies put exciting and unprecedented capabilities into the hands of the designer to develop, iterate, and manufacture products. In parallel with the growth of RP, computing power has grown by orders of magnitude and plummeted in price. Computer-aided design (CAD) applications that not so long ago required a $50K workstation running a proprietary operating system can now be run on a sub-$5000 computer and an inexpensive operating system (OS), with high-end graphics. Desktop replacement laptops are making this computing power portable. Affordable CAD solid modelers and high-speed Internet connections allow designers and engineers to work from any location and transmit files to in-house RP resources, or remote service bureaus, and receive parts quickly via courier service.

Key advantages of rapid prototyping are modeling directly from your three-dimensional data and the ability to quickly have a real part in your hands. Rapid tooling methods allow you to make preproduction, and sometimes even production, parts for testing and timely evaluation before moving to hard tooling.

Before rapid prototyping, to get a part required a detailed drawing that was then interpreted by a machinist or model maker to fabricate the part. Parts were designed to fit the limitations of machine tools, further limited to what could be communicated in a dimensioned drawing. Free form and complex surface parts can now be fabricated easily. Models took days or weeks and were expensive. RP can make parts that are nearly impossible to build from a drawing, with no drawings required. Nested assemblies are also possible, where objects may be built inside of other objects. Direct manufacturing is even emerging as a category where parts are built from data files, on demand, without tooling.

Rapid tooling is a growing technology that is RP, as applied to producing tooling used in high-volume manufacturing processes such as injection molding. This use of RP to produce patterns used in another process to produce tooling is sometimes referred to an indirect RP process.

Reverse engineering (RE) is a broad term for a process that may include starting with a physical object and using scanning and digitizing technology to produce a three-dimensional computer model of the object for reproduction. There are many important applications for RE, such as digitizing hand-sculpted models, the production of patient-specific prosthetics, scanning and reproduction of rare or fragile medical specimens, and the generation of CAD data from parts where CAD data are not available. Makers of digitizing equipment prefer to call this process reverse modeling rather than reverse engineering.

Together, computer numeric-controlled (CNC) machining, rapid prototyping, reverse engineering, rapid tooling, and direct manufacturing are a family of highly capable and flexible tools that get a part in your hands for evaluation, and in some cases can even generate the final product.

As good as three-dimensional CAD has become, there is still no substitute for seeing a real part in your hands and seeing how it really looks, feels, behaves, and fits with other parts. Rapid prototyping has become an essential tool in product development as well as scientific visualization. Rapid prototyping technology is also being adapted to numerous new medical applications, such as custom prosthetics, implants, and tissue engineering.

RAPID PROTOTYPE TECHNOLOGY

There are two basic types of rapid prototyping (RP) available, additive and subtractive. Additive modeling is like building a sculpture from clay, adding material until the final shape is produced. Subtractive modeling starts with a block of material, and a cutting tool removes material until the final shape is produced. This is a form of CNC machining. Roland DGA uses the term SRP™ (subtractive rapid prototyping) to describe its CNC machines and computer-aided manufacturing (CAM) systems that are optimized for prototyping, as opposed to industrial CNC for production machining.

Another term for rapid prototyping is the broader term *automated fabrication*. "Automated fabrication is a modern family of technologies that generate three-dimensional, solid objects under computer control."[1] As you can see from this definition, RP is a subset of the larger category, that of digitally controlled fabrication technologies. Automated fabrication, especially digitally controlled additive fabrication, is still relatively new. There exists a further category of direct manufacturing and manufacture-on-demand opportunities that has only begun to be explored. Another category of RP is referred to as automated forming, where a material is shaped and formed under computer control, without fixed tooling. Automated fabrication may also include new technologies for building engineered tissue scaffolds with RP and inkjet technology. Some of these applications are described at the end of this chapter.

Another category of RP technology is the use of reverse modeling and rapid prototyping in conjunction with one another. Case examples of this are included in the chapter.

Additive object modelers work in a similar ways. They assemble slices or layers of material to develop a three-dimensional object. Think of it as taking a cutting out of a series of flat paper dolls, then stacking them up to make a solid paper doll. Additive layered manufacturing methods use a variety of materials from photoreactive polymer, to plastic melted through a nozzle, to paper cut with a laser, to powders that are hardened layer by layer, and inkjet-style modelers to produce a free-form solid object. The resolution and surface finish of the model are controlled by how

---

[1] Burns, Marshall, *Automated Fabrication*, Prentice Hall, Englewood Cliffs, NJ, 1993.

each layer is, and the size of line or dot used to progressively harden the build material. Each RP method has its own advantages and limitations in prototyping and development of medical devices. RP additive modelers fall into two general categories: Industrial-grade rapid prototype machines, which can produce higher-accuracy parts, have large price tags ($75K to $250K and up) and require a special shop environment. The other are office-based three-dimensional printers. These are designed to be easy to use, can operate in an office, and are priced in the sub-$40K range.

Subtractive rapid prototyping (SRP™) is a term developed by Roland DGA, a maker of third- and fourth-axis CNC milling machines, to identify it in the rapid prototyping market. These machines are designed to be easy to operate by users not extensively trained as machinists. Many operations and functions, such as material setup, tool speed, and feed rates, are preprogrammed, and a tool path generation program is bundled with the machine to allow the user to perform a relatively simple setup and allow the machine to run unattended to produce a final CNC machined part.

In medical device product development, the RP technology used is not an end in itself. The designer needs to become familiar with the range of technologies available to make a rational decision based on the criteria important to the project. Some of these considerations are:

- Do we need RP models occasionally, or do we require a large number of iterations and models?
- Do we want to have an RP machine in-house, shared between a group of designers, or will we use a service bureau?
- If we bring it in-house, what are the costs of ownership?
- Will the vendor company be able to provide good support after the sale?
- What functions do the parts need to perform?
- Do we require parts that have the mechanical properties of the final material?
- Does the model need to be of medical-grade materials?
- Are we making parts that are especially large or small?
- How much detail do we need?
- What is the smallest feature size we are trying to build?
- What surface finish do we need to have?
- Does the model require built-in colors?
- What is our manufacturing workflow?
- How does the RP technology we choose best fit into that workflow?

These are some of the questions to ask when deciding which RP technology is appropriate for your needs.

Keep in mind that not every RP technology one can find in the literature is commercially available. There are actually relatively few major companies in the market. Some machines that were once marketed are no longer sold, and other technologies exist as research prototypes in various stages of development. When choosing a system that meets your needs for product development, it helps to filter out the various approaches that are not actually readily available, and focus on the ones that are. Then, narrow that list to a short list of technologies that meet your practical needs.

If your goal is to use RP technology in an innovative way, investigating the numerous methods that are either in development or have fallen by the wayside may provide the building blocks you need to deploy RP methods in entirely new areas. New RP technologies developed in universities may be available for license. Also, as some of the earlier technologies go off-patent, they can provide platforms for innovative new medical applications. In this chapter, there are several examples of innovative applications of RP technology that go beyond using RP to make prototype parts.

Here are some representative applications of RP technology in medical device R&D:

- A painted visual model for trade shows, investor presentations, internal review, or photo shoots
- Producing a pattern for making copies in soft tooling, e.g., casting in room-temperature vulcanate (RTV) molds
- Producing multiple copies of a visual model
- Producing models for fit and clearance checks
- Models for human factors and ergonomic studies
- A model used for bench tests where mechanical function is most important
- A prototype model that is to be used as part of an investigational device
- A model that is a master for a downstream manufacturing process such as investment casting
- A model that is large and bulky, such as an engine block or a museum model of an animal
- A model requiring very fine, jewelry-like detail, such as a small medical device
- A model that is optically clear and acts like a light pipe
- A model that is complex and would be difficult or impossible to machine
- A model that is in color and represents areas such as fluid flow patterns in a part or charged areas of a macromolecule
- Direct production of low volume or bridge tooling

- Direct manufacturing of a difficult-to-manufacture or low-volume part
- Packaging of RP and RE technology into an innovative combination to provide a product or service
- Some types of tissue engineering

All of these are possible with the appropriate use of RP technology.

Rapid prototyping is a way to cut steps and time out of the product development process. Iteration, the development of a product in evolutionary steps, is absolutely required for design and innovation. The more efficiently these iterations are produced, the more quickly decisions can be made to get to the next step in the process and identify the time to stop iterating and start producing. Every company, especially start-ups, has a "burn rate" and consumes money just standing still. It is imperative to pack the highest number of iterations into the shortest amount of time, with the least overhead expense. Another consideration: if you are working on an important problem, you can be sure other smart people are looking at the same problem, too. Rapid prototyping, properly used, is a tool to stay ahead of competition, quickly reduce your concepts to practice, and boil these concepts down into marketable products fast and first. Choosing the best RP technology for your needs moves the product development process forward the fastest, at the lowest cost, and with the results that you want. RP technology is a means to an end. Starting with clear goals in mind and having a basic understanding of the capabilities of competing RP technologies can help to efficiently sort through the array of approaches and marketing claims by RP manufacturers and vendors, and help you to choose the approach that best fits your business, engineering, and design needs. The RP field is evolving quickly, with new technologies and materials being introduced constantly.

This chapter gives an overview of materials and methods, as well as links to company websites. Links to websites covering the RP field in general and discussion groups are also included. These discussion groups can be important sources of information from actual users of RP machines and their capabilities and limitations in real-world use, and a place to find answers to specific questions. Numerous case study examples are included, both of RP in use and innovative applications of RP.

IN-HOUSE RP VS. SERVICE BUREAUS

Unless a company produces a large volume of parts, has a need for on-demand prototyping, needs to keep prototyping in-house for confidentiality reasons, has specialized needs, or uses RP as part of a manufacturing process, an outside service bureau may be an appropriate option.

RP Service Bureaus

Service bureaus vary widely in their range of services and whether they offer secondary operations, finishing, and additional services. Service bureaus range from solo operators with one RP machine to full-service model shops. Some of the larger service bureaus offer several RP technologies, e.g., SLA®, FDM™, SLS™, CNC, and three-dimensional printing, all under one roof, so it becomes easier to choose the right approach for a given job.

The value of service bureaus is that they make available to you the use of machinery that would be prohibitively expensive to own, as well as skilled operators. The other value service bureaus can offer is a package of services. They can make an RP prototype part and offer secondary operations, such as milling and drilling, light assembly, painting, RTV casting of less expensive copies in urethane, and painting. Many medical device companies do not want to bring these types of activities in-house; therefore, sending this work outside can be the most appropriate option. When looking for a service bureau, find a company that offers the right combination of services offered, price, quality, speed of delivery, and reliability.

Office-Based RP Machines

Some of the newer office-based RP machines are from 3D Systems (InVision™ multijet modeling (MJM)), Stratasys® (Prodigy Plus™), and Z Corporation (Z Printer 310). Some of these solutions bring in-office prototyping into the sub-$40K range. Solidscape sells its T66 model for under $50K, which is intended for production of smaller-size lost-wax investment casting masters. 3D Systems markets a similar system capable of producing wax masters, the InVision HR 3-D Printer. Roland sells its line of easy-to-use three-axis CNC milling machines from under $4K up to over $25K. These solutions make bringing RP in-house a more viable option. Your needs in terms of turnaround, part functionality, detail, surface finish, and volume of prototypes, and whether you need to do any secondary finishing operations in-house, will help determine if an office-based three-dimensional printing solution is right for your application. Do not forget to factor in the cost of consumables, maintenance, and the cost of a sufficiently skilled person to operate the machine. When looking for an in-house RP solution, consider whether the finished part from the RP machine is as close to the finished product you want as possible. Analyze whether you save money over the long run. How soon does the machine pay for itself in your situation? Do you need to protect confidential information? Can you split the cost by pooling this resource among several design and engineering groups? Do you have an existing manufacturing workflow where an RP machine can fit? These are some of the considerations and strategies for bringing RP in-house.

TYPES OF AVAILABLE RP TECHNOLOGIES

3D Systems: SLA®

SLA is a process invented by Charles Hull and developed by 3D Systems of Valencia, CA. The acronym SLA (stereolithography apparatus) comes from the name of the company's first machine, the SLA-1, introduced in 1988 and a registered trademark of 3D Systems (www.3Dsystems.com). SLA is the most common rapid prototyping system in use today. Numerous service bureaus offer SLA part production, competing on price, speed of delivery, and ease of ordering. Other companies, such as Sony, now also offer similar UV laser and photopolymer-based RP in their Solid Creation System (SCS®) line of RP machines (www.sonypt.com).

In stereolithography, a UV laser is used to trace the surface of a photoreactive polymer that hardens to produce a solid object based on a three-dimensional computer file, usually .STL (stereolithography) format. The stereolithography process builds the object in layers, as if you were building an object of stacked pieces of paper. A base on an elevator starts at the top of a tank of plastic and drops a small amount every time a new layer is laid down, and this "grows" the part. Support structures are required to support cantilevered areas of the part. These vertical supports are removed during finishing. When completed, the part is ready to remove from the tank. The part is then placed in a postcuring oven, where it is cured under a UV lamp to harden any uncured polymer. The part will have a characteristic stair-step finish equal to the per-slice resolution of the stereolithography machine. This stair-step finish is usually removed by sandblasting the parts, giving the parts a translucent frosted finish. Stereolithography machines require a controlled and vented shop environment.

Stereolithography machines are limited in the size of parts produced by the width and depth of the liquid material vat. Larger parts may be produced by making a large part (such as large instrument housings) in smaller sections, bonding the sections together with stereolithography resin.

Stereolithography machines are expensive pieces of capital equipment and require special setup and venting, as well as trained operators. Some larger corporations with specialized or high-volume prototype requirements have chosen to bring stereolithography in-house. Most start-ups, small companies, and consulting offices find using a service bureau vendor to get stereolithography parts to be quite convenient and cost-effective.

STEREOLITHOGRAPHY MATERIALS

Common materials for stereolithography rapid prototypes are the 3D Systems Accura® resins and the DSM Somos® line of resins (www.dsmsomos.com). DSM offers resins with expanded materials properties, such as flexibility or clarity. Newer composite SLA materials are being developed that are loaded with ceramic fillers for added strength. Huntsman Advanced Materials (www.renshape.com) offers a line of specialized SLA materials, including medical-grade resins, acrylonitrile–butadiene–styrene (ABS)-like materials, and selectively colorable resins. 3D Systems has recently announced its Accura Bluestone™ line of composite materials for high-heat applications.

SLA parts made from commodity prototyping resins are quite strong; however, they may fracture if overstressed, drilled, or milled. These parts can be milled and drilled with care. An advantage to the harder resins is that they are less prone to warping or sagging in thin unsupported sections, and take paint finishes very well. If snap fits are required, specify one the flexible stereolithography resins, e.g., DSM Somos. Check with your service bureau on the availability and properties of these resins.

The flexible grades are similar in properties to polypropylene; however, the parts may still break if flexed too much. Optically clear grades of stereolithography materials are also available, allowing the prototyping of light pipes and clear parts for evaluation of internal components and fluid flow tests.

SLA parts can be sensitive to heat and humidity. Thin or unsupported sections can warp and sag under heat and pressure, or from some paint solvents. Therefore, appropriate care must be taken in shipping and storing stereolithography parts.

Stereolithography parts range from clear amber in color to milky white or clear, depending on the material. The transparency of stereolithography parts can be an advantage when evaluating parts together in assemblies. Since it is a wet-build method, SLA gives one of the better surface finishes of the RP methods, with tolerances close to that of CNC machining. Feature sizes as small as 0.01 inch are achievable. The ultimate resolution depends on the beam size of the SLA machine and the step increment in the Z axis. The trade-off for more detail is slower build times, and therefore a more expensive part. Check with your vendor to find out the smallest feature its machine will produce.

Colored areas may also be built into stereolithography parts. This is often done with stereolithography models produced for surgical planning. With a colored area, the location of an area of special interest, such as nerves or tumors, may be highlighted to assist the surgeon planning an operation. To produce parts of a stereolithography model that are selectively colored, a special stereolithography material (available from Huntsman Advanced Materials) is used that contains a dye that activates at a higher energy level than that to cure the clear polymer. Two.STL files are produced, one with the normal anatomy and one with the areas of interest. The models are overlaid and run together, and the stereolithography machine is programmed to apply a higher-power setting to the laser that is curing the areas of surgical interest in that file. This results in a model where the normal anatomy is clear and the areas of interest are highlighted in pink or red.

Rapid prototyping stereolithography resins and machines are being constantly developed and improved. Visit industry websites regularly to learn of new developments in stereolithography technology. Be sure to look at the examples and applications sections to see examples of RP applied to medical device design and anatomical visualization.

At this time most stereolithography materials are not USP Class VI or medical grade. Stereolithography parts may be used for *in vitro* (benchtop) or preclinical testing; however, only parts fabricated from medical-grade materials are appropriate for clinical use. Huntsman Advanced Materials advertises USP Class VI resins for use in stereolithography machines (www.huntsman.com, www.renshape.com).

Another application of stereolithography technology is QuickCast™, developed by 3D Systems. This is where an SLA model is produced that is hollow inside, with a thin supporting lattice. This is to produce a model with as little material volume as possible. This model is used to produce an investment casting pattern, and the SLA material burns into a small volume of ash when the ceramic shell of the investment casting mold is fired.

SONY SCS™

SCS stands for Solid Creation System and is a stereolithography system made by Sony Precision Technology. It is similar to 3D Systems SLA in that it uses a UV laser to draw layers. Sony uses two laser beams and makes machines to build larger-size stereolithography parts (www.sonypt.com).

3D SYSTEMS: SLS™

SLS stands for selective laser sintering, a process patented by Carl Deckard in 1989 and a trademark of 3D Systems, which acquired the DTM Corporation of Austin, TX, and the SLS process in 2001. This is a process where a laser traces a beam onto the surface of a container of fusible powder. The laser heats the particles of powder and sinters them together into a solid section. An elevator drops by a small increment and another layer is sintered to the preceding layer. The process builds in layers, similar to stereolithography, except using dry powder instead of liquid polymer as a medium. The SLS process does not require the use of support structures as in stereolithography and FDM, as the part is supported by the uncured powder material as it is lowered into the powder chamber.

One advantage to the SLS process is its versatility. Almost any material that can be powdered and sintered may be used to produce a part. Parts made from sintered nylon, for example, are quite tough and flexible. SLS process build materials include glass-filled rigid plastics, elastomers, and metals. Since the SLS process allows the fabrication of sintered elastomers, making prototypes of rubber parts such as shoe soles and custom-shaped orthopedic brace padding is possible.

Another use of the SLS process is the production of injection mold tooling and tooling inserts. The SLS process allows the production of injection mold tools with built-in conformal cooling channels.

Another example for the SLS process in medical device design is fabrication of sintered metal parts such as laparoscopic grasper jaws that model the characteristics of powdered metal injection molded (MIM) parts. As-built SLS metal parts are green and require postcuring in a special oven to achieve full strength and density. SLS powdered metal parts may be infiltrated with bronze to increase strength and density and eliminate porosity.

SLS is an RP technology requiring specialized capital equipment and skilled operators. It is best to utilize this technology through a service bureau. The 3D Systems website provides links to a number of qualified service bureaus offering SLS part-building services.

STRATASYS: FDM

FDM stands for fused deposition modeling, a process invented by Scott Crump and developed and marketed by Stratasys corporation (www.stratasys.com) of Eden Prarie, MN. In this process a thin cord of plastic material is extruded through a nozzle, and strands of molten material are deposited layer by layer to produce a final part. The process is similar to building a model with a very small hot-glue gun. Since the part is being formed in air, cantilevered sections require a supporting structure to prevent sagging. This support structure is deposited during the build process, and broken away from the part when it is completed. Another method is to make the supports using water soluble material, which then allows the construction of complex details that are not damaged when the support material is removed. The FDM process is limited to those thermoplastic materials that may be formed into beads or cords, heated, and deposited. FDM materials are supplied by the manufacturer on preloaded spools. FDM material is typically lower in cost, relative to volume, than the SLA or SLS processes. FDM machines are also capable of producing parts from medical-grade materials. These materials are available in spools from the manufacturer. The most common build material is ABS plastic.

The cost of FDM machines has dropped significantly. At this time office-based FDM RP three-dimensional printers are available in the sub-$25K range, making them affordable to have in-house at a facility that produces enough volume of models to justify the purchase price, maintenance, and consumables costs. The lower-cost machines are limited in some of the features they offer, like water-soluble support deposition and the materials they can run.

RESOLUTION AND SURFACE FINISH

On the higher-end machines, resolution may be one of four settings. Maximum resolution is 0.005 inch. Accuracy is ±0.005 inch on models up to 5 inches. Accuracy is ±0.0015 per inch on models greater than 5 inches. On the lower-end office-based machines, maximum resolution is 0.010 inch.[2]

Surface finish is not as smooth as the wet processes like SLA or PolyJet. As-built FDM models are somewhat porous. However, since FDM parts can be made of plastics like ABS, they may be readily sanded, primed, and painted. FDM can also produce large parts up to 23 × 23 × 19 inches in the larger machines.

FDM models can be quite robust, and made from a number of engineering plastics, e.g., ABS, polycarbonate, and nylon. In the example, FDM parts were used to make a surgical tool based on surgeon input. Often, a surgeon will visit with the engineer, design a product in CAD based on the surgeon's input, and have a working model ready for evaluation the next day. (See Figure 6.1)

> Sofamor Danek engineers designed a ratcheting counter-torque surgical instrument using both prototyping technologies. The instrument is used to fasten set-screws to a corrective implant on a patient's vertebrae and to break off the screw heads at a preset torque level. The existing method required surgeons to use two separate tools, working them in opposing directions, using both hands. Engineers chose the FDM Titan™ for the ratcheting portion and the Eden PolyJet™ system for its extension assembly. The extension comprises two concentric tubes

---

[2] Specifications supplied by Stratasys, Inc.

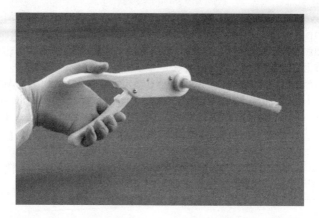

Figure 6.1 Figure shows a combination of polycarbonate FDM and Polyjet parts in a functioning surgical ratchet. (Courtesy of Stratasys and Medtronic Sofamor-Danek.)

or *cannulae,* one that slides inside the other. The Eden was used for this assembly because engineers wanted excellent detail on the inner and outer diameter and the smoothest possible surface finish. The FDM Titan produced a working, durable polycarbonate ratchet that withstood testing on steel set screws and required only one hand to control.[3]

FDM models may be used as masters for investment casting of orthopedic implants. In a case study from *Modern Casting Magazine*,[4] Biomet, Inc. (Warsaw, IN), engineers design an orthopedic implant in CAD, then review the design with the foundry to determine gate and vent locations. The model is saved as an .STL file and built in pattern wax using FDM. The model is smoothed, then mounted on a casting tree and dipped in ceramic slurry. The tree is processed at 1900°F to fire the ceramic and melt out the wax pattern. The fired investment shell is then ready for casting with steel. Using these RP processes, an implant in CoCr or stainless steel can go from design to casting in as little as 2 weeks. Once the design is tested and verified, the design is moved into quantity production with hard tooling.[5]

---

[3] Stratasys Corporation case study.
[4] *Modern Casting Magazine*, November 2001.
[5] Stratasys no longer supports the use of wax material in its machines. Wax masters may be produced with the Solidscape ModelMaker system, or the 3D Systems InVision system.

SOLIDSCAPE

Solidscape, Inc. (Merrimack, NH, www.solid-scape.com), manufactures the T66 Benchtop and T612 Benchtop systems. These systems are not rapid prototyping machines per se, as they are not intended to produce a functional part. Their purpose is to produce highly accurate master patterns for lost-wax (investment) casting or RTV molding. Because Solidscape's systems are able to build using extremely thin layers, models produced exhibit excellent surface finish and tight tolerances.

The maximum build platforms are somewhat smaller than most RP machines ($6 \times 6 \times 6$ inches on the T66 Benchtop and $6 \times 6 \times 12$ inches on the T612) and dictate the markets and applications that Solidscape targets. While patterns for toys, small medical devices, aerospace components, and consumer goods are commonly produced by Solidscape users, Solidscape systems are especially popular in the jewelry industry. This is because most jewelry consists of intricate designs that are traditionally cast using the lost-wax process.

The Solidscape system works by melting and depositing the build material (a wax-like thermoplastic) and a dissolvable wax support structure (to fill cavities and brace undercuts and cantilevered sections) in very small droplets through a piezo inkjet. The support material is dissolved using a heated solvent after the part is complete. After each layer build there is a milling step where the droplets are milled flat before the next layer is deposited. This contributes to the high accuracy of the process.

As mentioned above, the Solidscape system produce master patterns for lost-wax casting. One company that uses Solidscape systems in medical device manufacturing is Interpore Cross. Interpore Cross, a Biomet company, manufactures and markets spinal implant and orthobiologic devices. The Solidscape systems are used to produce the GEO™ Structure Vertebral Body Replacement implants. This spinal implant device is a latticed structure that comes in a variety of shapes and sizes. Interpore Cross is one of the largest installations of Solidscape systems, with over 30 machines in operation.

LOM™

LOM stands for laminated object modeling, a process originally developed by the Helisys Corporation. LOM uses a web of paper or other flexible sheet material and cuts this sheet material with a computer-controlled laser cutter. These sections are then laminated together with an adhesive to produce a final part. Excess material is sliced into blocks during the process and broken away from the part when finished. LOM was intended as a way to build large models from inexpensive materials. LOM has been used in pattern making for large castings and to produce large free-form models with thick wall sections. LOM has also been popular for producing architectural models. The technology had some early teething troubles, such as the laser causing the paper material to sometimes catch fire. Helisys ceased operations in 2000 and was succeeded by Cubic Technologies. The LOM process is currently marketed by the Stereoniks Corporation of Carson, CA.

Variations of the LOM process are seen in modelers from Solidimension (Israel), makers of the SD300 desktop three-dimensional printer. This modeler uses a LOM-type process laminating thin sheets of a polyvinylchloride (PVC) plastic material to produce models, with future plans to offer ABS and polycarbonate materials. Another variation of the LOM process is the Kira paper laminating process (PLT), which uses a knife to cut layers of material. The LOM process has a number of intriguing possibilities, as any material that can be supplied in sheet form, e.g., sheet metal, plastics, and composites that may be cut and laminated, is a candidate for LOM and related processes. Javelin 3D (Draper, UT) uses LOM-type technology in its MedLAM™ and CerLAM™ process to construct alumina–ceramic composite constructions in the shape of bones from computed tomography (CT) scan information, and other alumina ceramic objects.[6]

Z CORP.: THREE-DIMENSIONAL PRINTING

Z Corp. makes a line of machines referred to as three-dimensional printers.[7] Z Corp. three-dimensional printers use a powder-binder technology invented at and patented by the Massachusetts Institute of Technology (MIT). First, the three-dimensional printer spreads a thin layer of powder. Second, an inkjet print head prints a binder in the cross section of the part being created. Next, the build piston drops down, making room for the next layer, and the process is repeated. Once the part is finished, it is surrounded and supported by loose powder, which is then shaken loose from the finished part.[8] The low-end office-based machines sell for under $26K and uses inexpensive consumables. The build material may be either starch based or plaster based. The Z Corp. three-dimensional printers use Hewlett-Packard inkjet heads to deposit binders and food coloring-based dyes in layers on the build material. The surface finish of

---

[6] http://www.javelin3d.com/pdf/awards/BioceramicRP.pdf.
[7] Three-dimensional printeres are a general category of easy-to-use office-based machines for rapid protoyping.
[8] www.zcorp.com.

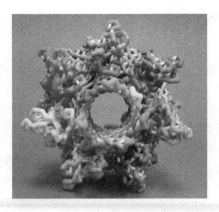

Figure 6.2 Hemolysin molecule. (Courtesy of Z Corp.)

the models is grainy, and the models are porous and somewhat fragile. The strength of the models may be increased by the use of infiltrants supplied by Z Corp. These are wax, rubber, cyanoacrylate, and epoxy materials, where the model is painted or dipped in these materials.

Due to the lower cost of materials, the Z Corp. three-dimensional printer is particularly suitable for the production of large, bulky models on their larger machines. The resolution of the process is less than that of other processes. The process has difficulty with small radii (>0.5 mm) and small feature sizes.

A recent development from Z Corp. is the Z-cast process. This is the process of producing a plaster casting mold directly, without the need for a lost-wax or sandbox casting pattern. The mold is printed using a plaster ceramic material. The material currently allows for the casting of low-melt-temperature metals such as aluminum, zinc, and magnesium. Tolerances and finish of the part are similar to sand casting.

A unique feature of the Z Corp. three-dimensional printing technology is the ability to print models in color. This is accomplished by adding a color print head to the system, and printing food color-based dyes on to the build material. This feature has become popular in the production of visual communication models such as models of fluid flow patterns, mold flow analysis, temperature maps, and stress pattern analysis. Figure 6.2 gives an example of the modeling of macromolecules with the Z Corp. Z810 three-dimensional printer.

POLYJET OBJET™ PRINTER

Polyjet is a technology developed by the Objet company (Rehovot, Israel, www.2objet.com). Objet makes the line of Eden™ RP machines, distrib-

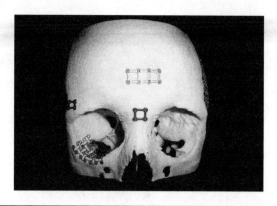

Figure 6.3 Three-dimensional printed model used for surgical planning. (Courtesy of Z Corp.)

uted in North America by Stratasys Corporation. PolyJet can be thought of as three-dimensional printing with stereolithography-like photopolymers. The Objet deposits a very thin layer of photopolymer with an inkjet-type print head that is cured with a UV lamp. A water-soluble gel support structure is built at the same time to support cantilevered areas of the model. This support is washed away when the model is complete.

The PolyJet is suitable for use in an office environment. The PolyJet is capable of very fine detail, with X, Y jet resolution of 600 × 300 dpi and a Z-axis layer of 16 microns (0.0006 inch). This has made the PolyJet popular with users making small objects requiring very fine detail and smooth surface finish. Material properties are similar to those of stereolithography parts.

DLP: ENVISIONTEC® PERFACTORY™

Digital light processing (DLP) is a photopolymer method to build parts. Envisiontec GmbH (Marl, Germany, www.envisiontec.de) markets this technology in its Perfactory system. In this process an entire image is projected onto the surface of a vat of photopolymer. The Perfactory lens system from Envisiontec is based on Texas Instruments DLP technology. In this method, a MEMS chip reflects an image off millions of mirrors through an optical engine into the surface of the resin to be cured. In this system a layer of material is exposed at one time, rather than traced with a single or dual laser. The system uses a visible light projector bulb to cure the resin, and therefore no UV laser or jetting technologies are involved.[9] The Perfactory is one of a new generation of RP machines

---

[9] http://rapid.lpt.fi/rp-ml-current/0082.html.

meant for in-house prototyping and the direct manufacturing market, suitable for nonshop environments.

SINTERING AND DIRECT METAL

A rapidly developing area using RP-layered manufacturing technology is the direct metal processes. These have matured from expensive and somewhat limited machines of a few years back to systems capable of direct manufacture of fully dense metals with properties and constructions difficult or impossible to achieve with conventional casting and machining methods.

Among the vendors for these direct metal systems is Arcam AB (Moldnal, Sweden, www.arcam.com), with its EBM (Electron Beam Melting) machine. EOS (Munich, Germany, www.eos.info) produces the EOSINT line of machines used in laser sintering of plastics, foundry sand, and direct metal applications.

Another very recent development has been the commercial release of the Solidica (www.solidica.com) system, a unique method of ultrasonically welding thin sheets of metal (e.g., aluminum) into a form, with an intermediate milling step between layer construction. The result is a metal matrix construction with finished milled features. This system is capable of laminating different metals into this metal matrix, as well as embedding functional elements such as embedded sensors, ceramics, and fiber optics. Solidica was founded by Dawn White, Ph.D. This construction method allows, for example, the production of aluminum injection mold tooling with conformal cooling channels for optimized cycle times. Also in this space is the Ex-One Corporation ProMetal™ process for layered manufacture of tooling (www.extrudehone.com). Artist Bathsheba Grossman (see later in this chapter) uses the ProMetal method to produce her sculptures.

RP APPLICATIONS IN PRODUCT DESIGN

The following are two examples of RP used to streamline and accelerate the product development process. In the example for Equilasers, a manufacturer of laser systems based in San Jose, CA, the company needed a design for the housing of a new Nd:YAG cosmetic laser system, the Equilase 30™.[10] The industrial and mechanical design was done, and the panels were fabricated from SLA parts. The size limitation on SLA parts was overcome by the parts being grown as smaller sections, then bonded together with SLA resin and painted. The project went from a clean-sheet concept design stage to a finished unit, ready to crate and ship to an

---

[10] www.equilasers.com.

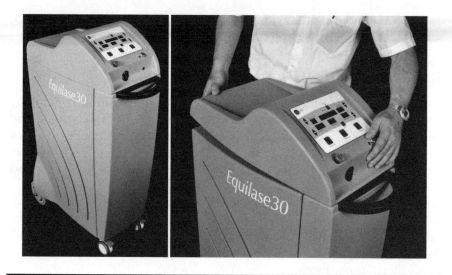

Figure 6.4 Large painted functional stereolithography RP panels. (Kucklick Design for Equilasers, Inc.)

overseas trade show in 4 weeks. The parts were designed as detachable panels with production in mind, and included all of the mounting hardware, wall thickness, and draft required when the parts were to be pressure formed. The parts were robust enough for functional testing and shipping.

In the example for Sleep Solutions, Inc.,[11] RP was used to iterate the product development and clinical testing process of the NovaSom QSG™ system. The original product was a test unit enclosed in a sheet metal project box, and needed to be redesigned for quantity production, as well as to have the look of a friendly, easy-to-use medical instrument for home use. The unit also had to be radio frequency interference (RFI) shielded and very durable for multiple shipping and reuse. Also, since the unit was to be very compact, design for assembly issues needed to be resolved before committing to hard tooling. An iteration of the design was produced in RP to test and debug the design. A final SLA master was produced, and several cast urethane duplicates were produced with RTV silicone tooling. The units were assembled using threaded inserts, as the final plastic parts would be. These units were used for mechanical and assembly testing and electronics package development, and also in final clinical validation while the injection mold tooling was in process. Once the tooling was done, injection molded parts were produced in a durable engineering plastic, with confidence in the fit and function of the final parts that had been verified with RP before the hard tooling

---

[11] www.sleep-solutions.com.

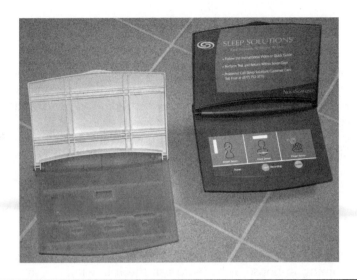

Figure 6.5 RP prototype (stereolithography and cast urethane) parts and injection molded final design of the NovaSom QSG™. (Kucklick Design for Sleep Solutions, Inc.)

was cut. RP was a useful tool to move this project forward quickly, and allowed several design and validation activities to proceed in parallel, with high levels of confidence in the final results.

CNC

Computer numerical control (CNC) machining was originally developed by John Parsons with the assistance of MIT, Wright-Patterson Air Force Base, and the U.S. Air Force around 1947. The original purpose was to machine very accurate curved objects that required complex jigs. Parsons originally conceived of the basis of the idea while working as a machine shop apprentice in 1929, and later while producing complex helicopter rotor blades at his own company for the military. The first CNC machine was built in 1949. In 1952 the first commercially available CNC machines were produced, and they were accepted into industrial use by 1957. One of the reasons CNC took so long to be accepted was that some of the companies involved (IBM and General Dynamics) saw "no application for it at all." In fact, a paper submitted by one of Parson's associates, Frank Stulen, to the American Helicopter Association on the use of CNC to produce helicopter rotor blades was rejected as "pure nonsense." CNC was also rejected at the time by the auto industry. It was finally the dogged persistence of John Parsons and his associates like Frank Stulen, and the intervention of the Air Force, by its purchasing a number of the first CNC machines and distributing them into the aircraft industry to help produce the new generation of advanced jet aircraft (the B-47), that finally led to the acceptance of CNC technology. CNC is now considered one of the cornerstones of the "Second Industrial Revolution."[12] CNC is but one of a number of revolutionary technologies (e.g., the personal computer, magnetic resonance imaging (MRI)) for which many experts originally saw no market or useful purpose.

There are numerous small CNC machines available that are driven by inexpensive personal computers. These range from light training models to smaller versions of industrial-grade machining centers. DesktopNC.com is a comprehensive resource of nearly every active (and inactive) manufacturer of small NC milling machines (www.desktopcnc.com/index.htm).

Given the reasonable cost of smaller CNC mills, as well as lower-cost domestic and import full-size machines, available new and used, it can be tempting to bring CNC machining in-house. When considering bringing CNC machining in-house, it helps to ask the following questions:

- Do we have a specific need to manufacture or prototype in-house?
- Are we willing to hire or train a skilled machinist to operate this machine?
- How much work could we get done outside for the cost of the machine, plus the cost of a skilled operator (or a skilled operator already on staff, taken away from his other responsibilities)?
- Does the small CNC machine we are considering have the power to machine all of the materials we need to work with (e.g., ferrous metals), or do our needs require a full-size machining center?
- Will the machine be used enough hours per day to justify the cost of the capital to purchase it, and the ongoing expenses of facility overhead, taxes, and maintenance?

Small start-up companies operating on investment capital can find that it is difficult to justify bringing CNC machining in-house, unless there is a specific reason for doing so. Some companies find that having a simple manual mill and lathe that can be operated by an engineer with sufficient skills can be adequate for proof-of-concept work, where it makes more sense to send out more complex or higher-volume jobs to a dedicated outside machine shop. Manual Bridgeport-type knee mills can also be retrofitted with two- and three-axis NC drives and controls, though this can make them more cumbersome to use as manual machines. The use

---

[12] For a more complete biography of John Parsons and the story of the birth of CNC, see the September 2001 *Metalworking Machine Mailer*, http://www.tadesite.com/parsons.mgi. Many of the historical details on CNC are cited from the article.

of the CNC function also requires special training, which can be difficult to retain for the casual or occasional user.

There are over 47 makers of desktop milling machines with nearly 100 models available, with prices ranging from under $5000 to over $40K. Machines listed as educational are meant to train machinists to operate larger machines. Rapid prototype and hobbyist machines are usually not suitable for cutting ferrous metals (iron, steel, and stainless steel) and are limited to machining jeweler's wax, modeling foam, chemical wood, and sometimes plastic. Some of the larger machines can handle machining brass and aluminum. When considering a desktop milling machine, carefully evaluate whether the machine will handle the types of materials you want to cut. Desktop machines also tend to use only one tool at a time, unlike the tool-changing capabilities found in full-size machining centers.

Roland (www.rolanddga.com) offers a line of easy-to-use desktop CNC machines marketed as subtractive rapid prototypers (SRP®). The smaller machines (MDX 15 and 20) are capable of machining wax, foam, and plastics at slow feed rates. The MDX 500 and MDX 650 machines are capable of milling nonferrous metals like brass and aluminum. A unique feature of the MDX 20 (about $5K) is that it is a combination lightweight tabletop three-axis mill and a three-dimensional scanner. The MDX 650 offers an optional tool changer for up to eight tools and an optional fourth-axis rotary material holder. They are bundled together with simple-to-use software, which allows a user with little or no previous machine shop experience to make parts. The drawback to these higher-end machines is their being limited in the materials they can machine, and their somewhat high cost (about $20K, not including optional accessories).

FULL-SIZE VMC CNC MACHINES

Haas Automation (Oxnard, CA), Fadal (Chatsworth, CA, a division of ThyssenKrupp, Germany), Mori Seiki (Japan), Mazak (Japan), Daewoo (Korea), and Chevalier (Taiwan) are manufacturers of CNC vertical machining centers (VMCs). Recently Haas and Fadal have both begun to offer tool room VMC CNC machines capable of both CNC and manual operation in the sub-$20K range, and mini-VMC machines in the sub-$30K range. These machines claim to be easy to use for operators not familiar with traditional CNC G-code programming. In contrast to the desktop machines mentioned previously, these VMCs require 230 V of single- or three-phase power. Industrial-grade CNC machines also require a separate computer program to generate tool paths, the series of cuts that the machine makes to produce a final shape from a block of material. Examples of these programs are Mastercam (www.mastercam.com), Surfcam (www.surfcam.com), and Gibbs CAM (www.Gibbscam.com). When looking for a

CAM package, it is important to determine how it will be used and how well it works with the CAD program you are using. A good place to start would be your CAD vendor, to see if it has a good CAM solution that works seamlessly inside of your current CAD program. Analyzing your requirements and streamlining your workflow are vitally important before you go through the time and expense of implementing an in-house CNC machining solution.

Full-size CNC VMCs have the advantage of being able to cut any machineable material. They also offer turrets that hold multiple tools. However, using these industrial CNC machines and the programs to run them requires an operator with a significant amount of machine shop knowledge and training. This is why many small start-up companies conserve their cash and send machine shop work out to skilled and reliable outside vendors.

MACHINABLE PROTOTYPE MATERIALS

For prototype models in inexpensive materials, there are a number of foam, chemical wood products, styling, and tooling board materials available.

The most popular and inexpensive is urethane, or surfboard foam. This can be easily hand shaped and sanded, and machined on any milling machine. The drawback of urethane foam is its porous surface and production of gritty foam dust residue when sanded. Another variation of this material is polystyrene surfboard foam. These materials are available at many hobby shops or surfboard supply shops.

Ren Shape® pattern-making materials are manufactured by Huntsman Advanced Materials. There are two basic types, styling boards and tooling boards. Styling boards are lower-density, lower-temperature materials designed for dimensional stability and ease of machining. Tooling boards are made for dimensional stability and heat resistance in the range of 232 to 496°F, for applications such as the production of vacuum-forming molds and other high-temperature pattern-making applications.

Machinable wax is used to produce tooling masters for lost-wax casting, or nonporous casting masters that release easily from RTV silicone rubber mold-making materials. Pattern-making wood includes medium-density fiberboard (MDF), plank pine, and chemical wood. Most of these materials are available from Freeman Manufacturing and Supply (www.freemansupply.com). Prototyping plastics commonly used and readily available for machining are Delrin® acetal (easy to machine, chemical and solvent resistant), ABS plastic (good general-purpose plastic, less expensive), polycarbonate (very tough and strong plastic, harder to machine with good surface finish), and acrylic (readily available at hobbyist plastic shops, hard, machines with good surface finish, can be polished). All of these materials except Delrin can be easily bonded with proper adhesives. These materials are available from any large plastics supply house. Two that I have used are Polymer Plastics Corporation (www.polymerplastics.com) and Port Plastics (www.portplastics.com). Ren Shape materials, machinable wax, and pattern-making wood products are available from Freeman Manufacturing and Supply (Avon, OH, www.freemansupply.com). Freeman also makes available online over 2 hours of excellent video tutorials on how to use various casting and prototyping materials, as well as sample kits of various molding, casting, and machinable materials. Prototype metals include easy-to-machine grades of brass and aluminum. Obomodulan® is a polyurethane prototyping board in several densities made by the Obo-Werke GmbH of Stadhagen, Germany (www.obo-werke.de).

For those who do not want to own a milling machine or even a CAD program, machined parts can be designed and purchased online at emachineshop.com. The site has a built-in draw program and an online quotation function for those who have an occasional need for machined parts and sheet metal prototypes.

RAPID TOOLING AND MOLDING

There have been several technologies developed to directly manufacture steel tooling for plastic injection molding. One of the barriers to acceptance is that the majority of methods rely on some form of laser sintering and require postprocessing to turn the sintered RP tool into a usable fully dense part. One potential advantage to RP tooling is in the free-form modeling capabilities inherent in RP. 3D Systems advertises its Laserform® material. This system allows the production of steel inserts for low-volume injection molding (20 to 50K shots.) One unique feature of the system is the ability to build into the tooling insert conformal cooling channels for specialized applications. Newer materials such as 3D Systems Laserform A6 can produce production-grade tools with good heat transfer characteristics.

Mold inserts may also be made from RP part masters by an electroforming process. Here, an RP part is used as a master, and a thick layer of copper is deposited on to the master, removed, and backed with epoxy. This is repeated until an A and B side of the mold is produced. The prototype core and cavity are then mounted into a mold base for prototype injection or compression molding. This service is offered by the Repliform company (www.repliforminc.com).

Another vendor who has entered the rapid tooling market is Protomold. By offering a defined set of mold-making services that are readily achievable within its CNC machining capabilities (part size, minimum feature size, minimum corner radius, limits on side actions, etc.) and an Internet storefront with online quoting, getting prototypes of many types of injection molded parts is fast, easy, and surprisingly inexpensive (www.protomold.com). Protomold keeps a fairly complete inventory of most types of molding plastics and can mold parts from customer-supplied material as well. Several other companies are also offering these types of rapid-turnaround injection molding services.

WHICH TECHNOLOGY IS BEST?

Every RP technology has it own strengths and limitations. There is no one RP approach that is best for every application. The best technology is the one that best meets the requirements for what you want to accomplish. Therefore, first determine which factors are most important: speed, size of parts, surface finish, minimum feature size, materials properties, in-house or outsourced, cost, and convenience. Is the model for visual evaluation? Will it be a master for other reproduction processes? Will it be used for mechanical testing? Will the RP part be used as a tool or mold? Does the part need to be made of a medical-grade material? Definitions of these factors will help you to make the best choice of the numerous RP technologies available to you. In practice, 3D Systems SLA and Stratasys FDM make up the majority of models made at service bureaus. Z Corp.'s three-dimensional printing system is a popular in-office system for those applications that can work with its surface finish and feature size limitations, and secondary operations requirements (wax, cyanoacrylate, and epoxy, and infiltration to strengthen the part). For parts that must be of a specific material, and not just a representation of it in an RP material, CNC machining is the best approach, though this may be more costly than RP, and you are limited to geometry that can be made with mill and lathe machine tools.

FILE PREPARATION

To produce an RP part requires a three-dimensional digital file of your part geometry, typically from a three-dimensional CAD or three-dimensional modeling program (e.g., SolidWorks™, Pro/Engineer™, Autocad™, Alias™, Rhino™, etc.) You must have a program capable of producing either a solid model or a closed-surface model. Two-dimensional drafting files (e.g., Autocad.dwg) will not work for processes such as SLA or FDM. Check your three-dimensional computer-aided design (CAD) software to be sure that you can export your three-dimensional model as an .STL file.

Three-dimensional scanners can also produce meshes that can be turned into .STL solid models. This is discussed in Chapter 7. The .STL files may also be produced from MRI and CT data. Mimics™ software from Materialise NV (Belgium) translates CT or MRI data into three-dimensional CAD, finite element meshes, or rapid prototyping data (www.materialise.com). Protomed, Inc., in Arvada, CO, specializes in producing stereolithography models for surgical planning from MRI and CT scan data (www.protomed.net). Two other programs for converting CT and MRI scans are VG Studio Max (Heidelberg, Germany, volume-graphics.com), a voxel-based modeler for animators, and Vitrea (Minnetonka, MN, vitalimages.com), a high-end solution for radiologists.

An .STL file is a polygon mesh surface file that is sliced up in the SLA machine's preprocessing software. This produces a series of outlines of part sections, or slices, that are then filled in by the SLA machine's UV laser. In a polygon mesh file a surface is described by a series of tessellated (tiled) triangles. The size and number of these triangles determine the resolution of the model. The higher the number of triangles, the higher the resolution and the smoother the model; however, this results in larger file sizes. Use the preview setting of your CAD program's .STL output function to see the effects of higher and lower triangle resolution settings, and how they affect the smoothness of the final .STL output file. If the file becomes overly large, try reducing the output resolution or compressing the file with a program such as WinZip™ before sending it to your service bureau.

OTHER FILE FORMATS

The majority of RP information is communicated in the .STL format. Some of the other more common neutral file formats available are:

- **PLY** format, or the Stanford triangle format. This is a simplified vertex and face description of a three-dimensional object. It is a simplified file format for the communication of three-dimensional surface models, usually acquired from three-dimensional scanners.
- **VRML** (virtual reality modeling format). Based on Silicon Graphics (Mountain View, CA) Open Inventor file format for use in Internet applications. Inventor is yet another file format that is a superset of the VRML networked graphics data format. VRML is useful with communication texture and color data along with three-dimensional object information. Other three-dimensional formats, such as STL and PLY, do not support this type of color and scene data.
- **IGES** (Initial Graphics Exchange Specification). An American national standard that is a neutral data format for the digital exchange of information among computer-aided design (CAD) systems and other applications. The standard is developed and maintained by the IGES/PDES Organization. IGES supports the representation of surfaces with smooth higher-order splines or nonlinear uniform rational B-splines (NURBS).

DXF (drawing interchange file). A file format developed by Autodesk, Inc. (Sausilito, CA) as a neutral file format for the communication of two- and three-dimensional vector information. DXF represents three-dimensional objects as polyface meshes, and not smooth surfaces or NURBS.

STEP (Standard for the Exchange of Product Mode Data). An ISO standard neutral file format for the communication of engineering solid model data generated from CAD programs.

For more information on the (numerous) three-dimensional file formats in existence, visit the Center for Machine Perception of the Czech Technical University department of Cybernetics (http://cmp.felk.cvut.cz).

RP COST-SAVING TIPS

The cost of SLA and other rapid prototype parts increases with the volume of the part. Larger-volume parts require higher expenses in machine time and materials costs. If a larger prototype is required, and cost is an issue, an RP method with lower material costs may be considered. A way to save cost with SLA, if a number of smaller parts are to be produced, is to run them all at one time, and incur only one setup cost or lot charge.

Another way to save costs is to produce only the part of the model that needs to be evaluated. For example, you may have only a connector interface that needs to be checked for function and fit. Save the part to a new CAD file and cut away the rest of the model so you are left only with the part of the model you want to evaluate. Save this section to an .STL file and send this to your service bureau for modeling. This will save the time and expense of producing the entire model in SLA.

If you are a company that operates globally, a way to speed product development and save time and costs with RP is to produce the CAD file in one country (e.g., the U.S.), then transmit the data file over the Internet to an RP service bureau in a distant country (e.g., Australia or Europe). Then, have the model delivered by the service bureau to the local person in that country who will use the model. This can avoid issues with customs and overseas courier services. You will want to establish a good working relationship with the overseas service bureau before trying this on a critical project. Some companies with international offices use this method, designing in one location, and transmitting CAD data to be fabricated by an in-house manufacturing operation in another country.

With RP machines capable of printing in color (Z Corp.), a model can be built as one part, with different components printed in a different color. The model can then be sectioned in CAD, or sawn apart to analyze how components fit together. This saves the time of building the model in separate parts and assembling them.

SECONDARY PROCESSES TO RP PARTS

Painting

The most obvious secondary finishing process to RP parts is painting. Stereolithography parts are the easiest to paint, requiring only finish sanding and primer. SLS parts can be painted, depending on the material. Stratasys FDM models can be painted, but require more finish work than stereolithography models. Z Corp. three-dimensional printed models can be painted, but require more finishing and sealing work.

Electroplating

Another secondary operation that can be performed on RP parts is electroplating or vacuum deposition. This gives RP parts the look of metal parts, or it can be used for EMI/RFI shielding. Consult the Thomas Register (www.thomasregister.com) for companies that offer these processes.

Machining

RP materials vary in their machinability. FDM models are readily milled and drilled; SLA parts can may be machined with care, though they may break easily.

Threaded Inserts

RP parts can be assembled with machine screws if bosses are designed into the part and threaded inserts are used. These are more accurate and reliable than attempting to drill and tap RP material, and they will duplicate the way the final molded parts are likely to be assembled. Threaded inserts are available from Penn Engineering Corporation, makers of PEM® inserts. (www.pennfast.com). These are inserts normally driven into infection molded plastic parts with an ultrasonic welder.

Installing the Inserts

One way to use these inserts in RP and cast urethane parts is to do the following: design the bosses in your part to the interference fit specifications given for the threaded insert when driven in with ultrasound. This information is available in the product literature for the insert. To install the inserts, use a soldering iron set to the melt temperature of the RP plastic that your part is made from. A pointed soldering iron tip that fits into the brass threaded insert works particularly well. Place the threaded insert into the boss until the insert's lead-in taper holds it in position. Place the hot soldering iron tip into the insert, and gently press the insert into the boss as the soldering iron melts the plastic. Remove the soldering iron tip from the insert. You now have a reliable and reusable assembly thread in your RP part.

UV CURE SEALING OF FOAM PARTS

When making urethane or styrene foam models either by hand or on a CNC mill, you will find that these models can be fragile in their thin sections, dusty, and not able to be painted. Sealing the model helps make it stronger as well as able to take paint. One method that has been tried is to use spackle or artist's gesso to seal the foam. The drawback to this method is that the gesso and spackle are heavy and can take a very long time to dry. A better solution is to use UV-curable surfboard polyester resin. These are low viscosity and easy to use and brush on the part. Putting the parts out in the sun for about an hour cures the resin. The result is a stronger, cleaner part. UV cure polyester is available from surfboard materials shops, or from Fiberglass Supply (Bingen, WA, www.fiberglasssupply.com).

RP CASTING PATTERNS

RP models may be used as masters to produce cast duplicates. Any casting method may be used, depending on the material to be cast. Room temperature-vulcanized (RTV) silicone rubber is the most common. Other casting materials such as dental alginate may be used also to produce wax patterns for making the plaster of dental stone molds.

When making a master for casting, do not forget to factor in the shrink of the casting material. Casting materials can shrink significantly as they harden. The percentage of shrink is different for each material. The data sheet from the supplier will provide this information. If the castings are being done at the same vendor as the RP master, the vendor will have this information on hand and can build the shrink factor into the master part for you. This means that dimensions are critical; a cast part made from a casting material with a 2% shrink factor will need to be scaled 2% larger than the master if the final part is to be the same size as the original CAD model.

Masters are usually done at a higher resolution than visual check or fit check parts. They are sanded and painted to ensure they release readily from the RTV mold and produce a smooth surface finish.

A twist on the use of RP casting masters is to use an RP model as a casting tool. SLA would work well, as it is not porous. If you have rubber grips or some other elastomer part to cast, try making the mold in RP, especially if you do not have access to a CNC mill. An RP mold, treated with mold release, can quickly produce a tool to cast silicone or urethane parts.

REVERSE ENGINEERING

Reverse engineering is a natural companion to RP. It uses three-dimensional scanning techniques to generate a CAD model to produce a copy of the object with RP techniques. Scanner vendors like to call this process reverse modeling. It is very similar to the older process of taking a clay impression or making a plaster "splash" mold to duplicate a part. There are a number of very useful and important applications for these methods. The subject of reverse engineering will be handled in more detail in Chapter 7.

INNOVATIVE APPLICATIONS OF RP

This last section is a digest of a number of innovative uses of rapid prototyping. Some of these are commonly used, others are in development, and yet others are a view into the future. Perhaps in one or more of them is the inspiration for your own groundbreaking innovation.

RP and Surgical Planning

RP has given surgeons powerful tools in planning high-risk complex surgeries. This is especially useful in cases presenting significant anatomical variations or damage, such as deformity or trauma.

For an interesting use of rapid prototyping using 3D Systems SLA process in surgical planning, see the November 2002 issue of *Designfax Magazine* online at www.designfax.net, "Conjoined Twins Separation a Model Surgery." RP models are now used routinely to plan these challenging surgeries.

When producing a model for surgical planning, it is often necessary to highlight areas of surgical interest or concern. To produce a stereolithography model that is selectively colored, use a stereolithography material containing a dye that activates at a higher energy level than that to cure the clear polymer.

Two stereolithography models are produced, one with the normal anatomy and one with the areas of interest. The models are run together, and the stereolithography machine is programmed to apply a higher-power setting to the laser curing the areas of surgical interest. This results in a model where the normal anatomy is clear and the areas of interest are highlighted in pink.

RP and Training Models

RP has found numerous applications in medical modeling. See "Rapid Prototyping of Temporal Bone for Surgical Training and Medical Education" in the May 2004 issue of *Acta Oto-Laryngologica* (vol. 124, pp. 400–402). Here, selective laser sintering is used to reproduce the temporal bone, and the malleus and incus of the middle ear. The model was cut and shaved using a surgical drill, burr, and suction irrigator in the same way as a real bone.

Molecular Modeling

Previously in this chapter was an example of a hemolysin molecule modeled in color with the Z Corp. three-dimensional printer. Bathsheba Grossman is a mathematician and artist in Santa Cruz, CA, who produces sculptures based on mathematical models and molecular information. Bathsheba was kind enough to share some of the details of how she prepares the molecule data set for burning into a glass block with CNC lasers:

> I get most of the glass done at precisionlaserart.com. To build a protein point cloud, I start with the PDB file, and my first aim is to turn it into a three-dimensional CAD model. The CAD software I use has a strong scripting language, so I do this by lexically converting the PDB into a script file. If ribbons or cartoons are required I use Kinemage as an intermediate step, since it writes a tractable ASCII format for these structures. If an electrostatic surface is required, I use GRASS (Graphical Representation and Analysis of Structure Server) to create the surface, and other software tools to smooth and condition it. Once I have the structure as a CAD file, I distribute points onto it. And lastly, I use some of my own software to dither these points, adding thickness to curves, and regulating the translucency of surfaces. So at the end of all this, I have a simple ASCII list of points, scaled to size, and that's what I send to the laser facility.[13]

---

[13] For more information on Bathsheba's sculptures, see www.bathsheba.com.

Rapid Prototyping for Medical Devices ■ 145

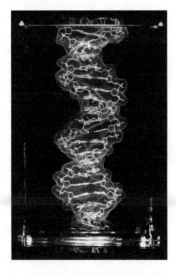

Figure 6.6 DNA model, laser engraved in glass. (Courtesy of Bathsheba Grossman.)

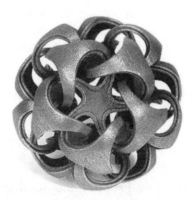

Figure 6.7 Quintron, metal print sculpture. Note the geometric complexity and nested shapes achievable with RP. (Courtesy of Bathsheba Grossman.)

RP-Produced Medical Products

Investment Cast Orthopedic Implants

Solidscape, Inc., recently announced that the company installed the 32nd of its ModelMaker™ RP systems in the production facility of Interpore Cross International. Interpore Cross is a medical device company with a complementary combination of spinal implant and orthobiologic technol-

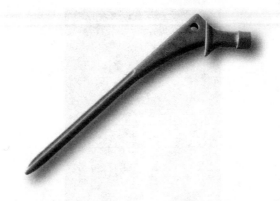

Figure 6.8 Hip implant stem casting master in wax. (Courtesy of Solidscape.)

ogies. The ModelMaker™ systems are used to produce the GEO™ Structure Vertebral Body Replacement implants, for which FDA clearance was recently received. This spinal implant device is a latticed structure that comes in a variety of shapes and sizes.

> "We evaluated a number of the RP systems available and determined the Solidscape technology to be the only system on the market capable of fabricating investment casting patterns that met the dimensional tolerances our products required," said R. Park Carmon, Vice President of Operations. "Application of advanced rapid prototype equipment to deliver production quantities is a good example of the innovative approach Interpore is taking to bring new products to the spinal market. The Solidscape system made that application possible."[14]

RP and RE Combined into a Product and Service

Crowns in One Visit

Sirona Dental Systems (Germany) makes the CEREC® system for the chairside production of dental crowns. Rather than taking a physical impression, drilling out the box for the crown, and sending the patient home with a temporary crown to come back in a week or two while a dental lab produces a crown from the impression, the CEREC system gives the patient a permanent crown in one visit. The way this is done is with a sophisticated three-dimensional scan of the tooth called a digital impression. The tooth is then drilled, and a second digital impression is taken of the box, or

---

[14] Solidscape, Inc., press release, May 29, 2002.

Rapid Prototyping for Medical Devices ■ 147

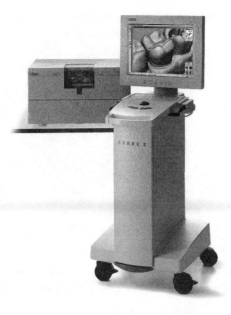

Figure 6.9 The CEREC system. (Courtesy of Sirona Dental Systems.)

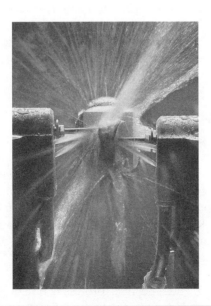

Figure 6.10 Milling the ceramic blank. (Courtesy of Sirona Dental Systems.)

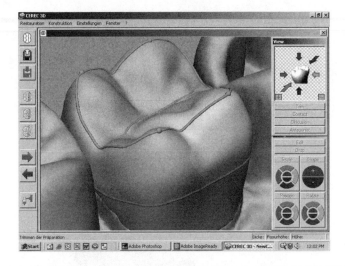

Figure 6.11 Three-dimensional data capture of a tooth. (Courtesy of Sirona Dental Systems.)

the cavity into which the crown will fit. The digital information from the scan of the intact tooth surface is combined with the box that the tooth implant will fit into. These data are then transmitted to a special milling machine that uses dental burrs to shape a blank of ceramic tooth crown material into the shape of the previous tooth surface and the box it is to fit into. The finished crown is then cemented in place, and the patient is sent home, with her permanent crown, precisely fitted, in one visit. This is an example of reverse engineering and rapid prototyping applied to a medical product and service.

RP and Tissue Engineering

Some of the greatest advances in technology have been the application of one technology redeployed into another area. An example is the combination of personal computers and Xerox® copier technology, which spawned the laser printer, and with it desktop publishing and graphics. Another is the adaptation of rapid prototyping technology to the areas of tissue engineering. RP is used to manufacture the framework onto which living cells attach and proliferate. A 1989 *Business Week* article gives a brief history and theory of tissue engineering:

> As early as 1979, Eugene Bell, professor emeritus of biology at MIT and the founder of Organogenesis, figured out how to grow skin in his lab. Since then, much of the field's progress stems

from a 20-year collaboration of two fast friends — Joseph Vacanti, a pediatric surgeon at Children's Hospital, and Robert S. Langer, a chemical engineering professor at MIT. Their lab "seeded the entire country with people doing this work," says Dr. Pamela Bassett, president of medical consultants BioTrend in New York.

The two, both 49, first met as researchers in the mid-1970s and started working on a way to grow tissue in the early 1980s. In 1986, they developed an elegantly simple concept that underlies most engineered tissue. Start with a scaffold, bent to any shape, made of an artificial, biodegradable polymer. Seed it with living cells, and bathe it in growth factors. The cells multiply, filling up the scaffold and growing into a three-dimensional tissue. Once implanted in the body, the cells are smart enough to recreate their proper tissue functions. Blood vessels attach themselves to the new tissue, the scaffold melts away, and the lab-grown tissue is eventually indistinguishable from its surroundings.[15]

As you can see, the basic theory is to make a tissue scaffold with the desired shape and characteristics, and deposit cells and growth medium on the scaffold to grow tissue in a directed way. This is the famous "ear on a mouse," where a scaffold made of human chondrocytes (cartilage) in the approximate shape of a human ear was attached to the back of a mouse, and tissue grew around it to resemble the shape of a human ear. This feat earned a fair bit of notoriety for the experimenter, Linda Griffith of MIT, and a fair bit of misunderstanding of the concept in the popular press.

Alternatively, the scaffold is implanted, and the body supplies the tissue to grow onto the scaffold. When the scaffold has served its purpose, it is then broken down and absorbed into the body. The difficulty in using this approach to build larger tissues and organs is providing tissues within the engineered construction with oxygen and nutrients. One of the difficulties to overcome is the 2-mm rule from physiology. This rule states that no living tissue in the body can be more than 2 mm away from a blood supply. This is one of the major obstacles in building implantable solid organs using tissue engineering.

---

[15] Arnst, Catherine and Carey, John, "Biotech Bodies," *Business Week*, July 27, 1998, http://www.businessweek.com/1998/30/b3588001.htm. See also "How to Grow a Human Heart: Advances in Tissue Engineering Are Bringing It Much Closer Than You Think," *MIT Technology Review Magazine*, April 2001.

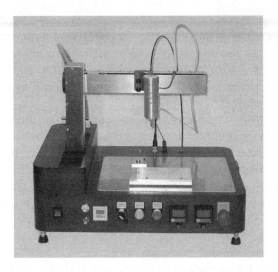

Figure 6.12 The Envisiontec Bioplotter. (Courtesy of Envisiontec GmbH.)

The Envisiontec Bioplotter

Envisiontec GmbH (Germany, www.envisiontec.de) makes the Bioplotter® to build scaffolds for tissue engineering. The Bioplotter acts in a similar way to a rapid prototyping machine and uses cell cultures to build new structures layer by layer.

The Bioplotter creates a digital data model of the structure to be built. It then dispenses cells, producing a three-dimensional arrangement of biological and biocompatible material.

Other work in this area is being conducted by Thomas Boland at Clemson University, SC, and Vladimir Mironov at the Medical University of South Carolina and the University of Missouri, Columbia:

> To print 3D structures, Boland and Mironov used a "thermo-reversible" gel recently developed by Anna Gutowska, research scientist at the Department of Energy Pacific Northwest National Laboratory. The non-toxic, biodegradable gel is liquid below 20°C and solidifies above 32°C. The team has done several experiments using easily available tissues such as hamster ovary cells. By printing alternate layers of the gel and clumps of cells onto glass slides, they have shown 3D structures such as tubes can be built up.[16]

---

[16] "Ink-Jet Printing Creates Tubes of Living Tissue," *The New Scientist*, January 22, 2003.

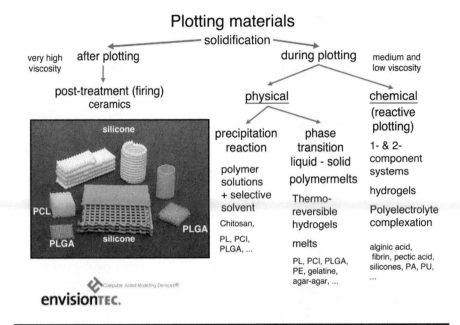

Figure 6.13 Tissue engineering plotting materials. (Courtesy of Envisiontec GmbH.)

The effect is evident when considering that similar to producing a colored document when a cartridge is filled with assorted ink colors, complex structures such as organs can be printed when a cartridge is replenished with different kinds of cells. However, that step requires the discovery of a method to produce circulatory networks that would furnish nutrients and oxygen to the deeply embedded cells. To make that a reality, Boland and Mironov aspire to print a whole system of veins, capillaries, and arteries that would support whole organs.[17]

In a *Business Week* article, Neil Gross reports:

> Doctors may one day use a variety of rapid prototyping techniques to build replacements for bones destroyed by injury or disease. The Office of Naval Research (ONR) in Arlington, Va., pioneered such techniques for making plastic, metal, and ceramic parts from digital designs. Biomedical engineers picked up the trend, making plastic plugs to replace pieces of damaged bone. Three years ago, the ONR teamed up with Advanced Ceramics Research Inc. in Tucson for more advanced applications.[18]

---

[17] "Desktop Printing of Living Tissue," *R&D Magazine*, March 2003.
[18] Gross, Neil, Ed., "Developments to Watch," *Business Week Online*, June 23, 2003.

Therics Corporation (Princeton, NJ, www.therics.com) applies RP methods to building bone graft material using RP technology.

For more information on the subject of tissue engineering and its current business and regulatory environment, see "Body by Science" by Aileen Constanz in the October 6, 2003 issue of *The Scientist*.

RP and Pharmeceuticals

RP may have applications in the packaging of pharmaceuticals: according to Ed Grenda's RP report website:

> Medical dosages forms which would be difficult if not impossible to make any other way are in development. Using rapid prototyping it's possible to fabricate pills with precise and complex time release characteristics or that dissolve almost instantly. A recent patent describes the interesting possibility of combining one drug with a second compound that synchronously counteracts the first drug's side-effects within the same pill. Medications can be made more effective and safer in this way and drug companies may be able to realize stronger revenue streams from older drugs that go "off-patent" by providing them in novel and beneficial dosage forms.[19]

RP and Analysis

Another novel application of RP is a using RP technology to facilitate an old analysis method: researchers at the University of Warwick have found a way of using a test devised in the 1930s, once used to gauge the stress on the superchargers in Spitfire fighter planes, to model the stress that surgical procedures would put on an aortic aneurysm. Rob Coppinger writes in *The Engineer*:

> Photoelasticity is a technique that has been used for decades in industry. It looks at the patterns of coloured light reflected from the surface of an object to gain a detailed understanding of the stresses on that object.
>
> Initially surgeons had tried placing mechanical strain gauges on an aortic aneurysm as they manipulated it but found that the gauges themselves placed an unwelcome additional physical strain on the aortic aneurysm.

---

[19] Grenda, Ed, http://home.att.net/~castleisland/ind_11.htm.

They turned to researchers at the University of Warwick led by Geoff Calvert who had an idea that would combine photoelastic stress analysis with the technology of rapid prototyping to solve the problem.

The University of Warwick and UCL researchers took a three-dimensional scan of the patient's actual aortic aneurysm and used rapid prototyping technology to produce an exact latex duplicate of the aneurysm. They then covered the duplicate with a reflective coating and used photoelastic stress analysis to examine the stress on the model aneurysm as the surgeon manipulated it.[20]

Programmable RP Molding

Saul Griffith, while a graduate student at MIT, developed a programmable "printer" for eyeglass lenses. This is a rapid prototype device that curves a membrane to form a mold cavity. The idea was to solve the problem of stocking an inventory of costly or inappropriate eyeglass lenses to serve the vision care needs of millions in the developing world who cannot afford standard prescription ground eyeglasses. A company, Low Cost Eyeglasses, has been formed to make this solution available to those who need it (www.lowcosteyeglasses.net).

Griffith's advances in low-cost lenses sprung from his interests in rapid prototyping technologies and efficient manufacturing. Using a process dubbed programmable molding, he created a portable device similar to a desktop printer that can produce any prescription lens from a single-mold surface in five to 10 minutes.

The device casts the lenses by applying pressure and constraints to a programmable membrane, which becomes the mold surface when under pressure. The current device uses car window tinting film for the membrane and a reservoir of baby oil for applying the correct pressure. A large range of lens types, covering the majority of prescriptions, can be cast from two such mold surfaces.[21]

---

[20] Coppinger, Rob, "Making Bones about It" and "From Spitfire to Surgery," *The Engineer*, August 4, 2004, http://www.e4engineering.com.
[21] Lemelson MIT Program press release, February 19, 2004.

Printed Food and Inkjet Proteins

Shimadzu Biotech, in conjunction with Proteome Systems, makes the Chemical Inkjet Printer (ChIP) to deliver precise picoliter volumes of reagents for microscale on membrane protein digestion. "The novel ChIP technology offers researchers a revolutionary new approach to automatic protein processing, identification, and characterization. Developed jointly by Shimadzu Biotech and Proteome Systems with financial support from the Australian Government's START Program, the ChIP is a unique technology platform for executing micro-scale on-membrane chemistry that will have widespread applications in biomedical research and biomarker discovery."[22]

Homaro Cantu is a chef at Moto restaurant in Chicago. He uses flavored inks printed onto edible paper.

> [His] maki look a lot like the sushi rolls served at other upscale restaurants: pristine, coin-size disks stuffed with lumps of fresh crab and rice and wrapped in shiny nori. They also taste like sushi. But the sushi often contains no fish. It is prepared on a Canon i560 inkjet printer rather than a cutting board. He prints images of maki on pieces of edible paper made of soybeans and cornstarch, using organic, food-based inks of his own concoction. He then flavors the back of the paper, which is ordinarily used to put images onto birthday cakes, with powdered soy and seaweed seasonings.[23]

This is yet another example of technology being redeployed in innovative ways for uses for which it was not originally designed.

Direct Manufacturing Freedom of Creation

Freedom of Creation (FOC) is based in Amsterdam, The Netherlands. This is a collaboration of two design school classmates who produce direct manufactured furniture and lighting using RP techniques. FOC also has been doing interesting work in the area of three-dimensional printed textiles, and is worth looking into for examples of innovative applications of RP (www.freedomofcreation.com). The work of the FOC team is available from Materialize, n.v. They sell a line of manufacture-on-demand

---

[22] Shimadzu Biotech and Proteome Systems Win R&D 100 Award for Novel Chemical Inkjet Printer (ChIP) Technology," http://www.shimadzu-biotech.net/pages/news/1/press_releases/2004_07_23_chip.php.

[23] Bernstein, David, "When the Sous-Chef Is an Inkjet," *New York Times*, February 3, 2005.

lamps and home furnishings using RP technology (http://www.materia-lise.com/made/MGXcollection2004.pdf).

Direct Manufacturing: The Center for Bits and Atoms

The Center for Bits and Atoms (CBA) is an initiative by the Massachusetts Institute of Technology (MIT) coordinated by Neil Gershenfeld and Bakhtiar Mikhak. The CBA seeks to explore innovative ways to deploy digital technology, including ubiquitous computing, digital programming of living systems, RP, and automated fabrication.[24] One interesting exploration is the use of personal fabrication, the use of digitally controlled rapid prototype technology to bring products and replacement parts to remote parts of the world without supply chain infrastructure. From the CBA mission statement:

> The Fab Lab program is part of the MIT's Center for Bits and Atoms (CBA), which broadly explores how the content of information relates to its physical representation.
>
> One of its grand-challenge research goals is to bring the programmability of the digital world to the physical world through the development of technologies to personalize fabrication rather than computation.[25]

The Fab Lab dream is to have technology that will allow a person to download a description of a product, send it to a general-purpose fabri-

---

[24] Perhaps the most dramatic example at CBA of programming nature comes from my colleagues Joe Jacobson, Shuguang Zhang, and Kim Hamad Schifferli, who showed how to take a protein and stick a 50-atom gold nanocluster onto it. For proteins, their shape is their function. If you use the little antenna to send radio energy into it you change the shape. That means that you can, for example, take a repressor protein that shuts off expression of a gene, and under a radio signal you can release it and let the gene be expressed, and then reattach it. The reason that is so important is that cells run programs to make things. When a cell fabricates, say, a flagellar motor, it's running a complex program, and more importantly it's error-correcting; it's doing logic. The antennas provide handles for programming those pathways. Cells are terrible as general-purpose computers, but they function based on this amazing ability to compute for fabrication....The real breakthrough may, in fact, be biological machinery that is programmable for fabrication. This may be the next manufacturing technology." Full text interview at the Edge Foundation website (the foundation's website has many such thought-provoking interviews and biographies and is worth visiting), http://www.edge.org/3rd_culture/gershenfeld03/gershenfeld_index.html.

[25] http://cba.mit.edu/projects/fablab/.

cation machine, and that machine will then produce a one-off example of the product, assembled, complete with functional parts and fabricated electronic circuitry.[26]

CONCLUSION

RP is a powerful way to accelerate product development when its capabilities and limitations are understood. While RP build materials can often mimic but not exactly duplicate the properties of the final production material, they can provide a close enough representation to enable a design and engineering decision, which is the purpose of a prototype, after all. It has been shown that RP is also an increasingly common aid in the planning and prepractice of complex surgeries.

RP technology can also be used in the direct manufacture of some parts where it is appropriate.

There are numerous technologies available, and it is the task of the design manager and innovator to evaluate these options and choose the technology or combination of technologies that best gets the job done.

Variations of RP and RE technologies are also being deployed and recombined in new and innovative ways such as for tissue engineering, and to accelerate product development and provide innovative new products and services to enhance human life.

RESOURCES

In-Print and Online Resources

Ed Grenda is president of the Castle Island Company and publishes a free online digest of RP technology. Of special interest is a page dedicated to the medical applications of rapid prototyping. This information is well researched, updated frequently, and free. Go to http://home.att.net/~castleisland/med_lks.htm#impl to visit the medical applications section.

For in-depth market and technical information on RP, Terry Wohlers publishes and sells his yearly **Wohler's Report** (http://www.wohlersassociates.com).

The book **Automated Fabrication** by Marshall Burns (Prentice Hall, Englewood Cliffs, NJ, 1993) gives some interesting history of RP and early innovative applications. The book is out of print, but it is readily available through Alibris.com.

Recently published is **Rapid Prototyping** by Andreas Gebhardt (Hanser-Gardener, Cincinnati, OH, 2003).

---

[26] Dunn, Katharine, "How to Make (Almost) Anything," *The Boston Globe*, January 30, 2005.

Also recently published is the ***User's Guide to Rapid Prototyping*** by Todd A. Grimm, available through the Society for Manufacturing Engineers (www.sme.org or www.tagrimm.com).

Prototype Magazine (England) is available for download in.pdf format at http://www.edaltd.co.uk/magdownloads/ and is part of the CADserver group of resources found at http://www.cadserver.co.uk/. *Prototype* is full of practical information and product specifications for RP.

Time Compression Technologies (U.S.) is an advertiser-supported publication covering the RP industry (www.timecompress.com).

The **Rapid Prototyping Mailing List (RPML)** is an ongoing conversation among 1500+ people. Edited and categorized archives can be found at the RPML site of Helsinki University of Technology (http://rapid.lpt.fi/.) The "Compleat RPML Archives" are the entire contents of all messages posted from September 11, 1995, to today. The list archives tens of thousands of pages of information, which can be used as a source of advice, case studies, contact information, expert individuals, and market data.

DesktopNC.com is a comprehensive resource of nearly every active (and inactive) manufacturer of small and desktop NC milling machines (http://www.desktopcnc.com/index.htm).

The **CAD/CAM Zone** (www.mmsonline.com) is an online discussion forum for working machinists. It is a good place to go to see discussions on CNC machinery and software from people who make their living in the manufacturing industry.

CADCAM Net is an online subscription-based service that tracks news and developments throughout the CADCAM and RP space (www.cadcam-net.com).

Fabbers.com (also see http://www.ennex.com/~fabbers/intro.asp) is a community of enthusiasts for direct manufacturing through RP technology. It is hosted by Marshall Burns (www.ennex.com).

The **Milwaukee School of Engineering** maintains a list of medical applications of RP (http://www.rpc.msoe.edu/medical.php).

The **Whole RP Family Tree** (http://ltk.hut.fi/~koukka/RP/rptree.html) is a compendium of RP that was, is, and is yet to be.

Professional Societies and Resources

Computer Aided Radiology and Surgery (CARS) Society: http://cars-int.de/index.htm
International Society for Computer Aided Surgery: http://igs.slu.edu/
Index of CARS Resources: http://homepage2.nifty.com/cas/casref.htm
International Society for Computer Assisted Orthopaedic Surgery (CAOS): http://www.caos-international.org/

Fabrication of Medical Models from Scan Data via Rapid Prototyping Techniques: K.L. Chelule, Dr. T. Coole, and D.G. Cheshire, School of Engineering and Advanced Technology, Staffordshire University, http://www.deskartes.com/news/fabrication_of_medical_models_fr.htm

Society of Manufacturing Engineers (SME): The SME organizes an annual event, the RAPID show, which is a tradeshow and symposium on all facets of the rapid prototyping and reverse engineering and modeling industry. It is a valuable event to attend if you have a special interest in this area (www.sme.org/rapid). This is the largest event of its kind in North America.

UNIVERSITIES AND ORGANIZATIONS

Many researchers refer to rapid prototyping by the name *solid freeform fabrication* and *functional freeform fabrication*. There are a number of projects underway in tissue engineering, bioceramics, advanced ceramic aerospace materials, direct manufacturing technologies and nanotechnology. This is a very quickly evolving field. Websites such as the DARPA (Defense Advanced Research Projects Agency) SFF site and the University of Texas, Austin SFF Laboratory are good places to look for links and breaking news. Here are a few of the universities and organizations working in this area:

The Annual SFF Conference. The 16th annual meeting was held in 2005 in Austin Texas, and hosted the leading researchers in this field.

Cornell University Functional Freeform Fabrication http://www.mae.cornell.edu/ccsl/research/sff/ and

The Golem Project (Genetically Organized Lifelike Electro Mechanics) http://www.mae.cornell.edu/ccsl/research/golem/index.html and http://helen.cs-i.brandeis.edu/golem/fabrication.html

The Bone Tissue and Engineering Center of the University of Pittsburgh (BTEC) http://www.btec.cmu.edu/research/engineering/sff/sff.htm and www.btec.cmu.edu

The Laboratory for Freeform Fabrication, University of Texas, Austin https://utwired.engr.utexas.edu/lff/about/index.cfm

The Laboratory for Freeform Fabrication and Advanced Ceramics, Rutgers University http://www.caip.rutgers.edu/sff/

University of Connecticut SFF Program http://www.ims.uconn.edu/~hmarcus/

DARPA Defense Science Office http://www.darpa.mil/dso/trans/sff.htm

Milwaukee School of Engineering http://www.msoe.edu/reu/ssf.shtml

University of Michigan SFF Laboratory

Stanford University
University of Dayton
MIT

ACKNOWLEDGMENTS

Thanks to Hendrik John (Envisiontec GmbH), Bathsheba Grossman, Joe Hiemenz (Stratasys), Jeroen Dille (Materialise n.v.), Bruce Lustig (Solidscape), Karen Kiffney (Z Corp.), Dr. Stefan Hehn (Sirona), Gary Sande (3D Systems), and Ed Grenda for their assistance and contributions to this chapter.

7

REVERSE ENGINEERING IN MEDICAL DEVICE DESIGN

Ted Kucklick

CONTENTS

The Value of Reverse Engineering in Patient Care 167
Reverse Engineering Methods 169
   Digitizing 169
      Case Example: Using a Low-Cost Scanner to Digitize
      a Vertebra 169
   Using a Flatbed Scanner for Three-Dimensional Reconstruction 173
   Cannibalizing an Existing Device 173
      Why Reinvent the Handle? 174
   Case Study: Building on an Existing Product for Higher
      Performance 174
      Case Example: Making Your Own Stent 176
Where to Find Used Medical Devices and Equipment 177
Three-Dimensional Reconstruction 179
   Common Three-Dimensional Capture File Formats and
      Terminology 180
Continuity 181
   Automated Touch Probe 183
   Light Beam Scanners 183
   Arm Probe Scanners 184
   Arm Probe Noncontact Scanners 185
   Three-Dimensional Image Reconstruction 185
Reverse Engineering and Inspection 186
Destructive Reverse Engineering 186
Reverse Modeling, Radiology, and Surgical Planning 186

Resources 187
　Used and Reconditioned Medical Equipment Vendors 187
　Bones and Bone Models 188
　Three-Dimensional Software 189
　Three-Dimensional Capture Equipment 190
　Three-Dimensional Service Bureaus 190
　MRI and CT Reconstruction and RP Modeling 190
　Three-Dimensional Scanning and Manufacturing Inspection 191
　Professional Societies and Resources 191
　　Society of Manufacturing Engineers (SME) 191
　　Three-Dimensional Information Websites 191
　　ACM Siggraph 191
　　Forensic Engineering 192

Reverse engineering (RE) is the process of taking something apart to see how it works and making a product that functions, in whole or part, like the original product, or as an intermediate step to an improvement on the original product. It is an attempt to recover as much of the "top level specification"[1] of a product as possible, and understand how and why a product works. Other related concepts to reverse engineering are reverse modeling and image reconstruction. In this chapter will be a discussion of the general subject of reverse engineering, case examples, and a list of resources.

　Reverse engineering to some is a negative word. It is, but only if it is being used to take the technology and intellectual property of others, claiming them as your own, and avoiding the work of making your own original contribution. Reverse engineering is a way to study what is already being done in order to make improvements, advancements, or new applications of existing technology. It is also a way to study existing products in order to develop compatible products or products that conform to standard clinical usage. Did you ever take things apart when you were growing up to see how they worked? (Most of the great inventors have.) Then you have engaged in reverse engineering. Reverse engineering, properly used, is an important tool, a textbook, for advancing the state of the art in clinical technology.

> Reverse engineering has long been held a legitimate form of discovery in both legislation and court opinions. The Supreme Court has confronted the issue of reverse engineering in mechanical technologies several times, upholding it under the

---

[1] Musker, David C., "Reverse Engineering," R.G.C. Jenkins Law Office, http://www.jenkins-ip.com/serv/serv_6.htm.

principles that it is an important method of the dissemination of ideas and that it encourages innovation in the marketplace. In *Kewanee Oil v. Bicron*, [the court called reverse engineering] "a fair and honest means of starting with the known product and working backwards to divine the process which aided in its development or manufacture."[2]

Companies that make scanning devices prefer the term *reverse modeling*, as they find the term *reverse engineering* to be negative, implying that their equipment enables the improper taking of the design work of others. Reverse modeling, or more properly digital geometry capture, is actually a subset activity of reverse engineering. It is a digital version of the "plaster splash" method of copying geometry, which was once common in the automotive aftermarket design business.

Reverse engineering serves an important function in the development of new medical device technology. Observing and studying accepted and proven technology is important when developing new products.

Reverse engineering for the purposes of learning and making your own original contribution is appropriate. However, plagiarizing, pirating, and purloining of product design and intellectual property is not. The German industrial designer Rido Busse developed the Plagiarius Award in 1977, in response to his designs being pirated by unscrupulous manufacturers.[3] The motto of Aktion-Plagiarius is "Innovation vs. Imitation." The German Industrial Designers Association now awards the prize, a black garden gnome with a gold nose, to the most egregious examples of design theft. "Winners" of this dubious distinction may be found at http://www.plagiarius.com/e_index.html. Reverse engineering properly done is an educational exercise that leads to innovation. You look at what is being done and find where it does and does not work, where it does not meet customer needs, and build upon this information to do better. We learn what is being done so that we can rise above the state of the art with our own original contribution.

The imitator dooms himself to hopeless mediocrity.

—**Ralph Waldo Emerson**[4]

---

[2] The website "Chilling Effects," a joint project of the Electronic Frontier Foundation and Harvard, Stanford, Berkeley, University of San Francisco, University of Maine, George Washington School of Law, and Santa Clara University School of Law clinics, has a detailed FAQ on the subject of reverse engineering: http://www.chillingeffects.org/reverse/faq.cgi#QID188.
[3] http://www.plagiarius.com/e_index.html.
[4] "Address to Divinity Students," *Harvard Classics*, Vol. 5, 1937, p. 39.

An even more serious abuse of reverse engineering is the production of counterfeit products with faked approval stamps. Such counterfeit products have shown up in aircraft parts and pharmaceuticals. Fake products can result in unfounded liability claims against the legitimate manufacturer, and damage to its branding and reputation. The industry needs to be vigilant against this dangerous criminal activity. This is not just pirating intellectual property; it is dangerous to public health and safety. MDDI Devicelink reports that "both finished goods and device parts have been successfully faked. For example, intra-aortic pumps worth $7 million were recalled after malfunctioning components were found to be counterfeit."[5] Recent news stories documented a medical device distributor prosecuted for selling fake hernia repair mesh, supposedly made by the Ethicon division of Johnson & Johnson.[6] Patients found to have received this fake product had to undergo revision surgery to remove the counterfeit product. Some of the larger medical device manufacturers have taken stringent measures to curb gray market trade in their products to prevent fakes from entering their distribution chain. The International Anti-Counterfeiting Coalition (www.iacc.org) and CSA International (www.csa-international.org) monitor activity in the trafficking of counterfeit products.

If you discover a technology by reverse engineering that is patented, you cannot use it anyway, unless it helps lead you to your own original invention, or you compensate the originator by way of an agreed-to license and royalty, or work around the patent. If it is a trade secret, and you are able to arrive at the know-how to make the product independently, you can use this information. If the information disclosed in the product is neither patented nor a trade secret, it is in the public domain and free for you to use, learn from, or build upon. Reverse engineering is also a way to discover what is already being done, and patent protected, so that you can avoid unintentional infringement. It is the responsibility of the designer and engineer to research prior art in the area they are working in. With the placement of the U.S. patent library online, this has become a much easier task than in the past. The searchable library of issued patents and published applications can be found at www.uspto.gov.

Another use of reverse engineering is the legitimate practice of studying a technology or method that is being applied in one area and redeploying and repurposing it for a different use. This is how many important clinical advances have occurred. One prolific inventor for one major medical device company often starts his invention process with a trip to the hardware store. It was his observation of how lead weights were clamped to a fishing line that inspired an idea for replacing intercorporeal suture

---

[5] http://www.devicelink.com/mddi/archive/03/01/021.html.
[6] Rick Dana Barlow, "Facts on Fakes," *Healthcare Purchasing News*, March 2004.

knots with a polymer bead clamped and melted to the suture. As many clinical innovations have probably come from the toy store and the tackle box as from the research lab. In another example, IDEO, an engineering and design consultancy based in Palo Alto, CA, keeps a library of interesting and clever mechanical devices from which its designers can study and draw inspiration.[7] Modifying and "hacking" existing technology have become popular pastimes. Two books on the subject of hardware hacking are *Hardware Hacking Projects for Geeks* by Scott Fullam (O'Reilly, Sebastopol, CA, 2003) and *Hardware Hacking: How to Have Fun While Voiding Your Warranty* by Joe Grand (Syngress, Rockland, MA, 2004).

There is also a term, *Macguyvering* (verb), for recombining and repurposing objects and technology at hand that has entered the popular slang lexicon.[8] Another term for this is *bricolage* (noun), an assemblage made or put together using whatever materials happen to be available. A *bricoleur* is one who invents his own tools and works with what is at hand. For example, the winning participants on the TV series *Junkyard Wars* are the bricoleurs most adept at macguyvering bricolage and show up the competition as mere bricklayers.

On the subject of reverse engineering, Pamela Samuelson writes the following:

> Reverse engineering is fundamentally directed to discovery and learning. Engineers learn the state of the art not just by reading printed publications, going to technical conferences, and working on projects for their firms, but also by reverse engineering others' products. Learning what has been done before often leads to new products and advances in know-how. Reverse engineering may be a slower and more expensive way for information to percolate through a technical community than patenting or publication, but it is nonetheless an effective source of information. Of necessity, reverse engineering is a form of dependent creation, but this does not taint it, for in truth, all innovators stand on the shoulders of both giants and midgets. Progress in science and the useful arts is advanced by dissemination of know-how, whether by publication, patenting or reverse engineering.[9]

---

[7] See Myerson, Jeremy, *IDEO: Masters of Innovation*, TeNeues, New York, 2001.

[8] *MacGyver* was a popular TV show in the 1980s about "the adventures of a secret agent armed with almost infinite scientific resourcefulness." *Macguyvering* is actually a word, which the author has even seen in a German technology lexicon.

[9] Samuelson, Pamela and Scotchmer, Suzanne, "The Law & Economics of Reverse Engineering," *Yale Law Journal*, April 2002, http://ist-socrates.berkeley.edu/~scotch/re.pdf.

Computer programs, software and firmware, as well as some circuitry are in a different category than physical parts when it comes to copying and reverse engineering. The software, electronics, and entertainment industries have erected a number of barriers against reverse engineering by use of copyright and licensing laws. Computer programs are copyrighted, and therefore copying any part of the program is prohibited. Also, computer programs are not sold to the end user; they are licensed. The end user does not take title to the program as property. As a condition of the license that is an agreement between the seller and buyer, the right to use the program is controlled by contract, and the licensee submits to a number of terms and restrictions, including an agreement not to reverse engineer or decompile the software. The Digital Millennium Copyright Act (DMCA) goes even farther by criminalizing the act of defeating anticopying locks and disseminating any copyrighted information thus obtained. To detect this, some software makers insert nonfunctional code and byte obfuscators into programs as markers to detect unauthorized copying. Software publishers have made it especially onerous for you to look under the hood and see how their software ticks.

Physical objects that are sold become the property of the purchaser. The owner is free to take apart his product to see how it works, unless the buyer and seller agree otherwise. Physical objects may be covered by copyrights and design patents. Boat hulls are subject to a special protection, from what is called the plug molding rule, or using a boat hull as a mold plug to make a duplicate of the hull.

Reverse engineering can involve taking an existing part, and without the original drawings or computer-aided design (CAD) model, producing a duplicate. This has an important application where drawings or a CAD model to your own part no longer exist, if they ever did. Three-dimensional scanning technologies and rapid prototyping (RP) have greatly simplified the process of reverse engineering these types of parts.

Reverse engineering tools also make possible the production of patient-matched and patient-specific prosthetics. With the availability of reverse engineering and rapid prototyping and manufacturing, this is more feasible all the time. In Chapter 6, a case study is given for the Sirona Dental GmbH Cerec® system, which uses digital tools to capture tooth information and build a final dental crown while the patient waits. The use of RP-produced anatomical models made from patient magnetic resonance imaging (MRI) and computer tomography (CT) scans to plan complex surgeries has become commonplace. Stanford University is taking this a step further, by building patient-specific computer analysis models that allow, for example, accurate modeling of blood flow in arteries, including fluid shear forces and vessel elasticity, which can help predict the results of vascular surgeries.[10]

Reverse engineering tools may also be used to verify the accuracy of your own manufactured parts. For example, a molded part is scanned in three dimensions, then overlaid with the three-dimensional CAD model to check for deviations between the manufactured part and the base CAD model data. A number of service bureaus offer this capability.[11]

THE VALUE OF REVERSE ENGINEERING IN PATIENT CARE

When designing surgical devices, product acceptance is sometimes based on how closely the device works like the devices the surgeon is familiar with already. Surgeons, especially ones that do a large volume of procedures, are very sensitive to anything that disrupts their workflow, even if it is a better-performing product. Many times surgeons will accept or reject a product based on how it feels in their hands. If the feel of your product is not what they have come to expect from a product of the type you are designing, they may reject the product.

In this process it is vitally important to actually observe what surgeons do, rather than rely only on what they tell you, or worse, relying only on descriptions in textbook literature. To rely only on textbook or verbal descriptions of a surgical procedure can lead to embarrassing and expensive design mistakes. Direct observation gives you a more complete and accurate picture of how a product is actually used, and why existing products work the way they do.

Physician preference is often based on their particular training. This will affect how surgical procedures evolve over time, and sometimes surgeons use procedures that seem counterintuitive to one who is not a practitioner. There is also not one way of doing things. Different surgeons that study under different mentors at different schools will do procedures in their own idiomatic way. There will be regional and national preferences. For example, electrosurgical pencils in the U.S. are sold with push buttons. Surgeons in Europe prefer hand pieces with rocker switches. This has to do with the differences in the way the instrument is held in the hand, and how the surgeon stands relative to the patient. Therefore, it is important to not just observe the handful of surgeons that are your close associates, but a larger sample outside of your immediate board of advisors.

---

[10] http://www-igl.stanford.edu/.
[11] http://www.laserdesign.com and http://www.scansite.com are two. Sculptors.org has information on art- and sculpture-based services.

If you are a medical device designer, it is your responsibility to learn and know as much as possible about the way your product is used, and the beneficial outcomes it is supposed to produce for the patient, as well as to be aware of any problems your device might cause. You need to talk to end users and have a deep understanding of their needs gained by direct observation. If you design surgical devices, this means observing surgeries. You also need to observe the patients your device will be used on. If you are a manager, this means sending your designers and engineers regularly into the OR. The smart managers know this and do this.

Managers, who keep their designers and engineers and product managers penned up in their cubicles, are doing a disservice to their workers, their company, the doctors and patients the company serves. The designers are not being given the tools they need to make knowledgeable contributions. (If you work for this kind of company, you may want to look for a better-managed place to work, with better training and growth opportunities.)

The practitioner and his support staff are motivated by patient care. This usually means providing the best care to the most patients at the most affordable cost. Look for ways that this has been achieved in existing products, and apply those lessons in your products.

Examining existing products, finding out how and why they developed, and carefully observing how they are used can help lead to innovative new products and procedures that will be accepted into the current surgical workflow.

Reverse engineering in medical device design can fall into the following categories:

- Digitizing a part in order to make a duplicate, if allowable
- Taking things apart to see how they work
- Using a mechanism from one product to use in a new way in another product prototype
- Competitive product analysis
- Prevention of unintentional infringement
- Detection of copying or infringement in a competitor's product
- Production of a replica or aftermarket part no longer supplied by a manufacturer
- Using an existing product as the basis of a new similar or compatible product
- Anatomical reconstruction for visualization
- Anatomical reconstruction to produce a fitted prosthesis
- Anatomical reconstruction to produce a replacement prosthesis

REVERSE ENGINEERING METHODS

Digitizing

Case Example: Using a Low-Cost Scanner to Digitize a Vertebra

The Roland MDX-20 is an inexpensive three-axis mill and three-dimensional scanner combination. While working on the design of an orthopedic implant, the reverse engineering capabilities of the MDX-20 made the design of a properly fitting implant possible.

One of the important features of an orthopedic implant is that it needs to fit closely to the bone where it is being placed in order for the bone to grow into the implant and anchor it in place. The product needs to fit closely to the lamina of the vertebral body for proper fixation. The lamina of the spine, however, is a complex surface for which it is difficult to make a model that fits to it properly.

Several attempts were made to look at spine vertebra models, measure landmarks with calipers, and build a model in CAD of an implant. Getting a rapid prototype implant to fit over the complex surfaces of the spine proved difficult and frustrating, resulting in several unsuccessful rapid prototype iterations.

When building an implant model from automotive styling clay onto a spine model, it became apparent that a digital "buck" or armature was needed to properly model the implant in CAD.

A spine model was obtained from Pacific Research Laboratories (Sawbones). This model was placed into the Roland MDX-20 and scanned. (See Figure 7.1.)

The MDX-20 has both a milling and scanning head. The cutting spindle head was removed, and the scanning sensor unit was mounted into the machine. The vertebra model was then mounted to the work area with adhesive clay. The surface of the model was scanned using the Roland's piezo needle touch probe scanning head. The MDX-20 is capable of scanning any firm object, such as metal, plastic, or clay. Parts that are made of rubber or do not have a firm surface cannot be scanned with the touch probe.

The Roland comes bundled with a simple-to-use program, Dr. Picza. (See Figure 7.2.) This program saves the scan data in a proprietary format (.PIX), which may then be exported as.DXF,.SAT, VRML, 3DMF, ACIS, or IGES.

In this example, the scan was exported as.IGES and opened in Rhino® (Robert McNeel Associates, Seattle, WA, www.Rhino3D.com). (See Figure 7.3.) Rhino was used to trim and clean up and cap the open side of the mesh. Rhino is a relatively inexpensive ($895), easy-to-use program for producing and editing high-quality meshes. Another strength of the program is its ability to act as a three-dimensional hub, which means it can open a

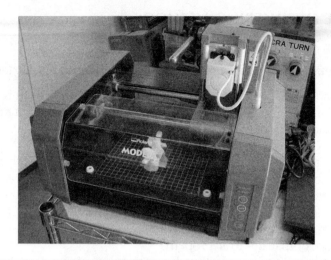

Figure 7.1 Setting up the spine model for scanning.

wide range of three-dimensional formats and export the edited mesh to yet another variety of formats. Rhino supports third-party plug-ins, including a plug-in to import Roland .PIX files directly into Rhino. This is useful for handling large, complex .PIX scan files from Roland DG scanners.

The inexpensive touch probe scanner shown here is useful for scanning one side of a surface at a time. You could scan two or more sides at a time and assemble the meshes in a three-dimensional editing program; however, this would be a lot of work. Roland makes a line of noncontact rotary laser scanners if you need to digitize a part "in the round." Another option for capturing geometry is digitizing probe arms from Faro and Immersion Corporation.

Producing a high-quality watertight mesh is important when importing into a CAD solid modeling program. This means that the mesh is free of gaps or discontinuities. This is important for the mesh to turn into a complete solid when imported, instead of a collection of fragmented surfaces. Using this method it may take a number of attempts to find the combination of file formats (.DXF,.IGES,.STEP,.SAT) that produces a solid model in your CAD program. (See Figure 7.4.)

This is a fairly simple demonstration of reverse modeling an anatomical specimen using inexpensive equipment and a mainstream engineering CAD program. This process of reverse modeling has been highly developed in the toy industry, where very complex models are sculpted, digitized, edited in a three-dimensional surfacing program, and output for prototyping and tooling.

Vendors can be an important resource for more sophisticated model production work. Programs such as Innovmetric's (Sainte-Foy, QC, Can-

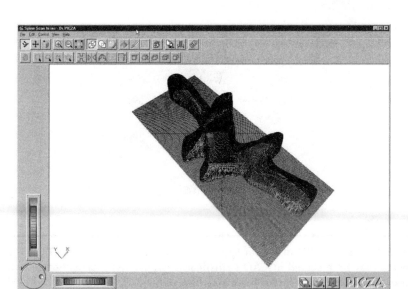

Figure 7.2 Scanned mesh in Dr. Picza capture program.

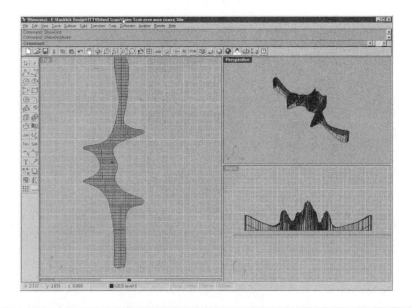

Figure 7.3 Editing three-dimensional mesh in Rhino.

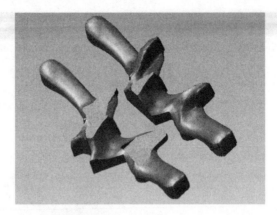

Figure 7.4 Solid CAD model of spine in SolidWorks. Features like the spinous process may be resected in CAD realistically. The lamina was sectioned with planes to extract curves for lofting a matching surface. (Example series T. Kucklick, Kucklick Design.)

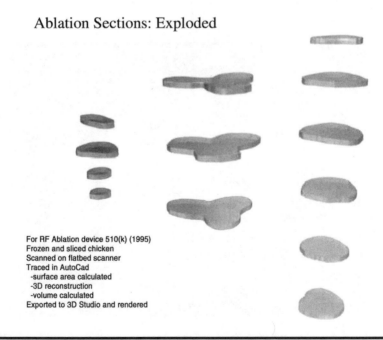

Figure 7.5 Three-dimensional tissue reconstruction using simple tools.

ada) PolyWorks™ offer sophisticated tools for handling and managing scanned point cloud data.

Using a Flatbed Scanner for Three-Dimensional Reconstruction

With so many tools at our disposal, we can combine them to quickly and easily solve problems. The tools may not be shrink-wrapped together into one package, but with a little imagination they can be used in innovative combinations.

I once had a need to determine the volume of tissue heated by a radio frequency (RF) ablation device I was working on. The purpose of the device was to produce RF ablations in solid organs to treat cancerous tumors. Since the ablations were being made with multiple electrodes and produced an irregular shape, calculating the volume of the ablations might have been a challenge.

To solve this problem, chicken breast was packed into a metal cup. The cup acted as the ground electrode. The ablation needle device was inserted into the solid mass of chicken meat, and the device delivered energy according to a time-and-temperature protocol.

The chicken was then frozen and sliced up to 3-mm sections with a commercial meat slicer. The slices were then put on letter-size overhead transparency plastic sheets. These were then placed on a flatbed scanner and, in order of the sections, scanned. The scans were saved as bitmap files and adjusted for brightness and contrast in Adobe Photoshop®. The scans were then imported into Corel Draw®, and the blanched, ablated area of the chicken was traced in the draw program. These outlines were exported as .DXF outlines and saved. These outlines were then imported into a CAD program (in this case Autocad®). The outlines were extruded into solid objects in the CAD program to a depth of 3 mm. Once the objects were generated in the CAD program, using the program's tools to calculate the volume of the ablation became a simple matter. To visualize the ablations, the sections were rendered in a three-dimensional program, 3D Studio®. (See Figure 7.5.) This allowed the use of the data for interpretation and presentations. This was done with a combination of simple-to-use and readily available tools.

Cannibalizing an Existing Device

One of the ways to develop new medical devices is to cannibalize a device that is already in use.

When working on a project for a client, I needed a robust flexible catheter with a steerable end for a proof-of-concept prototype. I could have built this from scratch; however, I would have had to locate materials, get them in-house, and build up this assembly. The cost in billable hours to build from scratch would be higher than locating and buying a used device and cannibalizing the part I needed. I suspected that what I wanted was readily available off the shelf, in some form. At first I tried to find replacement parts for small endoscopes, and found that these were limited in availability and quite expensive. I called one of my used equipment sources and found it had a pediatric bronchoscope from a German manufacturer with broken optics that was the right diameter and length for the device I wanted to prototype. The cost of this unit was about $600, which might sound like a lot, but a similar scope in good working order sells for over $2000. It was also less expensive than building the flexible component myself and charging the client for my time.

Getting the bronchoscope apart proved to be a little bit of a challenge. This unit was constructed to be watertight and quite resistant to disassembly. I had to resort to using a milling machine to carefully cut open the housing. Once I had the case open, I separated the flexible end of the bronchoscope from its case. Being able to cut open a piece of equipment like this was an education in itself, seeing how the device was constructed, how the fiber-optic bundles were laid out, how the steering actuation worked, and how it was engineered for reliability.

Once I had the flexible end of the device separated, I was able to concentrate on the more important part of the project, which was the connection mechanism between the flexible catheter and the actuation handle of the device that I was designing. This approach saved me time, gave me a reliable, high-quality steerable catheter quickly, got the device to proof-of-concept quickly, and saved the client money.

Why Reinvent the Handle?

Just cut off the part you do not want. When developing products there are a number of common handles and actuators that may be readily adapted to a device you are working on.

One example of a common actuator is the handle of a disposable wire grasper. The three loops of the actuator are for the thumb and middle and index fingers, and produce a pushing and retracting action. I have used this actuator for a number of projects. They are simple and inexpensive and are a convenient way to quickly and inexpensively build up a number of devices that require this type of actuator.

Case Study: Building on an Existing Product for Higher Performance

When making an incremental improvement to a product, there is often a part that is not proprietary, that had been in clinical use for decades.

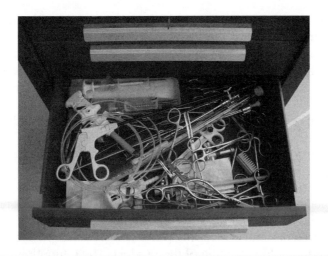

Figure 7.6 Assortment of medical devices for R&D.

Many times, surgical devices were originally borrowed from one type of surgical procedure and pressed into service in another specialty, thus becoming embedded into surgical practice by use and convention. This offers opportunity for improvement and innovation. A new feature can be added to this system that is higher performance, less invasive or less traumatic to the patient, and uses an existing instrument, familiar to the surgeon as a platform for a new technology. An example of this is the ClearVu™ flexible arthroscopic cannula. (See Figure 7.7.)

The ClearVu device was designed to overcome the problems with rigid inflow–outflow cannulae commonly used in three-portal knee arthroscopy. Rigid metal cannulae were borrowed from the Veress needle, originally used in general surgery. Bob Bruce, an orthopedic physicians assistant in San Jose, CA, saw a need for a better cannula while observing the shortcomings of the rigid metal cannula in surgical practice. In arthroscopy, the joint space is distended with water, and the viewing scope and instruments are inserted into the joint through small incisions, or portals. Surgical efficiency depends on the surgeon having a constant flow of clear water through the joint, or the surgical field quickly becomes murky and obscured with blood and surgical debris.

The knee also needs to be bent during surgery, and the metal cannula does not bend. This caused the distal end of the cannula to become clogged with soft tissue and the inflexible cannula shaft to make dents in the sensitive articular cartilage of the inside joint surfaces of the knee. The main disadvantage to the surgeon was that when the rigid cannula dug into soft tissue at the distal end, the flow of fluid through the knee stopped and the surgical field quickly became murky and obscured by blood, and the sharp end of the cannula often skived and damaged articular cartilage.

In the process of designing the flexible section of the cannula, Bob discovered a number of innovative solutions to keep the cannula from collapsing and kinking during a procedure. Being a former U.S. Army Special Forces medic and an avid outdoorsman, he noticed that fishing rods were tapered to keep them from breaking when flexed. Bob adapted this observation to develop a patented progressively flexible tapered cannula, purpose built and optimized for consistent fluid flow during arthroscopic procedures.

Bob, being sensitive to surgeons' resistance to the unfamiliar, used an existing metal cannula, cut off the front of the cannula, and replaced it with a flexible plastic cannula shaft of his improved design and the familiar stopcock proximal end. Once this prototype was accepted by surgeons, he produced a molded version of the product. The Cannuflow® ClearVu™ is now being marketed worldwide and is a less traumatic, high-performance replacement for metal cannulae in three-portal arthroscopy. From the patient's point of view, there is less trauma and pain during and after surgery, and the arthroscopic surgeon can see what he is doing, without the surgical field being clouded with blood and debris.

Case Example: Making Your Own Stent

There are times when using an off-the-shelf item may not be the best way to go, and making a home-brewed version is the better solution.

On a cardiac device project I worked on, a stent-like device was needed. The only way we knew of to get stents was to buy a stent-and-delivery catheter at retail. This gave us a stent that was not quite what we wanted and was very expensive (about $2000 each at that time). To save money, we took these precious devices and (carefully) cut them in half. Now they were only $1000 each. There had to be a better and more cost-effective solution.

The stent we needed did not have to be anything special. We were pushing it into a lumen in an open procedure in bench and preclinical tests; they did not need the flexibility and trackability of a commercially available stent.

We searched and found some companies that make stents and stent prototypes. We contacted one of these companies and found out the process of making a stent is really not that exotic. Stents are made by laser-cutting tubing, and there are vendors that specialize in this work. It was a relatively simple matter of deciding what open diameter we wanted and finding a thin-wall hypodermic tube of that diameter, which was an off-the-shelf item at a hypotube supplier. The vendor had a pattern for a

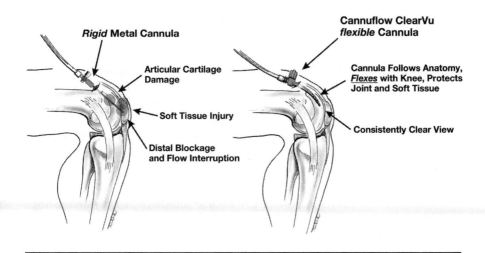

Figure 7.7 Example of using an existing product (a rigid metal cannula) as a platform for an improved version. (Illustration by T. Kucklick. Courtesy of Cannuflow, Inc.)

generic stent and cut a number of stents for us for a nominal lot charge. These stents were then collapsed down to their deployment size and used successfully in preclinical studies. The total cost per home-brewed stent was about $40 each.

WHERE TO FIND USED MEDICAL DEVICES AND EQUIPMENT

A lot of commonly used medical equipment is available for sale if you know where to find it. Buying used or refurbished equipment can be a cost-effective way to get equipment to work with. This equipment comes on the market by way of liquidation auctions and sale of equipment from facilities that are upgrading their hardware.

Purchasing directly from a manufacturer is sometimes difficult, especially if you do not have a doctor or medical facility purchasing for you. The other issue with buying from manufacturers is their understandable reluctance to sell their equipment into the industry or to a potential competitor. Some equipment companies tightly control their distribution, will not send you a catalog, or even let you browse their online catalog without you having to fill out a qualifying lead form.

If you have to have a particular piece of equipment that is not available on the used equipment market, it helps to have connections with a doctor or facility within that specialty to get it for you. Companies regularly purchase competitor's equipment through friendly surrogates.

Most used equipment dealers are good sources of capital and durable equipment such as RF generators, endoscopy units, arthroscopy units, and common surgical hardware like forceps and retractors. However, surgical disposables such as catheters, laparoscopic staplers, introducers, and so on, can be harder to find. The reason for this is that these items are packaged sterile and have a finite shelf life. Once the packaging expires, the device has little resale value to the reseller. This can be an advantage when looking for devices for parts. You may be able to buy expired disposables for a reasonable cost since you want to dissect them anyway. The disadvantage is that you are limited to whatever stock is on hand, when and if they have it.

The way resellers sometimes get their equipment is by purchasing a liquidation lot from a hospital that is closing or upgrading equipment. The reseller will buy a palette load or container load at auction, and some of these disposables can be part of the lot. Ask your reseller if it ever gets disposables like this bundled in a liquidation lot. Since the reseller may have a limited market for these, you may be able to get a good deal on them. An advantage to going through a reseller is that most devices are resold without many regulatory controls. You also do not need to deal with the sales and marketing departments of the manufacturer, who will want to know all about who you are before selling to you.

If you need a specific piece of equipment, especially a newer item, be prepared to use your network to get it and pay list price for it.

Another way to get equipment is from a doctor who has excess equipment or is upgrading. This is why it helps to have a physician on your board of advisors who is practicing in the specialty in which you are designing equipment. At least one member of your advisory board should be adept at getting for you whatever devices you need to study to do your product development.

Another way to get some types of new and used equipment is to see if the same or similar product is available for the veterinary market. Using these channels, you may find a device at lower cost, and with fewer restrictions when purchasing. For example, some manufacturers of endoscopes sell the same devices to the vet market as they do to hospitals.

Caution: When you purchase used equipment, purchase from an auction or from a practitioner; you do not know where the equipment has been. *Any device that has been used in contact with bodily fluids or mucous membranes is suspect and must be considered contaminated.* Most resellers are very good about providing clean and sanitary equipment, but some are not. I have seen both. If you have access to a sterilizer (steam, autoclave, Steris, etc.) and the device can be sterilized this way, *wear protective gloves, disassemble, clean, and sterilize used devices before using or handling them. Do not assume they are clean and sterile unless* the vendor has certified them as sanitary or sterile or you can verify that they have been cleaned and sterilized.

Another way to sanitize devices is to cold soak the device in Cidex® brand glutaraldehyde sterilant. Nooks, crannies, and valves in devices are places for organic gunk to hide. Endoscopes are especially prone to getting contaminated with biofilm and crud. Wear gloves, disassemble used equipment (as much as possible), always clean and sterilize before handling or using, and scrub yourself after handling by using the surgical scrub procedure. An exception to this is devices that are still in their factory packaging, where the packaging is intact and unopened.

Devices should also be carefully cleaned and sanitized or sterilized after bench tests with tissue or preclinical animal studies. To avoid the possibility of serious illness, always use careful sterile and sanitary techniques when working with medical devices. Remember, if you can smell it, it is alive (with germs) and needs to be decontaminated. If you can see blood, assume that it is contaminated with bloodborne pathogens (e.g., AIDS or hepatitis) and take appropriate precautions.

THREE-DIMENSIONAL RECONSTRUCTION

Some of the subject of three-dimensional reconstruction has been covered in Chapter 6. The process of three-dimensional reconstruction involves taking data from one three-dimensional object and bringing that information into a three-dimensional computer program, where the data may be used or manipulated and a three-dimensional object produced, based on the captured three-dimensional data set. This sounds simple in concept; however, as with most things, the challenge is in the details. One important thing to remember is that all of these data-capture methods yield some type of point cloud. This means a group of data points that are then interpolated by software to form a plane or surface. Once the surfaces are built, these can be closed to form a CAD solid. Once the points are captured and surfaces or solids are generated, they become "dumb" objects, as they were not built parametrically.

The other general concept to keep in mind is scan resolution. The higher the scan rate and the tighter the mesh, or number of triangles (polygons), the larger the file size. There is a trade-off between capturing enough data to produce a usable model and capturing too much and ending up with a large and cumbersome file size.

In each capture method, there is an art to getting a clean and usable data set. Sometimes it is simpler to just have a CAD draftsman use a set of calipers, take some measurements, and build a parametric solid model, instead of using automated data capture tools, especially if the desired end result is a feature-based CAD model.

Common Three-Dimensional Capture File Formats and Terminology

The majority of rapid prototype information is communicated in the .STL (stereolithography) format. Some of the other more common neutral file formats available are:

- **PLY** format, or the Stanford triangle format. This is a simplified vertex and face description of a three-dimensional object. It is a simplified file format for the communication of three-dimensional surface models, usually acquired from three-dimensional scanners.
- **VRML** (virtual reality modeling format). Based on Silicon Graphics (Mountain View, CA) Open Inventor file format for use in Internet applications. Inventor is yet another file format that is a superset of the VRML networked graphics data format. VRML is useful with communication texture and color data along with three-dimensional object information. Other three-dimensional formats, such as STL and PLY, do not support this type of color and scene data.
- **IGES** (Initial Graphics Exchange Specification). An American national standard that is a neutral data format for the digital exchange of information among computer-aided design (CAD) systems and other applications. The standard is developed and maintained by the IGES/PDES Organization. IGES supports the representation of surfaces with smooth higher-order splines or nonlinear uniform rational B-splines (NURBS).
- **DXF** (drawing interchange file). A file format developed by Autodesk, Inc. (Sausilito, CA) as a neutral file format for the communication of two- and three-dimensional vector information. DXF represents three-dimensional objects as polyface meshes, and not smooth surfaces or NURBS.
- **STEP** (Standard for the Exchange of Product Mode Data). An ISO standard neutral file format for the communication of engineering solid model data generated from CAD programs.

The basic difference between formats is this: DXF, STL, and PLY produce a polygon or *polyface mesh*. This means that a surface is made up of flat triangles that approximate the surface. A polygon mesh is a mathematically simpler way to describe a surface. DXF is a popular three-dimensional animation format, because a model is built using the smallest number of triangles to keep the three-dimensional file size small, and then the model is smoothed out visually when it is rendered in the animation software's shader. This works very well for animations that need to operate with limited hardware resources, like video game controllers. The results look smooth, but the underlying model may be roughly tessellated (faceted). Most three-dimensional programs can generate a .DXF file. NURBS produce a smooth surface and are more mathematically complex than a DXF polygon mesh. Higher-end surfacing programs can produce NURBS, e.g., Rhino and Alias®. *Parametric models* are feature-based solid models where the model is described by geometric features (extrusions, revolved profiles, fillets, etc.), and each of these features may be edited according to precise values. Parametric models are generated by engineering CAD programs, e.g., Pro/Engineer, SolidWorks, and AutoCAD.[12]

Digital Imaging and Communications in Medicine (DICOM) is not really a single-file format, but a way to organize radiology scan information under a common format. It contains information such as the CT or MRI image scans, their order, and slice thickness. A DICOM file is needed to then process through a software product like Materialise (Leuven, Belgium), Mimics®, and SimPlant® to produce an .STL file for the generation of a final three-dimensional physical model using rapid prototyping equipment.

CONTINUITY

The mathematical smoothness of a surface is described by its continuity. (See Figure 7.8.) C0 continuity is where two lines or surfaces meet, but are not curved or tangent. This is continuity by position only. C1 continuity is where a line or surface join and are curved, but not tangent (smooth). C2 continuity is where lines or surfaces meet and are both curved and smoothly tangent. Continuity becomes important when patching and cleaning up a captured mesh. Often, a captured mesh will have gaps where it lacks continuity and needs to be patched in a three-dimensional surfacing program. Sometimes the mesh will have kinks where there is a C0 or C1 continuity and a C2 smoothness is desired. This can be accomplished in a three-dimensional surfacing program; however, the time and expense in cleanup of the mesh should be allowed for in the project schedule and budget. Curve analysis tools in surfacing and CAD programs can help reveal creases and lack of desired continuity.

One difficulty in producing a rapid prototype model from captured point cloud data is ensuring a watertight mesh. This means that the surfaces may not have any gaps or lack of continuity. These gaps will result is an .STL file with holes and an unbuildable part. Sometimes mesh editing is required to patch up a model before it can be built successfully.

---

[12] For more information, see Griffin, Alair et al., Reverse Engineering: Practical Considerations for Rapid Prototyping, paper presented at AutoFact97, http://www.javelin3d.com/pdf/awards/ReverseEng.pdf.

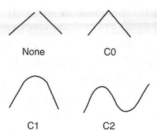

Figure 7.8 Types of continuity.

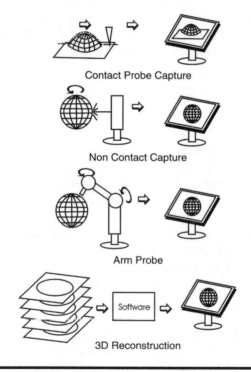

Figure 7.9 Methods of three-dimensional capture.

The four basic ways to achieve three-dimensional reconstruction are:

- Automated touch probe scanning
- Light beam scanning
- Arm probe capture
- Data set reconstruction

Automated Touch Probe

Automated touch probe scanners are a simple and convenient way to capture three-dimensional information. Inexpensive three-dimensional scanners like the MDX-20 described earlier in this chapter are available from Roland Corporation (Irvine, CA) and are bundled with capture software. Automated touch probe scanners of this type are limited to scanning one surface of an object at a time. (See Figure 7.9.)

Light Beam Scanners

Light beam scanners are noncontact probes that capture point cloud data. One type of scanner operates with a stationary beam, and the object is rotated to capture the point cloud. In the other, the object is stationary and the scanner moves to capture the image. One of the considerations in optical three-dimensional scanning is that the scanner requires a surface of uniform color and reflectivity to produce a clean scan. This may require that reflective parts be coated with powder. This can be a limitation, depending on the object to be scanned. If the object is, for example, a rare bone specimen or archeological object, the curator may object to having the object coated with nonreflective media. Also, for surfaces that require high-precision scanning (e.g., polished engine cylinder head surfaces), spray-on powders may actually produce a false picture of the geometry.[13]

Noncontact light beam scanners range from simpler models like the Roland LPX-250 to highly sophisticated (and expensive) models from Konica Minolta, Cyberware, and 3dMD. Noncontact light beam scanners work in similar ways, by projecting a beam of light to a surface and capturing Z-axis height information with very accurate range finding, and then building this information with software into a surface that accurately represents the scanned object.

Medical applications of three-dimensional scanning include a medically oriented hardware and software combination from 3dMD (www.3dmd.com) and a digital ear impression product for fitting hearing aids by Cyberware (Monterey, CA, www.cyberware.com). Cyberware is a pioneer in the high-end noncontact scanning industry, and its website provides numerous application examples. Cyberware noncontact scanners are an essential tool in movie digital special effects production. Other uses for noncontact digital scanning are in prosthetics, where a digital model is made of a residual limb for fitting, whole-body scanning for the

---

[13] See Shih, Albert, Three Dimensional Precision Optical Measurements, presentation to SME, May 9, 2005 (University of Michigan Engineering Research Center for Reconfigurable Manufacturing Systems).

video game industry, anthropometric studies, and the apparel industry. Polhemus (Colchester, VT, www.polhemus.com) specializes in digital motion capture and is an important technology in human factors gait analysis and realistic animation of video game characters. Polhemus also makes a device, the VisionTrak, for analysis of eye movements. This is used in human factors studies of vision, as well as in the advertising industry, where eye movements are tracked to study the effectiveness of advertisements and whether the viewer is reading the ad or just looking at the pictures.

An application for digitizing and reverse engineering is the production of burn masks. These are custom-fitted dressings that prevent the formation of disfiguring facial scars on burn victims. Total Contact Incorporated (Germantown, OH, http://www.totalcontact.com) specializes in the production of these masks.[14]

Arm Probe Scanners

Contact probe scanners are available from Faro (Lake Mary, FL, www.faro.com), Immersion (Microscribe) (San Jose, CA, www.microscribe.com), and Romer/CimCore (Farmington Hills, MI, www.cimcore.com).

Arm probe scanners are a way to digitize objects with a higher degree of user control than automated scanning methods. Arm probe scanners are popular in manufacturing environments such as automotive and aerospace. Arm probe scanners can plug directly into three-dimensional surfacing programs such as Rhino, where a user can trace an object and see the surfaces built in the computer. Arm probe scanners are also important as inspection equipment.

Arm probe scanners have found applications in medicine. Orthopedic surgeons often need accurate spatial information to place implants. Several three-dimensional systems have been developed and marketed to help the surgeon place joint prostheses (e.g., the BrainLab System, Munich, Germany). Some of these systems use noncontact three-dimensional positioning methods. Microscribe arms have been combined with Phillips CT scanners to provide more accurate biopsy needle track placement in a stereotactic application.[15]

---

[14] For more information on the use of fitted masks to prevent hypertrophic scarring, see Computerized manufacturing of transparent face masks for the treatment of facial scarring, *J. Burn Care Rehabil.*, 24, 91–96, 2003, and Integration of laser surface digitizing with CAD/CAM techniques for developing facial prostheses. Part 1. Design and fabrication of prosthesis replicas, *Int. J. Prosthodont.*, 16, 435–441, 2003. Several other articles on the subject are available from PubMed, http://www.ncbi.nlm.nih.gov.

[15] http://www.immersion.com/digitizer/case_study_gallery/Phillips_Case_Study_final.pdf.

Arm Probe Noncontact Scanners

These devices are a hybrid of a coordinate measuring machine (CMM) arm or articulated arm and a noncontact laser scanner head. One of the advantages of this type of device is that the arm probe orients the data capture scanning head in space and helps to organize the point cloud data, especially when in comes to knitting together captured surface patches. Scanners mounted on an articulating arm allow the user to "paint" the surface with the scanner and watch the surface develop on a computer screen. These devices are made by companies such as Metris, Perceptron, Laser Design, and Kreon.

Three-Dimensional Image Reconstruction

Another method of producing a three-dimensional data set is by taking a serialized two-dimensional data set, e.g., CT scans, and building this into a three-dimensional data set. Several companies offer this service, and can also provide a rapid prototype model for surgical planning and training. Using reverse engineering tools is also an important way to produce organ phantoms (training models) for surgical training.

One of the more ambitious three-dimensional image reconstruction projects is the Visible Human Project® of the National Library of Medicine. In 1993 researchers at Colorado State University took the cadaver of a Texas death row inmate, froze it, and sliced it into 1-mm sections. Each section was digitally photographed, and the resulting images were processed into a highly detailed three-dimensional database. Several more donated cadavers have since been processed and added to the database.[16]

Image reconstruction software to turn two-dimensional CT and MRI scans into three-dimensional data sets is available from Materialize, n.v. (Leuven, Belgium). Materialize sells its Mimics software to generate .STL files from CT scans. Materialize also offers a suite of applications for surgical planning and for editing and manipulating files in .STL format. These include Simplant, SAFE®, and SurgiGuide® products. Materialize also publishes numerous case surgical studies on its website (www.materialise.com).

Javelin3D (Salt Lake City, UT, www.javelin3D.com) offers its Velocity® software for MRI and CT scan three-dimensional reconstruction.

---

[16] For more information, see McCracken, Thomas, *New Atlas of Human Anatomy*, Metro Books, 1999, and http://www.nlm.nih.gov/research/visible/visible_gallery.html.

REVERSE ENGINEERING AND INSPECTION

One important use of reverse engineering/reverse modeling and data capture is in part validation and inspection. Traditionally, inspections are performed with gauges or coordinate measuring machines (CMMs). The limitation of these methods is the relatively small number of data points that may be inspected. Also, these types of inspections measure discrete points or line traces. Reverse modeling is a powerful method of part inspection. In this method, a finished part is scanned with high-accuracy three-dimensional digital capture tools, and then the scanned model is overlaid on the CAD file, which is theoretically accurate. The use of fiducial markers helps to align and register the scanned data set to the CAD data set. Inspection analysis software such as PolyWorks (www.innovmetric.com) is used to analyze the deviations between the CAD model and the manufactured part. The power of this method is the ability to apply geometric tolerancing analysis tools in software, as well as the ability to color map dimensional variances. This gives the ability to visualize not only discrete inspection points, but, for example, the flatness of a surface, with its high and low areas revealed.

DESTRUCTIVE REVERSE ENGINEERING

CGI Corporation (Capture Geometry Internally) makes a system for progressively milling and scanning an object, referred to as cross-sectional scanning. The part is obviously sacrificed in the process. However, this is one way to obtain the internal geometry of a part or product assembly (http://www.reverse-eng.com).

REVERSE MODELING, RADIOLOGY, AND SURGICAL PLANNING

Interesting work in the area of three-dimensional reconstruction and surgical planning is being done at Stanford University (Stanford, CA), where vascular procedures are preplanned for improved outcomes with the Advanced Surgical Planning Interactive Research Environment (ASPIRE) system. For example, a vascular graft procedure is planned by scanning the patient's anatomy and building a dynamic flow model that represents both the pulsatile flow of blood and the elasticity of the vessel wall. This allows the modeling of a vascular system and the ability to test different grafting approaches. This also allows the ability to choose the procedure that will produce the best flow with the least turbulence in the blood flow, to prevent thrombosis and improve outcomes.[17]

---

[17] http://www.acfnewsource.org/science/virtual_surgery.html.

On the electronics side of reverse engineering, there is a company near Colorado Springs, CO, Taeus International, founded by Arthur Nutter. Taeus is short for Tear Apart Everything under the Sun. Taeus is expert at dissecting electronics and microchips, looking for evidence of purloined technology in high-stakes patent litigation cases for clients such as Intel, HP, and Texas Instruments.[18]

Reverse engineering and modeling is an essential component in the toolbox of the medical device designer. Used properly, it helps to accelerate innovation, conserve capital, and produce devices that are compatible with standard surgical use and convention. It is an essential tool for competitive analysis. It is a way to learn accepted and successful design and assembly techniques. It helps to cross-pollinate technology from one field into a new area of application. It can be the seed and inspiration for your own original contribution.

Reverse engineering and modeling tools are becoming more powerful and less expensive all the time. Check with industry publications, informational websites, and industry conferences to keep up-to-date with the latest developments.

RESOURCES

Used and Reconditioned Medical Equipment Vendors

Whittemore Enterprises, Inc.
1114 Arrow Route
Rancho Cucamonga, CA 91730
Phone: 800-999-2452, 909-980-2452
Fax: 909-989-9976
E-mail: sales@wemed1.com
www.wemed1.com
Whittemore has a fully stocked showroom with a huge variety of surgical hardware and equipment. It is worth a visit just to browse for an afternoon.

United Endoscopy
10405 San Sevaine Way, Suite B

---

[18] Based on his experience in the patent litigation area, Mr. Nutter has an interesting rule of thumb on patent claims: "Most large technology companies sit on thousands of patents, but only a few claims are solid enough to hold up in court. Nutter can tell the good ones by using what he calls the "three-fingers" rule. 'If you cover up a claim with just three fingers, it's probably a pretty good claim,' he says. 'Claims that go on paragraph after paragraph are too vague and almost impossible to make stick.'" From Kellner, Tomas, "Silicon Strip Search," *Forbes Magazine*, March 28, 2005.

Mira Loma, CA 91752-1150
Phone: 951-360-0077, 800-899-4847
Fax: 951-360-0066
Good prices on used endoscopy equipment. Sometimes have in stock some disposables, e.g., laparoscopic staplers, etc.

Paragon Medical
P.O. Box 770187
Coral Springs, FL 33077
Phone: 800-780-5266, 954-345-3990
Fax: 954-340-2457

Arthroscopy and Medical Equipment International
7440 SW 50th Terrace #108
Miami, FL 33155
Phone: 305-662-2855
Fax: 305-662-1170
www.artroscopia.net
Source for new and used arthroscopes and orthopedic RF generators.

Medical Resources
550 Schrock Rd.
Columbus, OH 43229
Phone: 800-860-4716
Fax: 614-433-7387
Very broad range of supplies, good for some hard-to-find items.

Medical equipment is also available on eBay, though the selection for a particular use may be limited.

Bones and Bone Models

Pacific Research Laboratories (Sawbones)
10221 SW 188th St.
P.O. Box 409
Vashon, WA 98070
Phone: 206-463-5551
Fax: 206-463-2526
www.sawbones.com

The Bone Room
1569 Solano Ave.
Berkeley, CA 94707

Phone: 510-526-5252
http://www.boneroom.com
Natural bones and skeleton specimens of all kinds, animal and human.

Aptic Superbones
Phone: 866-265-BONE (2663)
www.discountbones.com
Synthetic bone models mimicking cortical and cancellous bone structure.

Three-Dimensional Software

Robert McNeel & Associates
3670 Woodland Park Ave. North
Seattle, WA 98103
Phone: 206-545-7000
Rhino 3D

Alias
www.alias.com
Makers of Alias and Maya® high-end surfacing and animation programs.

Materialise
Technologielaan 15
3001 Leuven, Belgium
Phone: +32 16 39 66 11
Fax: +32 16 39 66 00
www.materialise.com
Mimics®, Simplant® SAFE®, and SurgiGuide® software

3dMD
www.3dMD.com

VG Studio Max
Volume Graphics GmbH
Weiblinger Weg 92a
69123 Heidelberg
Germany

Vital Images, Inc.
5850 Opus Parkway
Suite 300
Minnetonka, MN 55343-4414

Phone: 952-487-9500
www.vitalimages.com

Three-Dimensional Capture Equipment

Faro
125 Technology Park
Lake Mary, FL 32746
Phone: 800-736-0234, 407-333-9911
www.faro.com

Cyberware, Inc.
2110 Del Monte Ave.
Monterey, CA 93940
Phone: 831-657-1450
www.Cyberware.com

Immersion Corporation
801 Fox Lane
San Jose, CA 95131
Phone: 408-467-1900
Fax: 408-467-1901
www.microscribe.com

Roland DGA
15363 Barranca Pkwy.
Irvine, CA 92618-2216
http://www.rolanddga.com

Three-Dimensional Service Bureaus

Javelin 3D
www.javelin3D.com

MRI and CT Reconstruction and RP Modeling

Protomed
www.protomed.com

Biomedical Modeling, Inc.
www.biomodel.com

Three-Dimensional Scanning and Manufacturing Inspection

CavLab
www.cavlab.com
One of the largest service bureaus offering three-dimensional modeling and inspection.

Professional Societies and Resources

Society of Manufacturing Engineers (SME)

The SME organizes an annual event, the RAPID show, which is a trade show and symposium on all facets of the rapid prototyping and reverse engineering and modeling industry. It is a valuable event to attend if you have a special interest in this area (www.sme.org/rapid). This is the largest event of its kind in North America.

Three-Dimensional Information Websites

> Computer Aided Radiology and Surgery (CARS) Society: http://cars-int.de/index.htm
> International Society for Computer Aided Surgery: http://igs.slu.edu/
> Index of CARS Resources: http://homepage2.nifty.com/cas/casref.htm
> International Society for Computer Assisted Orthopaedic Surgery (CAOS): http://www.caos-international.org/
> 3DLinks.com: A very useful compendium of information on three-dimensional capture devices and three-dimensional products.
> Ed Grenda's Castle Island site: http://home.att.net/~castleisland/scn_08.htmhttp://home.att.net/~castleisland/scn_08.htm. This site has a great comparison chart of three-dimensional scanning technologies and vendors. It is a good idea to check this site for the latest developments, as this is a technology that is changing and improving very quickly.

ACM Siggraph

ACM Siggraph (www.siggraph.org) is the computer graphics special interest group of the Association for Computing Machinery (ACM). Siggraph puts on an annual conference and trade show that is one of the more important events for anyone working in the computer graphics and three-dimensional modeling field. Any piece of equipment or vendor you can think of exhibits at this huge event (the 2004 attendance was 27,000+).

Forensic Engineering

Brown, Sam, *Forensic Engineering: An Introduction to the Investigation, Analysis, Reconstruction, Causality, Risk, Consequence, and Legal Aspects of the Failure of Engineered Products*, ISI Publications, Humble, TX, 1993.

8

USING MEDICAL ILLUSTRATION IN MEDICAL DEVICE R&D

Ted Kucklick

CONTENTS

The Value of Medical Illustration to Medical Device R&D 194
A Short History of Medical Illustration 196
Types of Medical Illustration 203
    Textbook Illustration 203
    Surgical Approach Planning 203
    Rendering from CAD Programs 204
    Layer Technique in Photoshop 204
    The Blue Screen Trick 204
Device Development 205
Intellectual Property Development (Utility and Method) 206
Regulatory 206
Investor Presentations 209
Marketing, Physician Training, and Patient Information 209
Medical-Legal 210
Medical Teaching and Training Models 210
Three-Dimensional Animation 212
The Medical Illustration Bookshelf 213
    Other Books 214
    Artistic Anatomy 215
Finding and Using Medical Illustration 215
    Licensed Use vs. Buyout 215
Commercially Available Resources to Find Medical Illustrators 216

THE VALUE OF MEDICAL ILLUSTRATION TO MEDICAL DEVICE R&D

Most people that even know what medical illustration is think that it is only for marketing and textbooks. However, medical illustration can be an important way to conceptualize and communicate medical device design ideas. Medical illustration is a highly developed specialty that has been an important adjunct to the understanding of anatomy and biological systems, as well as a way to conceptualize and visualize the interaction of medical devices with anatomy and pathology. Medical illustration can help engineers and designers understand the anatomy they are designing a device to treat, to help plan appropriate surgical approaches, to help conceptualize new devices, to document designs and inventions, and to clearly communicate these device ideas to others.

This chapter will give a short history of medical illustration, the key role it has played in the development of medicine, how it is used now, and how to integrate it into the product development process. A number of practical and timesaving tools will also be explained that show how to get engineering data and medical illustration to work together efficiently.

When a surgeon is trained, he studies anatomy. From this training a proficient surgeon develops the ability to picture in his mind what the patient will look like on the inside, before starting the procedure. Medical illustration in textbooks, surgical atlases, and training models, as well as gross and regional anatomy training, are essential tools to develop this skill.

When an engineer or designer is given the task to develop a medical device, she is often trained and skilled in design and engineering, but may lack detailed knowledge of the anatomy or pathology that the device is intended to treat. Studying anatomical atlases is a good way to begin to understand relevant anatomy. Studying a number of good printed reference materials is a good start. However, there is no substitute for a basic knowledge of gross anatomy, physiology, and detailed understanding of the regional anatomy in the area you are working with.

The engineer and designer, like the surgeon, can develop the ability to picture in their mind and sketch and represent how a medical device will interact with the anatomy and structures to be treated. The designer will be able to picture and sketch, for example, how a catheter will enter through the femoral artery, thread through the abdominal aorta, and enter the heart via the aortic arch and into one of the coronary arteries in the aortic ostium. The ability to sketch out this type of approach, as well as describe it, can help to produce better medical device design decisions, determine feasible and infeasible surgical approaches, and conceptualize novel ways to perform a surgical intervention. It helps to answer the question "Can we get there from here?"

A trained medical illustrator can work with design and engineering to help the advising surgeon communicate his therapeutic concepts to the design team, and work with the design team to understand and communicate how the device will work in anatomy. Engineers and designers can also learn and use the skills and techniques developed by medical illustrators in their own concept generation and communication of design ideas. Medical illustration has developed numerous ways to communicate complex anatomical information in a clear and understandable way. This can help to make the product clear and understandable to management, investors, regulators, patent counsel and patent examiners, and patients.

As important as seeing a good picture reference is to understanding anatomy and physiology, there is no substitute for working with and handling actual tissue and observing actual surgeries relevant to the area in which you are working.[1] This will help you to understand how tissues react, how they feel, how tough or fragile they are, and any number of other features that a textbook cannot adequately communicate. In medical illustration there are a number of pictorial conventions, or common ways to represent information that may not correspond with real anatomy, but are a way to filter and modify visual information and emphasize what is relevant. One of the most obvious is that arteries are often rendered in red and veins in blue. If you have ever seen the inside of a real person, you know that these structures are not so conveniently color coded. If you think of a medical illustration as having a relationship to real anatomy somewhat like a wiring diagram has to actual wiring, then this can help you to understand how these conventions work. The other thing about medical illustration is that the structures are usually shown clean, and not bloody, as they might be in real life.

Another important distinction with illustration, medical photography, and studying anatomy is that an illustration and a photograph will render the visual information quite differently. In studying real anatomy, live tissue, fresh cadaver tissue, and cadaver tissue preserved in formalin all look and behave very differently. Living perfused tissue is different in color, the structures are inflated with blood, the tissue draws heat away from thermal ablation devices and has a different texture. Further, it is different in a number of important ways from even fresh cadaver tissue. Fresh cadaver tissue obviously does not bleed, has no muscle tone, and is usually less elastic than living tissue. It also goes immediately into some stage of decomposition. Preserved cadaver tissue in formalin is relatively

---

[1] "In collecting the evidence upon any medical subject there are but three sources from which we can hope to obtain it: that is from living subjects, from examination of the dead and from experiments upon living animals" (Sir Astley Cooper, 1768–1841).

tough and leathery compared to fresh cadaver tissue. This is because the formalin cross-links the proteins in the tissue. This also changes the color of the tissue. Fixed tissue tends to have less color than fresh cadaver tissue or living tissue.[2]

Illustrations, photographs, and tissue studies are all important tools to conceptualize, design, refine, and communicate in medical device development. In all of this it is important to remember that we are designing products to be used on real living people, patients, not pictures.[3]

A SHORT HISTORY OF MEDICAL ILLUSTRATION

Medical illustration has served a vital role in developing and communicating accurate information about the human body and its physiology. The development of medical illustration has grown together with changing beliefs about the nature of the physical body, the role of learning by observation, the development of the sciences and medicine, and the development of printing technology and electronic communication media.

For most of human history, the workings of the human body have been of great interest; however, until recently, comparatively little information was systematically compiled, preserved, and communicated.

Learning in the ancient Western world centered in Alexandria, Egypt. The first textbooks of medicine and anatomy, *The Usefulness of Parts* and *On Anatomical Procedures*, were produced by Galen, between 130 and 200 A.D. For various reasons, dissection of cadavers was considered a violation of a corpse back in ancient Greek times. Vivisection of animals was considered inhumane and virtually unknown. Dissections were likely done (along with chance observations from various injuries) and recorded by Homeric and Hippocratic Greek physicians. However, the practice of dissection was frowned upon by the culture of the time.[4] Little in the way

---

[2] "In dissecting cadavers there may be some fear and discomfort associated with looking at and handling a dead body. First of all, cadaver tissue fixed in formalin is sterile, and not an infection risk, though gloves are strongly recommended. (Fresh cadaver tissue needs to be handled with the same high level of caution as living tissue and blood)" (Dr. D.R. Johnson, Centre for Human Biology, University of Leeds).

[3] When participating in my first dissection of a cadaver arm when designing an orthopedic surgical device, I was doubly uncomfortable that it was cadaver tissue and dismembered at that. I had to work at keeping images from bad B movies out of my mind. The thing that got me over my initial squeamishness was thinking of Ps. 139:14 — that the human body is fearfully and wonderfully made — and that I was going to have a privileged opportunity to examine this marvelous work. This helped me get over the initial discomfort, and after the dissection helped build a deep and lasting appreciation for the design and structure of the human body. —TRK

[4] Edelstein, Ludwig, *Ancient Medicine*, Johns Hopkins University Press, Baltimore, 1994, pp. 247–301.

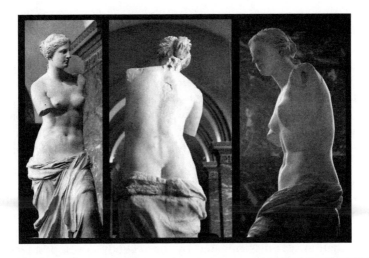

Figure 8.1 The Venus Di Milo, the Louvre, Paris. A masterful classical handling of surface anatomy. (Photos by T. Kucklick.)

of detailed anatomic knowledge was recorded and transmitted in the ancient world. One reason was the culture, another was the difficulty is distributing visual information, and yet another was the lack of a common nomenclature for describing anatomy. Classical sculptors produced masterful works of the surface anatomy of the exterior of the body, but comparatively little was depicted of the inside.

Recorded learning of the ancients (not destroyed by fires) passed into the hands of the Arabs with the capture of Alexandria in 642 A.D. Texts from Alexandria and works that were preserved in Christian monasteries, such as one in Jundi Shapur, Iraq, which fell into conquered territory, were translated by Averroes, Albumazen, and Al-Kwarizmi, and eventually transmitted to Europe in the Middle Ages in Latin translations by way of Spain.[5]

The forces of the Renaissance, the Reformation, the Enlightenment, and the development of printing technology revolutionized the understanding of science and medicine, and the dissemination of more accurate knowledge of the human body.

The modern understanding of the structure and function of the human body began with medical illustration. Leonardo da Vinci recorded numerous observations of the dissected human body in his notebooks. These illustrations, however, were not discovered until the end of the 18th century. A near contemporary of Leonardo, Andreas Vesalius (1514–1564),

---

[5] Burke, James, *Connections*, Little Brown & Co., Boston, 1978, pp. 21–22.

produced the most significant and influential work in the understanding of the human body.

Vesalius, born in Belgium in 1514, studied medicine and settled in Padua, Italy, becoming a respected anatomist. Vesalius produced the landmark *De Humani Corporis Fabrica*, which translates to *On the Structure of the Human Body*, in 1543.

One result of Vesalius's work was to overturn the accepted, but erroneous, understanding of anatomy based on the work of Galen[6] and embedded into the universities through the structure of scholasticism. Vesalius is considered the father not only of modern anatomy, but also of medical illustration.[7]

Not only did Vesalius compile systematic and detailed information on the human body derived from observation, but he also developed ways to realistically present this information by way of engravings and drawings. This information was disseminated by the recently developed technology of printing and made possible an unprecedented understanding of the human body by both scientists and artists.

Work by anatomist artists like Bernard Siegfried Albinus (1697–1770), professor of anatomy at Leiden and an extraordinary illustrator, contributed to the further understanding and visual depiction of the human body.

A link from Vesalius to another landmark discovery in medicine was through the work of William Harvey.[8] Harvey, the discoverer of the mechanism of blood circulation, was trained in Padua by Gabriello Fallopio (1523–1562), for whom the Fallopian tubes are named. Fallopio had been a student of Vesalius and was teacher of Fabricus ab Aquapendente (1537–1619), an influential instructor at Padua, who in turn instructed Harvey.[9] *Exercitato de Motu Cordis et Sanguinus in Animalbus*, his treatise on the circulation of blood, is one of the most important works in medicine and biology and is illustrated with numerous woodcuts.[10]

Another medical pioneer was William Hunter (1718–1783), who made extensive and systematic studies of anatomy and is the father of modern

---

[6] McCracken, Thomas, Gen. Ed., *New Atlas of Human Anatomy*, Metro Books, 1999, p. 15.

[7] Much of the controversy between the Roman church and authorities like Aquinas and Albertus Magnus, and investigators like Vesalius and Galileo, had to do with the upsetting of the carefully crafted medieval system of scholasticism, an amalgam of tenets from classical authorities like Galen, Plato, Aristotle, and Ptolemy and Roman church precepts.

[8] In his work, Harvey dissected both his father and his sister.

[9] Lyons, Petrucelli, et al., *Medicine: An Illustrated History*, Abradale Press, 1978, p. 433.

[10] Which was a theory proposed by Michael Servetus some 85 years earlier, but whose work was cut short by a fatal disagreement with John Calvin over Servetus's Arianism.

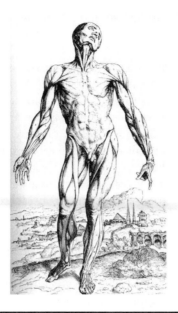

Figure 8.2 Vesalius's "Flayed Man." (From *De Humani Corporis Fabrica*, 1543.)

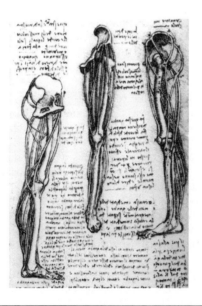

Figure 8.3 Da Vinci, dissection notebook page.

obstetrics. Hunter wrote and illustrated *The Anatomy of the Human Gravid Uterus, Exhibited in Figures* (1774), "one of the finest anatomical monographs ever produced."[11]

Despite this impressive record of progress, procurement of cadavers for study in Britain was a thorny problem.[12] A distinct fear through the end of the 19th century was that if one were to die and their corpse were violated, they would thus be denied a proper Christian burial. Parliament passed an act that allowed the dissection of convicted murderers in 1752. Prior to this, Henry the VIII allowed a limited number of hanged criminals to be thus examined. Prior to the more secular 20th century, cadavers were obtained from the ranks of these criminals or the poor who expired in hospitals at public expense (and thus considered public property). As the profession of surgery developed, and with it the demand for anatomical specimens, the practice of grave robbing and body snatching helped serve the needs of the surgical colleges. There is the nefarious case of Burke and Hare, who procured anatomic specimens for a Dr. Robert Knox in Edinburgh, Scotland, in the 1820s.[13] Typically, cadavers were procured from persons that that been executed or had expired naturally; however, Burke and Hare accelerated the process with some 16 victims in and around the Hare rooming house.[14] These were sold to Dr. Knox, who did not inquire very closely where these bodies came from. The resulting scandal and riots in Aberdeen helped lead to the Anatomy Act of 1832. This legislation, promoted by the Utilitarian philosopher Jeremy Bentham, finally provided a regular and legal source of cadavers for scientific study and also established guidelines for their ethical and considerate use.

---

[11] William Hunter was elder brother to John Hunter (1728–1793), founder of pathological anatomy and known for his fiery temper. He coined many of the terms used today to describe dental anatomy. William is considered the founder of the scientific approach to surgery. Students of William included Edward Jenner, inventor of vaccination, and Sir Astley Cooper, anatomist (Cooper's ligament) and pioneer in vascular surgery. These students, following William's principles, carried out pioneering experimental research and applied their findings to the clinical needs of patients. http://www.hoslink.com/pioneers3.htm and http://www.hunteriansociety.org.uk.

[12] For an interesting history on the subject of the procurement of cadavers for anatomical study in Britain, see Johnson, D.R., Introductory Anatomy, Centre for Human Biology, University of Leeds, http://www.leeds.ac.uk/chb/lectures/anatomy1.html.

[13] http://www.edinburgh.gov.uk/libraries/historysphere/burkeandhare/burkeandhare.html. The city of Edinburgh Burke and Hare "Midnight Tour" is a popular contemporary tourist attraction.

[14] "Up the close and down the stair, In the house with Burke and Hare. Burke's the butcher, Hare's the thief; Knox, the man who buys the beef."

Bentham was also one of the first to willingly donate his body for dissection, a now common practice.[15]

Another landmark work in the dissemination of understanding of the human body and its systems was the publication of *Anatomy Descriptive and Surgical* by Henry Gray, in 1858, commonly known as *Gray's Anatomy*. *Gray's Anatomy* took a further step of teaching a form of anatomy useful to medical students and practicing doctors.

Work by 19th-century anatomists and illustrators such as Johannes Sobotta of Germany and Eduard Pernkopf of Austria introduced color illustration and a clean and idealized representation of the dissected body. J.C.B. Grant produced another type of work, *Grant's Anatomy*, which focused on documenting and explaining the relationship of organ systems.

Another medical illustrator worthy of note is Max Broedel, considered the father of modern medical illustration. Broedel was a mostly self-taught medical illustrator. Broedel was driven to understand, not just render his subjects. This led Broedel to make important contributions to medical technology and procedure in his own right.[16] He founded the Johns Hopkins Department of Art as Applied to Medicine in 1911, the oldest medical illustration program in the U.S.[17]

One of the best-known modern medical illustrators is Frank Netter, M.D. Dr. Netter was both a medical doctor and a trained commercial artist and produced a prodigious volume of work, especially in his volumes for the Ciba-Geigy Corporation. Netter's work for the Ciba Clinical Symposia

---

[15] "The riots, the murders and public opinion meant that something had to be done and the outcome was the 1832 Anatomy Act, which was a key issue in the election of 1832. A key figure behind this was Jeremy Bentham, founder of University College London. His idea was essentially that anyone applying to a hospital for treatment was in effect giving permission for the use of their body, in the event of a poor result, being available for dissection, followed by Christian burial. Although forgoing a Christian burial Bentham was publicly dissected at University College in 1828." Johnson, D.R., Introductory Anatomy, Centre for Human Biology, University of Leeds, http://www.leeds.ac.uk/chb/lectures/anatomy1.html.

[16] "Broedel's determination to understand completely what he was drawing led to his becoming an investigator — and even devising some new surgical approaches. For instance, he recommended that surgeons start fishing for kidney stones from the avascular part of the kidney, in order to limit damage to the organ's filtering mechanisms, which are in the vascular areas. This insight, and a sturdy, triangular stitch still known as Broedel's suture, developed from the artist's in-depth study of a kidney in the autopsy room" (http://www.hopkinsmedicine.org/about/history/history7.html).

[17] "The curly-headed character also was a bon vivant, a member of the Saturday Night Club, which included some of Baltimore's best conversationalists and beer drinkers, including his close friend, H.L. Mencken" (www.hopkinsmedicine.org).

illustrated numerous new medical technologies such as those in the rapidly developing field of cardiology. Dr. Netter was one of the founders of the Association of Medical Illustrators (AMI) in 1945.

One of the important developments in the depiction and understanding of the human body is the advent of digital tools for three-dimensional reconstruction. The Visible Human Project® of the National Library of Medicine has produced a digital data set of anatomy based on the reconstruction of sliced sections of donated cadavers. This has made possible a virtual human that may be dissected any number of ways, and any number of structures or systems studied. One of the more important features of this data set is the ability to rotate the virtual specimen in space to any viewing angle, and the ability to subtract away structures quickly and easily, leaving other structures in the model intact. Previously, this process required laborious and painstaking dissection of structures, especially in delicate organs like the brain. This work was done by a team of computer modelers and programmers, as well as a number of medical illustrators, including Thomas McCracken.

One of the important advances resulting from digital reconstruction of anatomy is the depiction of anatomical variation. Medical illustration, by its nature, usually chooses an ideal, average, or representative depiction of an anatomical structure. However, in real life there is significant variation in body types, as well as tortuosity of blood vessels and any number of other features. Digital reconstruction from actual anatomy helps to map and document these variations.

Computer-aided radiology and surgery (CARS) is an important tool in surgical planning and detection of variations in anatomy prior to a procedure. This is especially important in challenging procedures such as neurosurgery, where a variation in the location of a blood vessel and hitting it by mistake can be a potentially devastating complication in a craniotomy. Low-cost computing power has made this a more affordable tool in the hands of physicians for procedures, and CARS is beginning to make a difference in the noninvasive screening and detection of disease. The information learned and compiled from CARS is contributing in a revolutionary way to our understanding of anatomy.

Another recent development in the study and popularizing of anatomy is Gunter von Hagens' *Korperwelt* (Bodyworlds). These are donated cadavers that Hagens has taken dissected and has plastinated (preserved in plastic). These cadavers are then placed in life-like poses and publicly displayed.[18]

---

[18] "Anatomical dissection gives the human mind an opportunity to compare the dead with the living, things severed with things intact, things destroyed with things evolving, and opens up the profoundness of nature to us more than any other endeavor or consideration" (Goethe, from the body donor solicitation card, Institute for Plastination).

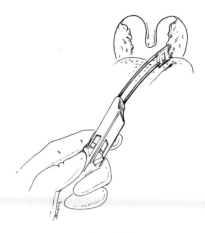

Figure 8.4 Example of pen-and-ink procedure training textbook illustration.

This work is both fascinating and controversial. For more information on von Hagens and Bodyworlds, see www.korperwelten.de or www.bodyworlds.com.[19]

TYPES OF MEDICAL ILLUSTRATION

Textbook Illustration

This is the type of illustration most people are familiar with. These are illustrations that show a surgical procedure. Often these are done in pen and ink for clarity. The illustrator usually works with the surgeon writing a book chapter to produce these drawings. These illustrations help in understanding pathology and treatment of conditions. They are a very useful guide to existing and accepted procedures, and can help the designer when developing an improved surgical device and method.

Surgical Approach Planning

Medical illustration can be quite useful in developing a new surgical approach. Some medical illustrators specialize in anatomical regions and

---

[19] Having recently attended the Bodyworlds2 exhibit in Cleveland, OH, the exhibit is quite remarkable. There were 20 whole bodies and over 200 anatomical specimens. For anyone who has either seen or done dissections, the amount of work that went into the exhibit is impressive. There are sectioned cadavers, ones mounted in lifelike poses, such as skiers, skaters, and skateboarders, and specimens of pathology such as cancers, stroke, myocardial infarction, and examples of dissections with orthopedic implants. It is as close as you can get to a dissection without doing it yourself and having to smell the formalin.

procedures, such as gynecology or cardiology. A medical illustrator with expertise in the area in which you are working can be an asset in "coming up to speed" on the details of an anatomical region, as well as a source of information for existing clinical practice. The illustrator can produce custom illustrations of the anatomical region and, if the illustrator has the skills, produce accurate three-dimensional models that can be imported into CAD programs to test ideas.

Rendering from CAD Programs

Most CAD programs have a built-in or accessory realistic rendering program. This allows the designer to apply realistic materials and finishes to a part, and render the result as an image. Check the documentation of your particular program for information on its renderer.

CAD models, both detailed and rough representative models, can be rendered and then easily trimmed and made into a separate object. Another way to quickly grab an image is to use the <Print Screen> key (on a PC). This saves an image on the screen to memory. This can then be pasted in to a bitmap image editing program like Photoshop® by using the <Control+N> "New file" command, then the <Contol + V> "Paste" command. This makes a new file at the size of the screen-rendered image in memory. "Paste" places the image, where it can then be cleaned up.

Layer Technique in Photoshop

The layers in Photoshop are a powerful tool for editing and presenting graphics. An illustration of anatomy can be produced, and each structure placed on a different layer, as if on separate sheets of acetate. The layers can then be adjusted for transparency and be made to appear to recede in space. Layers may also be turned on and off. A series of illustrations, showing, for example, a catheter threading up an artery, can be illustrated on different layers and progressively turned off and on, and the resulting image saved to a .JPEG file. These can be used to produce a flip book animation, which can be made into a digital movie or used as sequential slides in a presentation program such as Powerpoint™.

The Blue Screen Trick

A simple way to trim a rendered object is to render it on a contrasting background, such as magenta or blue. This way the Photoshop "magic wand" tool can be used to select the background, and then the selection can be inversed to select the rendered object. Once the object is selected, use the <Control + X> command to cut the object from the background,

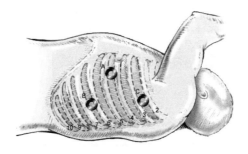

Figure 8.5 Thorascopic approach planning illustration.

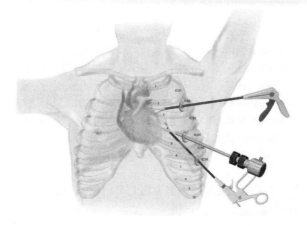

Figure 8.6 Surgical approach planning illustration with CAD models and layered illustration.

use <Contol + N> to open a new file, and then use <Control + V> to paste the object. This places the object in a new file, as a separate object, where it can be easily moved and manipulated in a layered illustration. See Figure 8.6 for an example of this type of illustration.

Using these techniques, CAD data can easily be combined with hand-rendered illustrations, scanned illustrations, or photographs to produce illustrations that show the medical device in an anatomic setting. For a guide to exchanging rendered CAD data from three-dimensional programs to two-dimensional image editing and animation programs, see Figure 8.8.

DEVICE DEVELOPMENT

Medical illustration is useful when conceptualizing a device and its usage. It is also a useful part of the design history record (DHR) and design

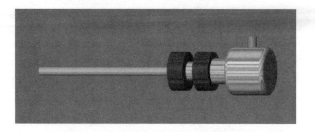

Figure 8.7 Rendered CAD model on contrasting background for use in image editing software.

controls, when establishing and documenting user requirements and resulting device designs. In this, Adobe Photoshop or some other good bitmap editing program like Corel Painter™ is quite useful. In the vascular device example, the original drawing was sketched in pencil, then scanned into a computer and opened in the editing program. The drawing was used as an underlay, and color was added to the illustration in separate layers. Finally, captions and the company logo were added. This method of starting in hand-drawn media and transitioning to digital media can be a time-saver over producing the entire work digitally, and it is a method used by many professional medical illustrators.

INTELLECTUAL PROPERTY DEVELOPMENT (UTILITY AND METHOD)

When recording lab notebook information, supporting anatomical illustrations can help clarify and explain complex procedures, and help document and establish claims for both devices and methods. Good, clear lab notebook illustrations can also save time and expense when producing patent drawings. Black-and-white cartooning techniques can work very well to generate clear, direct, interesting lab book drawings. If the lab drawings are good enough, they might be used as is, or with minimal cleanup in a patent application. This saves the expense of a patent draftsman having to redo this work. Lab notebook illustrations can capture utility disclosures and claims, and also document novel ways to use a device in concept form or discovered in preclinical and clinical testing.

REGULATORY

Medical illustration can help to clarify device concepts and use to regulatory bodies, such as the Food and Drug Administration (FDA). For example, this can be part of the documentation to claim substantial equivalence in a 510(k) application.

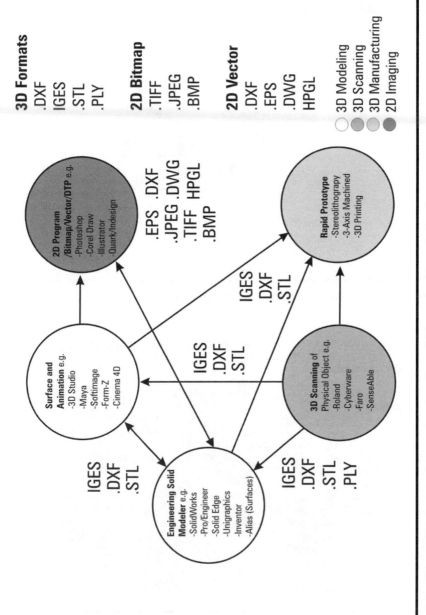

Figure 8.8 File exchange map for moving data from CAD to graphics applications.

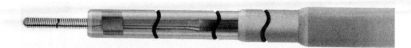

Figure 8.9 Catheter illustration.

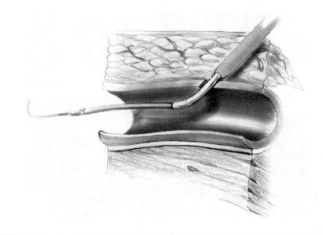

Figure 8.10 Vascular closure device concept sketch.

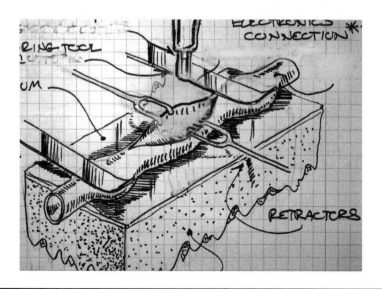

Figure 8.11 Lab notebook illustration example.

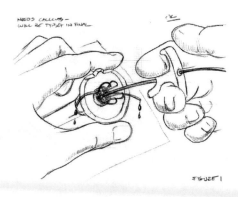

Figure 8.12 Drawing for 510(k) regulatory application for a medical device showing function.

INVESTOR PRESENTATIONS

An old saw in the investment world is "don't invest in what you don't understand." Good technical and medical illustration can help to clearly communicate sometimes arcane medical information in a compact and compelling way to potential investors. If they can clearly grasp the concept and the value of what you are presenting, and they can see a clear, plausible path to execution, they may be more inclined to invest in your company. In the accompanying example, a CAD solid model of the device and a Foley balloon was composited with a two-dimensional digital illustration of anatomy for an investor presentation. This helped to communicate the device concept and the company was successfully funded. (See Figure 8.13.)

MARKETING, PHYSICIAN TRAINING, AND PATIENT INFORMATION

Medical illustration is common in trade show exhibits, medical journal ads, physician training materials, and instructions for use (IFUs). Good medical illustration is not that expensive, especially relative to the cost of space in medical and trade journals, and the cost of attending a trade show. Some medical illustration I have seen in some major journals and at major trade shows is of low quality. The image and the reputation of your company are being displayed in the quality of what you put into your graphics. If you are going to take the time and spned the money to put illustration into your marketing and training materials, at least make sure it is quality work done by a competent professional.

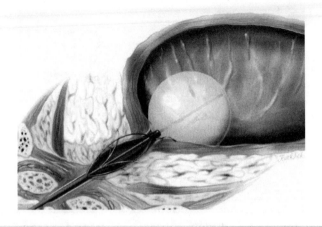

Figure 8.13 Illustration combining a CAD model of a medical device and a two-dimensional illustration for an investor presentation.

MEDICAL-LEGAL

One established subset of the medical illustration profession is medical-legal. There are medical illustrators who specialize in producing courtroom illustration and are familiar with the procedures and protocol involved with these presentations. This is usually used by the plaintiff to establish claims of medical malpractice, personal injury, or product liability. This type of illustration may also be useful when arguing a defense in a product liability case.

MEDICAL TEACHING AND TRAINING MODELS

Another area of medical illustration is the production of medical models. There are numerous varieties of medical models, from the purely visual, to those for training, to those purely for engineering. Rapid prototype models have become a common tool for planning complex surgeries. Examples of these are shown in Chapter 6. Training models mimic some features of a surgical procedure, such as the retraction of tissue for an open procedure, the trackabilty of a catheter, or the insertion force of an introducer. SOMSO Models (Marcus Sommer Somso-Modelle) has been manufacturing medical models in Sonnenburg and Coburg, Germany, since 1876, and has been in the Sommer family for five generations. SOMSO makes models of nearly all human anatomy and many zoological and botanical models, and can be purchased in the U.S. from Holt Anatomical (Miami, FL), the Anatomical Chart Company, and many medical college bookstores. Companies like Pacific Research (www.sawbones.com) pro-

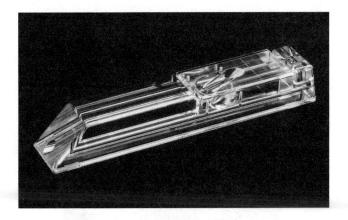

Figure 8.14   Femoral artery access training model.

duce bone models for demonstration and training purposes, as well as carbon fiber bones for realistic engineering testing. Laerdal Corporation (formerly Medical Plastics Laboratory) makes a wide range of medical teaching and training models, specializing in training models for EMS and resuscitation. Kilgore International (www.kilgoreinternational.com) specializes in dental and skull models. Simulab (www.simulab.com) makes models for training surgeons on a variety of procedures. Farlow's Scientific Glassblowing (www.farlowsci.com) makes glass vasculature models for testing catheters and other medical devices. Phantoms mimic some characteristic of an organ where radiology is applied.[20] These can be calibration phantoms or imaging phantoms.[21] CIRS, Inc. (www.cirs.com), specializes in radiology phantoms.

---

[20] The International Commission on Radiation Units and Measurements (ICRU) defines a tissue substitute as any material that simulates a body of tissue in its interaction with ionizing radiation, and a phantom as any structure that contains one or more tissue substitutes and is used to simulate radiation interactions in the human body (http://www.cirsinc.com/overview.html).

[21] "**Calibration Phantoms:** are used to establish the response of radiation detectors and for correcting quantitative information derived from digital images. **Imaging Phantoms:** are used for the assessment of image quality. Within these functional categories phantoms can be further defined: **Body Phantoms:** have the shape and composition of the human body or part of it. They are also referred to as anthropomorphic phantoms. Phantoms that are used for standardization and inter-comparison of various radiation conditions are often referred to as Standards. **Reference Phantoms:** include phantoms used to derive radiation dose calculations, mineral density equivalences or other similar type measurements. They can further be defined by their intended modality such as Ultrasound, Mammography, MRI and Computed Tomography (CT)" (http://www.cirsinc.com).

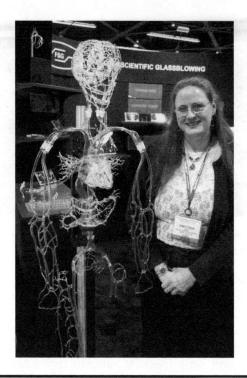

Figure 8.15 One of Farlow's glass vascular training models.

THREE-DIMENSIONAL ANIMATION

Whether threading a catheter, deploying a device, or expanding a stent, three-dimensional animation is a powerful communication tool. One caveat: three-dimensional animation can be expensive. There is the cost of building the three-dimensional model (especially complex anatomy like the heart) and the cost of rendering the final result to video. Three-dimensional animators typically charge per hour for model building, and a per-minute charge for finished video. Importing existing CAD data whenever possible can save some of the expense of three-dimensional model making. Also, there are companies that sell three-dimensional clip models of body parts, so that some of this work does not need to be done from scratch. Three-dimensional animation is usually reserved for marketing applications where the return on investment (ROI) from increased sales offsets the expense of the animation. Three-dimensional animation is a specialty all its own requiring expensive specialized equipment to render the animation file to tape, and specialized software like Softimage®, Maya®, or 3DStudio® to produce the animation files. It is important to find an animator that has these skills and has a comprehensive understanding of medical illustration and anatomy when looking for an illustrator to do this work.

THE MEDICAL ILLUSTRATION BOOKSHELF

Medical device designers can benefit from having a complete library of good anatomical reference material. The question is: What is good reference material? A number of years ago, the Association of Medical Illustrators[22] published a suggested reference bookshelf, and some of those recommendations are reflected in this list.

There is no one atlas that covers every structure in the way and in the detail you might require. It is a good idea to go to a school of medicine bookstore and look at each one of these books to see which is most appropriate for your needs. If you buy only one atlas, *Netters Atlas of Human Anatomy* is probably the best single volume. A recommendation is that you have at least more than one, and over time, acquire several. Comparing the approach and presentation between two or more references will help to build a better understanding of the structures you are studying. Also, there are a number of specialized atlases in areas like cardiology, neurology, urology, and so on (e.g., *Netter's Atlas of Human Neuroscience*), if you need even more detailed information. It is best to start with a good shelf of the general atlases, and purchase an expensive specialized atlas if you have a specific need for one.

Frank Netter and John T. Hansen's *Atlas of Human Anatomy*, third edition (Icon Learning Systems, Teterboro, NJ) is the most popular anatomical atlas in print. Icon Learning Systems purchased the Netter collection of work from Novartis in 2000, and publishes and licenses his work (www.netterart.com).

Carmine D. Clemente's *Clemente Anatomy: A Regional Atlas of the Human Body*, fourth edition (Williams & Wilkins, Baltimore, 1997) is another excellent and popular anatomical atlas. This atlas was originally published in Germany, and the illustrations are done mostly by a number of German medical illustrators, with a more naturalistic rendering style than Netter's. A companion volume is *Clemente's Anatomy Dissector*.

Johannes Rohen, Chihiro Yokochi, and Elke Lutjen-Drecoll's *Color Atlas of Anatomy*, fourth edition (Williams & Wilkins, Baltimore, 1997) is a comprehensive photographic atlas of careful and skillful cadaver dissections. This is a good companion to have to the illustrated atlases, as it shows real tissues and not just idealized representations.

---

[22] www.ami.org.

P.H. Abrahams, Sandy C. Marks, and Ralph Hutchings' *McMinn's Color Atlas of Human Anatomy*, fifth edition (Mosby International, St. Louis, MO, 2003) is another well-done and comprehensive photographic atlas of gross anatomy dissections.

Richard Drake, Wayne Vogl, Adam Mitchell, *Gray's Anatomy for Students* (Churchill Livingston Publishers, 2004). Richard Drake, Ph.D., director of anatomy, Cleveland Clinic Lerner College of Medicine, Cleveland, OH, worked with a team of authors and illustrators to produce an updated version of *Gray's Anatomy* for medical students. The atlas is different than Netter's or Clemente's, as all of the illustrations were done by one group of artists especially for the book, and thus have more structure and consistency as a group.

Other Books

Gray's Anatomy and *Grant's Anatomy* are the original modern anatomy books. Grant's had recently had a major revision. *Grant's Dissector* is a companion volume to the *Anatomy*.

Thomas O. McCracken's *New Atlas of Human Anatomy* is a showcase of computer renderings from the Visible Human Project for a popular audience. It is instructive to compare these renderings to the illustrations and photographs in the academically oriented atlases.

The Anatomical Chart Company makes numerous charts describing nearly every important bodily structure and many pathologies, as well as distributing anatomical medical models and books.

Anatomical Chart Company
4711 Golf Rd., Suite 650
Skokie, IL 60076
Phone: 847-679-4700
Fax: 847-674-0211
http://anatomical.com/

Staywell/Krames Communications produces a wide range of patient education pamphlets that are well researched and well illustrated. If you have been in a doctor's office, you have probably seen them.

Krames
780 Township Line Rd.
Yardley, PA 19067
www.krames.com
www.staywell.com
Phone: 800-333-3032

Artistic Anatomy

For designers that need to illustrate the external human form, and other structures like heads, hands, and feet, artistic anatomy references can be helpful. Here are some of the better ones:

> *Anatomy for the Artist*, Jeno Barcasy, Octopus Books, London
> *Anatomy Lessons from the Great Masters*, Robert Beverly Hale and Terrence Coyle (Hale was the dean of figure-drawing instructors), Watson-Guptil, New York
> *Anatomy for the Artist*, Sarah Simblett (numerous photographs and overlays), DK Publishing, New York
> *Human Anatomy for Artists*, Eliot Goldfinger (a classic), Oxford University Press, New York
> *Strength Training Anatomy*, Frederic Delavier (may be useful if you are designing exercise equipment), Sportstech Books, Victoria, Australia
> *The Art of Figure Drawing*, Clem Robins (Robins was a student of Hale and Coyle; a good introduction to life-like figure drawing), Northlight Books, Cincinnati, OH

FINDING AND USING MEDICAL ILLUSTRATION

Licensed Use vs. Buyout

When hiring a medical illustrator, there are two basic ways to obtain rights to the work. One is a license for a specified use, and the other is a buyout, where the buyer obtains all rights to a work and possession of the original art or file.

The issue of buyouts is a hot topic among illustrators. Traditionally, illustrators are reluctant to sell work outright, unless it was a piece specific to the client. Buyouts are available, but at a higher cost than a license. Illustrators over their career build a library of stock art and license these out. (This is how illustrators are able to even out their income stream and make a decent living.) If you are looking for an illustration of an anatomical structure, there are probably numerous stock examples immediately available from the artist. The artist can also modify the work to meet your specific needs. A professional medical illustrator can be an important partner to an engineering team, if he or she has in-depth knowledge of the anatomy in the area you are working in.

One issue that may need to be clarified with the illustrator is the practice of assigning any intellectual property and inventions to the company. Some medical illustrators have detailed and valuable experience in medical specialties and can make inventive contributions, but may not be familiar with customary intellectual property (IP) arrangements in engineering groups. To not clarify this issue up front, and assume the illustrator is "just an artist" and not in a position to make an inventive contribution, may invite potentially acrimonious disagreements over IP ownership.

COMMERCIALLY AVAILABLE RESOURCES TO FIND MEDICAL ILLUSTRATORS

The Association of Medical Illustrators Sourcebook (Serbin Press, Santa Barbara, CA) is an annual publication with ad pages from working medical and natural science illustrators. If you are a qualified buyer of medical illustration, you can call Serbin and ask to be on its distribution list, or purchase a copy when available. Serbin has a limited number of back issues of the *Sourcebook* occasionally available.
Serbin Communications
511 Olive St.
Santa Barbara, CA 93101
Phone: 800-876-6425
Fax: 805-965-0496
E-mail: admin@serbin.com
Sourcebook online: http://www.medillsb.com/

Indexed Visuals (IV) is an online source for medical illustration. IV is an online catalog of thousands of pieces of stock art and ad pages by illustrators. The artists may be contacted directly to negotiate fees for a particular piece of artwork. Go to www.indexedvisuals.com.

The Association of Medical Illustrators is a professional group of medical illustrators founded in 1945.
Association of Medical Illustrators
245 1st St., Suite 1800
Cambridge, MA 02142
Phone: 617-395-8186
HQ@ami.org

9

BRIEF INTRODUCTION TO PRECLINICAL RESEARCH

James Swick, Ph.D.

CONTENTS

Overview 217
In Vitro Testing 218
    The Animal Models 218
    The Project 219
The *In Vivo* Study 219
    Data Collection 220
    The Team 220
    Good Laboratory Practices 220
Summary 221

OVERVIEW

Medical devices must be tested in a living system (*in vivo* testing) in order for them to be approved by the Food and Drug Administration (FDA) for clinical trials. This can be a daunting task to some. In order to minimize the fear and trepidation that comes with this aspect of device development, I will lay out a guide that will allow the reader to map out a schedule for success and minimize chances for failure.

    Once your device has undergone all the rigors of bench-top testing, it is wise to see how it performs *in vitro*. What I mean by this is to procure explanted tissue in order to identify any modifications that may need to be made prior to the *in vivo* phase. There are several sources for obtaining the necessary organ/tissue, which I will discuss later on.

The most important aspect of preclinical work is identifying where to perform the testing. The right lab is critical to your success. A lab with inexperienced personnel who lack the knowledge to help with the intra-operative portion of your procedure can be frustrating and costly. Therefore, it is extremely important to explore all the options open to you before committing to any one facility or group.

If your device is novel and requires submission for independent device exemption, you may also want to consider working with a lab or consultant knowledgeable in good laboratory practices (GLP).

IN VITRO TESTING

When you feel your device is ready for prime time, there a few things you must keep in mind. First is the organ system you will be targeting. A good example is an intravascular stent with delivery system. You may want to test its mechanical characteristics in explanted tissue. There are several places where you can procure arterial sections, e.g., butcher shop, meat packing plant, universities, or an independent lab. In the case of coronary stents, you will need an explanted heart.

This holds true for other organ systems as well. The least expensive route (butcher shop and meat packing plant) is not always the best, however. The tissue may not be in the best condition. If at all possible, you should try and get your samples from an independent lab or university. The latter two sources will give you tissue that has been removed by someone with surgical skill and kept as fresh as possible.

Once you have the tissue, you may need to set up an artificial environment to mimic blood flow, etc. As a physiologist, I cannot help you with this, but you engineering folks should be able to figure this part out.

If you need an artificial circulatory system, there are companies and independent model makers who can provide a plastic or glass model that works very well. Some of these can be a bit pricey, but you can use them over and over. They are also very nice to demonstrate your device to potential investors or end users.

The Animal Models

You must always be mindful that working with live animals is a privilege and should never be taken lightly. The U.S. Department of Agriculture (USDA) regulates the use of animals for research purposes through the Animal Welfare Act (you can find this on its website, www.usda.gov).

The right animal model for your *in vivo* phase of development is truly the most important decision you will make. You need to take into consideration what others have used in the past, as well as which particular species is the most similar to human anatomy. You can get direction from the medical literature as well as by talking to researchers knowledgeable in your specific area of interest.

Some good questions to ask include:

- How many animals will I need?
- What organ system is your focus?
- What have others used?
- What species will give the most human-like anatomy?

The Project

The next step is to develop the project itself. You will need to consider how to begin, i.e., survival vs. terminal. I always recommend that new projects begin with terminal procedures in order to develop technique (surgical or interventional) as well as to determine what the device will do to the animal physiologically. You may need to incorporate specific medications in order to ward off complications.

What equipment will be required? If your procedure is interventional, you will need the proper imaging equipment, i.e., fluoroscopy or ultrasound.

What physiological parameters will need to be measured? You will need to collect the appropriate data for your final submission. It is wise to check any guidance the FDA may have regarding your particular area of interest. Also check with clinicians to find out what physiological parameters they want to see measured, i.e., hemodynamics, clinical chemistry, etc. If you do not plan all aspects of your procedure up front, you may find that you have wasted precious time and money. Not having all the data for your submission to the FDA may require that you go back to the lab or, at worst, start over. I cannot stress this point enough. You must plan every detail of your project and evaluate your progress along the way. If things do not go as planned, be prepared to stop and reevaluate before going forward.

THE *IN VIVO* STUDY

Once you have developed your plan of attack and have formalized it in a protocol, submit this to the Institutional Animal Care and Use Committee (IACUC) of the test facility you have chosen for the study. Most preclinical labs have their own template for this submission. After it has been reviewed and approved, you will be ready to begin.

There are a myriad of variables you need to take into consideration here:

- What specialty equipment will you need, i.e., fluoroscopy, ultrasound, etc.?

- Will you need surgical or interventional expertise, and who will provide this?
- How much time will be required for the study?
- What kind of support can you expect from the test facility?
- Will this be a survival procedure or terminal?

In most cases it is recommended to begin with your first animal being terminal. This is so that you can work out any problem areas that may not have been accounted for. By doing this you will be able to develop the surgical or interventional technique so that you will know what to expect going forward.

Data Collection

You will need to establish all the parameters you want to evaluate prior to starting your study. Items such as histology, clinical pathology, angiography, etc., must be determined so that you can glean pertinent data from the outset. If you do not plan this aspect of the study, you may find yourself wasting precious time and money. If hemodynamic values are of interest, it is usually helpful to develop a data collection document so that you can have all the relevant information in one place.

The Team

The personnel who will be responsible for making your project successful are critical to having a good result. Be certain that everyone on your side of the team knows what their responsibilities and duties are prior to beginning the procedure. The personnel from the test facility must also know ahead of time what is expected of them as well. You, as the study sponsor, are ultimately responsible for making sure that there is a direct line of ongoing communication between your staff and the staff at the test facility.

Good Laboratory Practices

Good Laboratory Practices (GLP) refers to the U.S. Food and Drug Administration's guidelines for submitting data for review by the FDA in order to receive investigational device exemption (IDE) or premarket approval (PMA) for clinical trials. Inasmuch as this discussion is meant to be an introduction to preclinical research, I will refrain from any dialogue on this particular subject. There have been volumes written on GLP and how to approach this type of data collection. All I will say is that once you are ready to enter this realm, be prepared to work very closely with the regulatory department of the chosen test facility. The paper trail here can be daunting. Make sure that the facility you choose has a proven track record before beginning your work. This is a very high bar indeed, and it requires extreme attention to detail and can be very costly.

SUMMARY

In summary, I would like to stress two very important points. First, plan, plan, plan and continue planning prior to beginning any *in vivo* work. Discuss your project with the test facility staff and get their input, as these are the folks with the most experience. The other vital point is data collection. Do your homework and know precisely which parameters will be necessary for your final assessment.

10

REGULATORY AFFAIRS: MEDICAL DEVICES

Thom Wehman

CONTENTS

Introduction 225
   Regulatory Requirements Are Enforced by Law 225
   Make Regulatory Affairs Cost-Effective 225
   Regulatory Requirements Improve Device Safety and
      Effectiveness 225
   Regulatory Affairs Requires Good Judgment 226
FDA Overview and Authority 226
   Important FDA Jurisdiction Acts, History, and Assistance 227
   Online Assistance 227
The Basics: Short Discussion of Establishment Registration,
Device Submissions, Device Listing, and Device
Classification 228
   Establishment Registration 228
   Device Listing 228
   Device Classification 229
   Device Functional Classification 230
   510(k) Premarket Notification 230
   Substantial Equivalence 231
   Premarket Approval Submission 232
   Investigational Device Exemption and Supporting Studies 232
   Third-Party Submission Review by Accredited Parties 233
   Importing into the U.S. 234
      Initial Importers 234

Exporting Devices 234
    Certificates for Foreign Government 235
    Additional Regulations by Different States 235
Special Considerations 236
    Exemptions from 510(k) and GMP Requirements 236
        Class I Devices 236
        Class II Devices 236
    Special 510(k) 237
    Abbreviated 510(k) 238
    De Novo 238
    Product Development Protocol 239
    Humanitarian Use Device/Humanitarian Device Exemption 239
Good Quality and Procedural Practices 240
    Quality System Regulations (QSR) 240
    Quality System Inspection Technique (QSIT) 241
    Good Clinical Practice 241
    Good Laboratory Practices 242
        Regulations 242
    Preclinical Studies 242
Summary of Title 21 of the Code of Federal Regulations,
Parts 800 to 1299, for Medical Devices 243
    Part 800: General Requirements 243
    Part 801: Labeling 243
    Part 803: Medical Device Reporting (MDR) 244
    Part 806: Medical Devices: Reports of Corrections
    and Removals 246
    Part 807: Establishment Registration and Device Listing for
    Manufacturer and Individual Importers of Devices 246
    Part 808: Exemptions from Federal Preemption of State and
    Local Medical Device Requirements 248
    Part 809: *In Vitro* Diagnostic Products for Human Use 248
    Part 810: Medical Device Recall Authority 249
    Part 812: Investigational Device Exemptions 250
    Part 820: Quality System Regulation 257
    Part 821: Medical Device Tracking Requirements 259
    Part 822: Postmarket Surveillance 261
    Part 860: Medical Device Classification Procedures 262
    Part 861: Procedures for Performance Standards
    Development 263
    Parts 862 to 1050 264
Abbreviations 265
    International and National Standard Abbreviations 265
    Regulatory Abbreviations 265

INTRODUCTION

Regulatory Requirements Are Enforced by Law

The first rule of regulatory affairs is that it is based on regulation; that is, it is a legal obligation. From a business point of view, it is expense, and it does contribute to the cost of doing business. Thus, for the sake of maintaining a profitable business while still providing for necessary safety and effectiveness of a medical device, regulatory affairs must be a well-planned function and not just improvised as the need arises. For a medical device start-up company, regulatory affairs strategy and implementation must be addressed from the very beginning.

Make Regulatory Affairs Cost-Effective

The discussion in this chapter focuses on meeting all regulatory needs for a company in a cost-effective fashion. The emphasis on cost-effective leads to the second rule of regulatory affairs: more is not better. Good regulatory control requires good documentation, but it does not require an ever-growing set of instructions and procedures. Adherence to documented procedures is of paramount importance. Thus, if documents become too complex or too numerous, adherence may suffer.

The Medical Device User Fee and Modernization Act of October 2002 increased the cost of doing business for any company wishing to sell medical devices in the U.S. by imposing device submission fees. The fees, as of May 2005, which underscore the need for good device development and regulation planning, are listed in the table below:

Submission Type	Standard Fee	Small-Business Fee
Premarket approval (PMA)	$206,811	$78,588
180-day PMA supplement	$44,464	$16,896
510(k)	$3,480	$2,784

Regulatory Requirements Improve Device Safety and Effectiveness

Medical device regulations were implemented and are enforced to ensure that the best possible safety and effectiveness will be obtained from an Food and Drug Administration (FDA)-cleared or -approved device. It is the companies' management responsibility to provide continued safety and effectiveness after a device is released for sale by employing a good-quality validation and reliability program. The U.S. FDA program Quality System Regulation (QSR) is described in the "Summary of Title 21 of the Code of Federal Regulations, Part 820: Good Manufacturing Practices" section of this chapter. Similar international quality systems (ISO 9000), specifically for medical devices (ISO 13485), are beyond the scope of this chapter.

Regulatory Affairs Requires Good Judgment

The reader will note that immediately following the text in each section is a short list of bullet points of what was covered. The intent is to quickly visualize the essence of each regulation. The goal of this chapter is to make the reader aware of requirements and options so that he or she can speak knowledgeably with regulatory affairs professionals in order to exercise good judgment. Only study, training, and experience will lead to a full grasp of regulatory complexity in order to exercise good judgment.

- Regulations are enforced by law.
- More documentation is not always better.
- Adhering to all regulations does not guarantee that there will not be any adverse events, but it will lessen the likelihood of punitive damages.
- FDA medical device regulations were implemented to ensure safety and effectiveness.
- Start regulatory affairs strategies immediately after funding of company.

FDA OVERVIEW AND AUTHORITY

The FDA is comprised of six different centers and two offices:

Centers
- Center for Food Safety and Applied Nutrition (CFSAN)
- Center for Drug Evaluation and Research (CDER)
- Center for Devices and Radiological Health (CDRH)
- Center for Biologics Evaluation and Research (CBER)
- Center for Veterinary Medicine (CVR)
- National Center for Toxicological Research (NCTR)

Offices
- Office of the Commissioner (OC)
- Office of Regulatory Affairs (ORA)

The division that deals with medical devices is CDRH. If a device has some other component, such as drugs or biological products, the FDA decides which is the primary mode of action and assigns review responsibility accordingly.

Important FDA Jurisdiction Acts, History, and Assistance

FDA reorganization 1930: There was a sweeping expansion of FDA to include coverage of new drugs, devices and cosmetics. Also, FDA was given increased court jurisdiction.

The Federal Food, Drug and Cosmetics Act (FD & C) of 1938: The FDA was expanded to regulate cosmetics and therapeutic devices and additional regulation of food and drugs.

The Medical Device Amendments of 1976: Added provisions governing device/facility registration and listing, classifications, premarket notification (510(k)), premarket approval (PMA), investigational device exemption (IDE), good manufacturing practice (GMP), medical device reports (MDR), and other controls. This expansion was so extensive that over time devices are referred to as pre-amendment or post-amendment.

The Safe Medical Devices Act of 1990: Comprehensive changes to include device recall, preproduction design validation, expanding authority to surgical hospitals and nursing homes, and establishing biological divisions to include devices that contain drugs and biological products (CBER).

FDA Export Reform and Enhancement Act of 1996: Substantially reduces many regulatory obstacles for exporting unapproved drugs, biologics, and devices.

1997 FDA Modernization Act (FDAMA): Significantly reduced time frame and work required for clinical studies, clearances, approvals, and device manufacture and design requirements.

2002 Medical Device User Fee Modernization Act (MDUFMA): Instigated user fees for device submissions, third-party inspections, reprocessed single-use devices, and other provisions.

Online Assistance

Division of Small Manufacturers, International and Consumer Assistance (DSMICA): This is a special group within FDA that was set up to answer questions from the medical device industry. It can be contacted via its website: http://www.fda.gov/cdrh/dsmamain.html.

International regulations: To obtain medical regulations for other countries listed in *International Organizations and Foreign Government Agencies*, go to http://www.fda.gov/oia/agencies.htm.

- FDA has multiple divisions to ensure health and safety for food, drugs, and devices.

- There are multiple levels of device classification to meet different levels of risk.
- There have been many FDA amendments and acts to improve safety and reduce regulatory obstacles.

THE BASICS: SHORT DISCUSSION OF ESTABLISHMENT REGISTRATION, DEVICE SUBMISSIONS, DEVICE LISTING, AND DEVICE CLASSIFICATION[1]

Establishment Registration

Establishments involved in the production and distribution of medical devices intended for marketing or leasing (commercial distribution) in the U.S. are required to register with the FDA. Registration provides the FDA with the location of medical device manufacturing facilities and importers. No registration fee is required. An establishment means any place of business under one management at one physical location at which a device is manufactured, assembled, or otherwise processed for commercial distribution. The owner/operator of the establishment is responsible for registration. Owner/operator means the corporation, subsidiary, affiliated company, partnership, or proprietor directly responsible for the activities of the registering establishment.

Device Listing

Most medical device establishments required to register with the FDA must list the devices they have in commercial distribution, including devices produced exclusively for export. This process is a means of keeping the FDA advised of the generic categories of devices an establishment is marketing. Each generic category is represented by a separate classification regulation found in Title 21 of the Code of Federal Regulations (CFR), Parts 862 to 892, or FDA-assigned device name. Each regulation number or device name is associated with one or more product codes. Regulation numbers with more than one product code identify the product in further detail. For example, "Manual Surgical Instruments for General Use," 21 CFR 878.4800, contains several product codes, including GAB (disposable suturing needle), GDX (scalpel), HTD (forceps), and HRQ (hemostat).

---

[1] Also see additional details in the CFR discussions in the "Summary of Title 21 of the Code of Federal Regulations, Parts 800 to 1299, for Medical Devices" section. Some of the text in this section and following sections are taken directly from FDA Title 21.

Listing of a medical device is not approval of the establishment or a device by the FDA. Unless exempt, a premarket clearance (510(k)) or a premarket approval (PMA) is required before a device can be marketed or placed into commercial distribution in the U.S. No listing fee is required.

Device Classification

The FDA has established classifications for approximately 1700 different generic types of devices and grouped them into 16 medical specialties, referred to as panels. Each of these generic types of devices is assigned to one of three regulatory classes based on the level of control necessary to ensure the safety and effectiveness of the device. The three classes and the requirements that apply to them are:

1. Class I: General Controls
   a. With exemptions
   b. Without exemptions
2. Class II: General and Special Controls
   a. With exemptions
   b. Without exemptions
3. Class III: General Controls and Premarket Approval

The class to which your device is assigned determines, among other things, the type of premarketing submission/application required for FDA clearance to market. If your device is classified as Class I or II, and if it is not exempt, a 510(k) will be required for marketing. All devices classified as exempt are subject to the limitations on exemptions. Limitations of device exemptions are covered under 21 CFR xxx.9, where xxx refers to Parts 862–892. For Class III devices, a premarket approval (PMA) application will be required unless the device is a preamendments device (on the market prior to the passage of the medical device amendments in 1976, or substantially equivalent to such a device) and the device has not been designated a PMA. In that case, a 510(k) will be the route to market.

Device classification depends on the *intended use* of the device and also upon *indications for use*. For example, a scalpel's intended use is to cut tissue. A subset of intended use arises when a more specialized indication is added in the device's labeling, such as "for making incisions in the cornea." Indications for use can be found in the device's labeling, but may also be conveyed orally during sale of the product. A discussion of the meaning of intended use is contained in *Premarket Notification Review Program K86-3*.

In addition, classification is risk based; that is, the risk the device poses to the patient or the user is a major factor in the class it is assigned. Class

I includes devices with the lowest risk, and Class III includes those with the greatest risk.

Device Functional Classification

As mentioned above, the FDA has established classifications for over 1700 types of devices and has categorized them into 16 medical specialties, referred to as panels. Experts from the different panels are often called upon to review regulatory requirements or rulings for specific devices. Panel numbers and panels are:

- 868 Anesthesiology
- 870 Cardiovascular
- 862 Clinical Chemistry and Clinical Toxicology
- 872 Dental
- 874 Ear, Nose and Throat
- 876 Gastroenterology and Urology
- 878 General and Plastic Surgery
- 880 General Hospital and Personal Use
- 864 Hematology and Pathology
- 866 Immunology and Microbiology
- 882 Neurology
- 884 Obstetrical and Gynecological
- 886 Ophthalmic
- 888 Orthopedic
- 890 Physical Medicine
- 892 Radiology

510(k) Premarket Notification

The designation 510(k) refers to section 510(k) of the 1976 Medical Device Amendment Act.

Each company that wants to market Class I, II, and some III devices intended for human use in the U.S. must submit a 510(k) to the FDA at least 90 days before marketing unless the device is exempt from 510(k) requirements. There is no 510(k) form, but instead a format for the submission is described in 21 CFR 807.

A 510(k) is a premarketing submission made to the FDA to demonstrate that the device to be marketed is as safe and effective, that is, substantially equivalent (SE), to a legally marketed device that is not subject to premarket approval (PMA). Applicants must compare their 510(k) device to one or more similar devices currently on the U.S. market and make and support their substantial equivalency claims. A legally marketed device is a device that was legally marketed prior to May 28, 1976 (preamendments device), or a device that has been reclassified from Class III to Class II or I, a device that has been found to be substantially equivalent to such a device through the 510(k) process, or one established through the evaluation of automatic Class III definition. The legally marketed device to which equivalence is drawn is known as the predicate device.

Applicants must submit descriptive data and, when necessary, performance data to establish that their device is SE to a predicate device. Again, the data in a 510(k) is to show comparability, that is, substantial equivalency (SE), of a new device to a predicate device. The data need not show superiority to the predicate device.

Substantial Equivalence

Unlike PMA, which requires demonstration of reasonable safety and effectiveness, 510(k) requires demonstration of substantial equivalence. Substantial equivalence (SE) means that the new device is as safe and effective as the predicate device.

A device is SE if, in comparison to a predicate device, it:

- Has the same intended use as the predicate device *and*
- Has the same technological characteristics as the predicate device *or*
- Has different technological characteristics that do not raise new questions of safety and effectiveness, and the sponsor demonstrates that the device is as safe and effective as the legally marketed device. A claim of substantial equivalence does not mean the new and predicate devices must be identical. Substantial equivalence is established with respect to intended use, design, energy used or delivered, materials, performance, safety, effectiveness, labeling, biocompatibility, standards, and other applicable characteristics. Detailed information on how FDA determines substantial equivalence can be found in the *Premarket Notification Review Program 6/30/86 (K86-3)* blue book memorandum.

Until the applicant receives an order declaring a device SE and a 501(k) clearance, he may not proceed to market the device. Once the device is determined to be SE, it can then be marketed in the U.S. If the FDA determines that a device is *not* SE, the applicant may resubmit another 510(k) with new data, file a reclassification petition, or submit a premarket approval (PMA) application. The SE determination is usually made within 90 days and is made based on the information submitted by the applicant.

Premarket Approval Submission

Premarket approval (PMA) is the FDA process of scientific and regulatory review to evaluate the safety and effectiveness of Class III medical devices. Class III devices are those that support or sustain human life, are of substantial importance in preventing impairment of human health, or that present a potential, unreasonable risk of illness or injury. Due to the level of risk associated with Class III devices, the FDA has determined that general and special controls alone are insufficient to ensure the safety and effectiveness of Class III devices. Please note that some Class III preamendment devices may require a Class III 510(k). See the historical background section below for additional information.

A PMA is the most stringent type of device marketing application required by the FDA. The applicant must receive FDA approval of its PMA application prior to marketing the device. PMA approval is based on a determination by the FDA that the PMA contains sufficient valid scientific evidence to ensure that the device is safe and effective for its intended use. An approved PMA is, in effect, a private license granting the applicant (or owner) permission to market the device.

The PMA applicant is usually the person who owns the rights, or otherwise has authorized access, to the data and other information to be submitted in support of FDA approval. This person may be an individual, partnership, corporation, association, scientific or academic establishment, government agency or organizational unit, or other legal entity. The applicant is often the inventor/developer and ultimately the manufacturer.

FDA regulations provide 180 days to review the PMA and make a determination. In reality, the review time is normally longer. Before approving or denying a PMA, the appropriate FDA advisory committee may review the PMA at a public meeting and provide the FDA with the committee's recommendation on whether the FDA should approve the submission. After the FDA notifies the applicant that the PMA has been approved or denied, a notice is published on the Internet (1) announcing the data on which the decision is based and (2) providing interested persons an opportunity to petition the FDA within 30 days for reconsideration of the decision.

The regulation governing premarket approval is located in 21 CFR 814, "Premarket Approval." A Class III device that fails to meet PMA requirements is considered to be adulterated under Section 501(f) of the FD&C Act and cannot be marketed.

Investigational Device Exemption and Supporting Studies

An investigational device exemption (IDE) allows the investigational device to be used in a clinical study in order to collect safety and effectiveness data required to support a PMA application or a premarket notification (510(k)) submission to the FDA. Clinical studies are most often conducted to support a PMA. Only a small percentage of 510(k)s require clinical data to support the application. Investigational use also includes clinical evaluation of certain modifications or new intended uses of legally marketed devices. All clinical evaluations of investigational devices, unless exempt, must have an approved IDE *before* the study is initiated, either from an institutional review board (IRB) for a nonsignificant risk device or an IRB and the FDA for a significant risk device.

Clinical evaluation of devices that have not been cleared for marketing requires:

- An IDE approved by an IRB. If the study involves a significant risk device, the IDE must also be approved by the FDA.
- Informed consent from all patients.
- Labeling for investigational use only.
- Monitoring of the study.
- Required records and reports.

An approved IDE permits a device to be shipped lawfully for the purpose of conducting investigations of the device without complying with other requirements of the Food, Drug, and Cosmetic Act (Act) that would apply to devices in commercial distribution. Sponsors need not submit a PMA or Premarket Notification 510(k), register their establishment, or list the device while the device is under investigation. Sponsors of IDE's are also exempt from the Quality System Regulation (QSR) except for the requirements for design control.

Third-Party Submission Review by Accredited Parties

The purpose of the Accredited Persons Program is to conduct the initial review of 510(k)s for selected low- to moderate-risk devices in order to reduce workload and backlog. Thus, it enables the FDA to use its scientific review resources for higher-risk devices, while maintaining a high degree of confidence in the review of low- to moderate-risk devices, and provides manufacturers of eligible devices an alternative review process that may yield more rapid 510(k) decisions.

Specifically, an accredited person may not review any Class III device, or Class II devices that are permanently implantable, life supporting, life sustaining, or for which clinical data are required. The FDA also sets limits on the number of Class II devices that may be ineligible for accredited person review because clinical data are required.

On September 23, 1998, the FDA published a list of persons accredited to conduct 510(k) reviews for certain devices, which is available at http://www.fda.gov/cdrh/thirdparty. Accredited persons were eligible to begin reviewing applications after they successfully completed a training session. On November 21, 1998, the agency began accepting 510(k) reviews from accredited persons and terminated the Third Party Review Pilot Program that began on August 1, 1996.

Importing into the U.S.

Foreign manufacturers must meet applicable U.S. medical device regulations in order to import devices into the U.S., even if the product is authorized for marketing in another country. These requirements include registration of establishment, listing of devices, manufacturing in accordance with the quality system regulation, medical device reporting of adverse events, and premarket notification 510(k) or premarket approval, if applicable. In addition, the foreign manufacturers must designate a U.S. agent. As with domestic manufacturers, foreign manufacturing sites are subject to FDA inspection.

Initial Importers

An initial importer is any importer who furthers the marketing of a device from a foreign manufacturer to the person who makes the final delivery or sale of the device to the ultimate consumer or user, but does not repackage or otherwise change the container, wrapper, or labeling of the device or device package. The initial importer of the device must register its establishment with the FDA. Registration information, including the registration form FDA-2891, can be found under "Establishment Registration" on the FDA website.

Initial importers are also subject to medical device reporting (MDR) under 21 CFR 803, "Reports of Corrections and Removals" under 21 CFR 806, and "Medical Device Tracking" under 21 CFR 821, if applicable. Under the MDR regulations importers are required to report incidents in which a device may have caused or contributed to a death or serious injury, as well as report certain malfunctions. The importers must maintain an MDR event file for each adverse event. All product complaints (MDR and non-MDR events) must be forwarded to the manufacturer. Under medical device tracking requirements, certain devices must be tracked through the distribution chain.

Exporting Devices

Any medical device that is legally cleared or approved by the FDA in the U.S. may be exported anywhere in the world without prior FDA notification or approval. The export provisions of the FD&C Act only apply to unapproved devices. For a device to be legally in commercial distribution in the U.S., the following requirements must be met:

- The manufacturing facility must be registered with the FDA on Form FDA-2891.
- The device must be listed on Form FDA-2892 with the FDA.
- The device must have a cleared premarket notification 510(k) or premarket approval unless exempted by regulation, or if the device was on the market prior to May 28, 1976 (before the medical device amendments to the FD&C Act).
- The device must meet the labeling requirements of 21 CFR 801 and 809, if applicable.
- The device must be manufactured in accordance with the Quality Systems Regulation (QSR) of 21 CFR 820 (also known as good manufacturing practices), unless exempted by regulation.

In addition, the U.S. exporter must comply with the laws of the importing country.

Certificates for Foreign Government

While the FDA does not place any restrictions on the export of these devices, certain countries may require written certification that a firm or its devices are in compliance with U.S. law. In such instances, the FDA will accommodate U.S. firms by providing a certificate for foreign government (CFG). These export certifications were formerly referred to as a certificate for products for export or certificate of free sale. The CFG is a self-certification process that is used to speed the processing of requests. Original certificates will be provided on special counterfeit-resistant paper with an embossed gold foil seal.

As of May 2005, CDRH requires an initial fee of $175 per certificate and $15 per certificate for additional certificates issued for the same products in the same letter of request. Original certificates will be provided on special counterfeit-resistant paper with an embossed gold foil seal.

Additional Regulations by Different States

Each state should be contacted for its specific medical regulations; here is an example for California's FDB:

The Food and Drug Branch (FDB) mission is to protect and improve the health of all California residents by ensuring that foods, drugs, medical devices, cosmetics, and certain other consumer products are safe and are not adulterated, misbranded, or falsely advertised, and that drugs and medical devices are effective.

- They accomplish their mission through sound investigations and inspections, based on valid scientific principles and specific legal authority, and effective industry and consumer education.
- They strive to regulate fairly and without unduly burdening California businesses.
- They do this by helping businesses understand the public health basis for regulatory requirements, encouraging businesses to voluntarily correct deficiencies, and uniformly enforcing regulatory requirements to prevent unfair competition.
- This success is crucial to the health of California residents and the economic vitality of the industries we regulate.

- The above discussion on basics applies to all medical devices and medical device companies in the U.S.

SPECIAL CONSIDERATIONS

Exemptions from 510(k) and GMP Requirements

Class I Devices

The FDA has exempted almost all Class I devices (with the exception of reserved devices from the premarket notification requirement, including those devices that were exempted by final regulation published in the *Federal Registers* of December 7, 1994, and January 16, 1996. It is important to confirm the exempt status and any limitations that apply with 21 CFR 862 to 892.

If a manufacturer's device falls into a generic category of exempted Class I devices, a premarket notification application and FDA clearance is not required before marketing the device in the U.S. However, these manufacturers are required to register their establishment by submitting Form FDA 2891, "Initial Registration of Device Establishment," and list the generic category or classification name of the device by submitting Form FDA 2892, "Device Listing."

Class II Devices

The FDA has also published a list of Class II (special controls) devices, subject to certain limitations, that are now exempt from the premarket notification requirements under the Food and Drug Administration Modernization Act of 1997. The FDA believes that these exemptions will relieve manufacturers from the need to submit premarket notification submissions for these devices and will enable the FDA to redirect the resources that would be spent on reviewing such submissions to more significant public health issues. The FDA is taking this action in order to meet a requirement of the Modernization Act. Class II devices are annotated II. Please note that Class II devices are *not* exempt from GMP requirements.

Special 510(k)

Since design control requirements are now in effect and require the manufacturer to conduct verification and validation studies of a type that have traditionally been included in 510(k) submissions, the agency believes that it may be appropriate to forgo a detailed review of the underlying data normally required in 510(k)s. For this reason, the FDA is allowing an alternative to the traditional method of demonstrating substantial equivalence for certain device modifications. For these well-defined modifications, the agency believes that the rigorous design control procedure requirements produce highly reliable results that can form, in addition to the other 510(k) content requirements, a basis for the substantial equivalence determination. Under the Quality Systems Regulation, data that are generated as a result of the design control procedures must be maintained by the manufacturer and be available for FDA inspection.

For a Special 510(k) submission, a manufacturer should refer to 21 CFR 807.81(a)(3) and the FDA guidance document entitled "Deciding When to Submit a 510(k) for a Change to an Existing Device" to decide if a device modification may be implemented without submission of a new 510(k). If a new 510(k) is needed for the modification, and if the modification does not affect the intended use of the device or alter the fundamental scientific technology of the device, then summary information that results from the design control process can serve as the basis for clearing the application.

Thus, a manufacturer who is intending to modify his or her own legally marketed device will conduct the risk analysis and the necessary verification and validation activities to demonstrate that the design outputs of the modified device meet the design input requirements. Once the manufacturer has ensured the satisfactory completion of this process, a "Special 510(k): Device Modification" form may be submitted. While the basic content requirements of the 510(k) (21 CFR 807.87) will remain the same, this type of submission should also reference the already cleared 510(k) number and contain a declaration of conformity with design control requirements. Refer to http://www.fda.gov/cdrh/ode/parad510.html for the contents of a "Special 510(k): Device Modification" form with a declaration of conformity to design controls.

Abbreviated 510(k)

Device manufacturers may choose to submit an abbreviated 510(k) when (1) guidance documents exist, (2) a special control has been established, or (3) the FDA has recognized a relevant consensus standard. An abbreviated 510(k) submission must include the required elements identified in 21 CFR 807.87. In addition, manufacturers submitting an abbreviated 510(k) that relies on a guidance document or special controls should include a summary report that describes how the guidance document or special controls were used during device development and testing. The summary report should include information regarding the manufacturer's efforts to conform to the guidance document or special controls and should outline any deviations. Persons submitting an abbreviated 510(k) that relies on a recognized standard should provide the necessary information and a declaration of conformity to the recognized standard. Such persons should also refer to the agency's guidance entitled "Guidance on the Recognition and Use of Consensus Standards." While abbreviated submissions will compete with traditional 510(k) submissions, it is anticipated that their review will be more efficient than that of traditional submissions.

In an abbreviated 510(k), a manufacturer will also have the option of using a third party to assess conformance with the recognized standard. Under this scenario, the third party will perform a conformance assessment to the standard for the device manufacturer and should provide the manufacturer with a statement to this effect. Like a special 510(k), the application should include a declaration of conformity signed by the manufacturer, while the statement from the third party should be maintained in the device master record (DMR) pursuant to the Quality System Regulation. Responsibility for conformance with the recognized standard, however, rests with the manufacturer, not the third party.

The incentive for manufacturers to elect to provide summary reports on the use of guidance documents or special controls or declarations of conformity to recognized standards will be an expedited review of their submissions.

De Novo

This provision, which is referred to as the evaluation of automatic Class III designation provision (also known as *de novo* or risk-based classification), is intended to apply to low-risk products that have been classified as Class III because they were found not substantially equivalent (NSE) to any identifiable predicate device.

Under this provision, within 30 days of receiving a not substantially equivalent determination (which places the device into Class III), the person receiving the classification order may request that a risk-based classification determination be made for the device. The request must provide a description of the device and detailed information and reasons for any recommended classification. FDA will then classify the device.

Not later than 60 days after the date of the submission of such a request, the FDA must make a classification determination by written order, placing the device into one of the three statutory device classes. A device placed into Class I or II in this written order can then be commercially distributed. A device classified into Class III may not be marketed based on the classification order and will require an approved PMA or completed product development protocol (PDP) before commercial distribution can commence. Any clinical studies performed with a Class III device must be performed in accordance with an investigational device exemption (IDE). A device classified into Class I or II under this provision becomes a predicate device for future premarket notification submissions, which means that any manufacturer may show that a new device is substantially equivalent to this predicate.

Product Development Protocol

In the product development protocol (PDP) method for gaining marketing approval, the clinical evaluation of a device and the development of necessary information for marketing approval are merged into one regulatory mechanism. Ideal candidates for the PDP process are those devices in which the technology is well established in industry. The PDP process provides the manufacturer with the advantage of predictability once the agreement has been reached with the FDA.

The PDP allows a sponsor to come to early agreement with the FDA as to what would be done to demonstrate the safety and effectiveness of a new device. Early interaction in the development cycle of a device allows a sponsor to address the concerns of the FDA before expensive and time-consuming resources are expended.

The PDP is essentially a contract that describes the agreed-upon details of design and development activities, the outputs of these activities, and acceptance criteria for these outputs. It establishes reporting milestones that convey important data to the FDA as they are generated, where they can be reviewed and responded to in a timely manner. The sponsor would be able to execute its PDP at its own pace, keeping the FDA informed of its progress with these milestone reports. A PDP that has been declared completed by the FDA is considered to have an approved premarket approval.

Humanitarian Use Device/Humanitarian Device Exemption

The regulation provides for the submission of a humanitarian device exemption (HDE) application, which is similar in both form and content to a premarket approval application, but is exempt from the effectiveness requirements of a PMA. An HDE application is not required to contain the results of scientifically valid clinical investigations demonstrating that the device is effective for its intended purpose. The application, however, must contain sufficient information for the FDA to determine that the device does not pose an unreasonable or significant risk of illness or injury, and that the probable benefit to health outweighs the risk of injury or illness from its use, taking into account the probable risks and benefits of currently available devices or alternative forms of treatment. Additionally, the applicant must demonstrate that no comparable devices are available to treat or diagnose the disease or condition, and that they could not otherwise bring the device to market.

An approved HDE authorizes marketing of the humanitarian use device (HUD). However, an HUD may only be used after institutional review board (IRB) approval has been obtained for the use of the device for the FDA-approved indication. The labeling for an HUD must state that the device is a humanitarian use device and that although the device is authorized by federal law, the effectiveness of the device for the specific indication has not been demonstrated.

- The above discussion on special considerations and methodology applies only in exceptional circumstances.

GOOD QUALITY AND PROCEDURAL PRACTICES

Quality System Regulations (QSR)

The current good manufacturing practice (GMP, or sometimes referred to as cGMP) requirements set forth in the Quality System Regulation (QSR) require that domestic or foreign manufacturers have a quality system for the design, manufacture, packaging, labeling, storage, installation, and servicing of finished medical devices intended for commercial distribution in the U.S. The regulation requires that various specifications and controls be established for devices, that devices be designed under a quality system to meet these specification, that devices be manufactured under a quality system, that finished devices meet these specifications, that devices be correctly installed, checked, and serviced, that quality data be analyzed to identify and correct quality problems, and that complaints be processed.

Thus, the QSR helps ensure that medical devices are safe and effective for their intended use. The Food and Drug Administration monitors device problem data and inspects the operations and records of device developers and manufacturers to determine compliance with the GMP requirements in the QSR. The QSR is contained in Title 21 CFR 820. The "Good

Manufacturing Practice (GMP)/Quality System Regulation" page has a link to the *Medical Device Quality Systems Manual: A Small Entity Compliance Guide*, which details the requirements of the new QSR and provides detailed guidance in the following areas.

Quality System Inspection Technique (QSIT)

The guide was prepared by the FDA Office of Regulatory Affairs (ORA) and the Center for Devices and Radiological Health (CDRH). It provides guidance to the FDA field staff for inspecting medical device manufacturers against the Quality System Regulation (21 CFR 820) and related regulations. It serves as a guide for a company to prepare for a site inspection by the FDA. Field investigators may conduct an efficient and effective comprehensive inspection using this guidance material, which will help them focus on key elements of a firm's quality system.

This process for inspections is based on a top-down approach to inspecting. The subsystem approach is designed to provide the key objectives that can help determine a firm's state of compliance. The process was designed to account for the time constraints placed on field investigators when performing device quality system inspections.

Good Clinical Practice

Good clinical practice (GCP) is a standard for the design, conduct, performance, monitoring, auditing, recording, analysis, and reporting of clinical trials. It is comprised of the regulations and requirements that must be complied with while conducting a clinical study. Specifically, these regulations apply to the manufacturers, sponsors, clinical investigators, institutional review boards, and medical devices. The primary regulations that govern the conduct of clinical studies are included in Title 21 of the Code of Federal Regulations (21 CFR):

- **21 CFR 812**, "Investigational Device Exemptions," covers the procedures for the conduct of clinical studies with medical devices, including application, responsibilities of sponsors and investigators, labeling, records, and reports.
- **21 CFR 50**, "Protection of Human Subjects," provides the requirements and general elements of informed consent.
- **21 CFR 56**, "Institutional Review Boards," covers the procedures and responsibilities for an IRB that approves clinical investigations protocols.
- **21 CFR 54**, "Financial Disclosure by Clinical Investigators," covers the disclosure of financial compensation to clinical investigators that are part of the FDA's assessment of the reliability of the clinical data.

21 CFR 820 Subpart C, "Design Controls of the Quality System Regulation," provides the requirement for procedures to control the design of the device in order to ensure that the specified design requirements are met.

Good Laboratory Practices

Good laboratory practices (GLP) under 21 CFR 58 apply to nonclinical laboratory studies (safety studies) that are intended to support applications for research and marketing permits, including investigational device exemption and premarket approval applications. Compliance with this part is intended to ensure the quality and integrity of safety data obtained from studies such as animal studies submitted to the FDA.

If information on nonclinical laboratory studies is provided in the IDE application as part of the report of prior investigations, a statement that all such studies have been conducted in compliance with applicable requirements in the good laboratory practice regulations in Part 58 must be provided. If any study was not conducted in compliance with the GLP regulations, a brief statement of the reason for the noncompliance must be provided.

Regulations

21 CFR 58, "Good Laboratory Practice for Non-clinical Laboratory Studies," http://www.accessdata.fda.gov/scripts/cdrh/cfdocs/cfcfr/showCFR.cfm/CFRPart=58.

Preclinical Studies

Preclinical studies are conducted primarily for safety purposes, although they can show effectiveness in a nonclinical setting. There are two major categories of preclinical studies: *in vitro* (bench top) and *in vivo* (animal model or cadavers). *In vitro* studies can utilize excised tissue and organs, or just use simulated equipment to demonstrate effects. *In vivo* studies may either be GLP or non-GLP.

There is a third type of study, which is not utilized very often but is still allowed to demonstrate safety: non-IDE, outside-the-U.S. human studies. As may be seen from introductory section above, every country has its own regulatory requirements.

- This section is the most important for demonstrating that a device has been designed to be effective and safe. It also describes procedures that will ensure continued good quality, reliability, and cost-effectiveness (good quality is free).

SUMMARY OF TITLE 21 OF THE CODE OF FEDERAL REGULATIONS, PARTS 800 TO 1299, FOR MEDICAL DEVICES

Note: This summary is intended only as an overview since only highlights of the sections have been discussed. Answers to specific questions and detailed information should be obtained directly from Title 21 of the CFR, or online at http://www.fda.gov/cdrh.

Part 800: General Requirements

This part of the CFR describes requirements for specific medical devices (Subpart B) and administrative practices and procedures (Subpart C).

Subpart A: Reserved for the FDA's future use
Subpart B: Requirements for specific medical devices
1. Contact lens solutions
2. Patient examination gloves and surgical gloves, sample plans and test method for leakage defects (due to great demand for examination and surgical gloves)

Subpart C: Administrative practices and procedures
Administrative detention of device that is considered altered or mishandled during an FDA audit:
1. A written detention order is given that the devices are not used, moved, or tampered with during the detention period (maximum 20 days unless extended). A detention order may be appealed and a hearing requested. Records of the detention order and the release must be retained by the company for at least 2 years.

Part 801: Labeling

Subpart A: General provisions
1. Name and place of business or manufacturer, packer, or distributor. The name shall be qualified by a phrase that describes the connection with the device, such as "manufactured for," "distributed by," or any other expression of the facts.
2. Similar phrases may be used, such as "indication" or "intended for" to describe the intended use. *Caution*: Any representation of a device to be used for something other than its approved intended use, including misleading statements, is considered misbranding and may result in recall and fines.
3. Directions must be adequate so that a layman can use a device safely and for the purpose for which it was intended, even though the device is intended to be used by a skilled practitioner.

4. Misleading statements can be considered misbranding, a serious offense.
   5. Labeling must be readable. This requirement, as anyone who has struggled to read the fine print on a label can attest, is difficult to fulfill because of all the information that sometimes is required to be added to the labeling. The simplest way to meet this requirement is to have a package insert.
   6. For distribution in the Commonwealth of Puerto Rico, labels must be in Spanish.
   7. The label that is most prominent in an over-the-counter device must display the principal feature of the device in bold.
   8. The most prominent part of the label must report the contents of the package.
Subpart B: Reserved
Subpart C: Labeling requirements for over-the-counter devices
   1. The panel to be displayed, the principal display panel, must be large enough to accommodate all mandatory information.
   2. The most prominent part of the label must have a statement of identity.
   3. There must be a declaration of net quantity of contents.
   4. The label must contain a warning if the device contains any ozone-depleting substances.
Subpart D: Exemption from adequate direction for use
   Specific direction for use may be exempted from placement on a label if the device requires a unique skill set for use, such as a physician, dentist, or any other licensed practitioner. In that case, the following wording must be applied to the label: "Caution: Federal law restricts this device to sale by or on the order of a healthcare professional (physician, dentist, etc.)."
Subpart E: Other exemptions
   Medical devices, processing, labeling, or repackaging exemptions are discussed.
Subparts F and G: Reserved
Subpart H: Special requirements for specific devices
   Requirements for impact resistant lenses, maximum levels of ozone and chlorofluorocarbon propellants, hearing aids, menstrual tampons, latex, and nature rubber products are discussed.

Part 803: Medical Device Reporting (MDR)

Subpart A: General procedures
   1. Device user facilities, importers, and manufacturers must report to the FDA deaths and serious injuries to which a device has or

may have caused or contributed. Also, files must be established and maintained for adverse events, including device malfunctions. Specific follow-up and summary reports must be submitted to the FDA.
2. These reports must be available to the public.
3. Reports must follow the instructions and format outlined in CFR Sections 803.10 through 803.11. Further instructions concerning reports are contained in CFR Sections 803.12 through 803.19.

Subpart B: Generally applicable requirements for individual adverse event reports
1. Medwatch forms described in Section 803.20 must be used, including reporting codes in CFR Section 803.21.
2. User facilities must submit an MDR report to device manufacture and the FDA within 10 days.
3. Importers must submit reports to the manufacturer and the FDA within 30 days.
4. Manufacturers are required to submit MDR reports to the FDA within 30 days.
5. Manufacturers are required to submit MDRs within 5 days if there are indications (e.g., trend analysis) that necessitate remedial action or if the FDA has made a written request for a 5-day reporting.

Subpart C: User facility reporting requirements
1. The user facility has 10 days to report to the FDA on Form 3500A.
2. Detailed information in Form 3500A is described in CFR Section 803.32 for individual adverse event report data elements.
3. Annual reports must be written and submitted to the FDA.

Subpart D: Importer reporting requirements
1. Importer must file FDA Form 3500A within 30 days of the event.
2. Detailed information needed for Form 3500A is given in CFR Section 803.42.

Subpart E: Manufacturer reporting requirements
1. Manufacturers must file Form 3500A within 30 days.
2. Detailed information is given in CFR Section 803.52.
3. Reports, which require 5 days for notification, are described in Subpart B above.
4. A manufacturer must submit an annual baseline report on FDA Form 3417 or its electronic equivalent.
5. Supplemental reports must be submitted if information was not known or was not available when the initial report was written.
6. Foreign manufacturer: Every foreign manufacturer must designate a U.S. agent to be responsible for reporting MDRs. The manufacturer has 5 days to report a change of the designated agent.

Part 806: Medical Devices: Reports of Corrections and Removals

Subpart A: General provisions
1. Manufacturers and importers must maintain records of all corrections and removals whether they are required to be reported to the FDA or not.
2. Exemptions to reporting requirements that may improve the performance or quality but do not reduce risk to health are listed below:
    - Market withdrawals
    - Routine servicing
    - Stock recoveries

Subpart B: Reports and records
1. Information to be reported is described in Section 806.10 of CFR.
2. Detailed records must be kept of all corrections and removals that need not be reported to the FDA, as well as those that must be reported.
3. All reports that were submitted to the FDA are available to the public after personnel and trade secret information is removed.

Part 807: Establishment Registration and Device Listing for Manufacturer and Individual Importers of Devices

Note: Only frequently addressed definitions are listed here. See CFR 807 for additional definitions.

Subpart A: General provisions
1. **Commercial distribution**: Distribution of any device intended for human use.
2. **Establishment**: Place of business under one management at one general physical location at which a device is manufactured, assembled, or processed.
3. **Manufacturer**: Place where preparation, propagation, compounding, assembly, processing or repackaging, importation, or initiation of specification for manufacturing of a device occurs.
4. **Official correspondent**: Person designated by operator of establishment to correspond with the FDA.
5. **Classification name**: Term used by panel to describe the device.
6. **510(k) summary**: Summary of information regarding safety and effectiveness of device described in 510(k).
7. **510(k) statement**: Statement made in 510(k) that all safety and effectiveness data will be made available within 30 days of the request.

Subpart B: Procedure for device establishment
1. All owners or operators of an establishment, which is not designated exempt (see Subpart B below), engaged in the manufacture of a device intended for human use shall register with the FDA, Form 2891. Annual registration is done with Form 2891A.
2. Listing must be within 30 days of the time of first manufacture, repackaging of the final device design.
3. Initial listing of each device for sale must be done on a separate Form 2892 sheet.
4. Exact information required for registration may be seen in CFR Section 807.35.
5. See Sections 807.26 through 807.37 for discussions on amendments, updating, notification, and inspection of registrations.
6. Establishment or device registration does not in any way denote approval or clearance of the establishment or products.

Subpart C: Registration procedure for foreign device establishments
1. An establishment within any foreign country engaged in manufacturing a medical device for sale in the U.S. must register with the FDA. All information shall be in English.
2. All imported devices must be listed with the FDA. All information shall be in English.
3. Each foreign establishment must appoint a U.S. agent who maintains a place of business in the U.S. Any changes in agent must be reported within 10 days to the FDA.
4. All imported devices must go through appropriate FDA regulation clearances or approvals before sale in the U.S.
5. This restriction does not apply to devices imported for investigative use (IDE; see CFR 812).

Subpart D: Exemptions
Subcontractors, veterinary devices, general-purpose chemical and laboratory equipment, licensed practitioners, and others are exempted per CFR Section 807.65.

Subpart E: Premarket notification procedure (510(k))
1. All devices that require a premarket notification must have one submitted 90 days prior to introduction of it is for commercial distribution. Commercial distribution or sale cannot start until the FDA clears the premarket notification.
2. A device is exempt from premarket notification if it is:
   - Listed by the FDA as an exempt device classification
   - The device was in commercial distribution before May 28, 1976
   - The device requires a premarket approval (PMA)

3. A list of information required in a premarket notification submission is given in CFR Section 807.87. The format of a premarket submission, the content and format of 510(k) summary, and the 510(k) statement are given in Sections 807.90, 807.92, and 807.93, respectively, or can be found on the FDA website.
4. Substantial equivalence to a device already cleared for sale must be demonstrated. Confidentiality of information can be obtained.
5. Any representation that the FDA has approved a 510(k) cleared device is considered misbranding.
6. After the premarket notification is reviewed, the FDA can:
    - Issue an order that the device is substantially equivalent and clear it
    - Issue an order that it is not substantially equivalent
    - Request additional information
    - Advise the applicant that a 510(k) is not necessary

Part 808: Exemptions from Federal Preemption of State and Local Medical Device Requirements

Subpart A: General provisions
   This section contains special provisions governing the regulation of devices by states and localities.
Subpart B: Exemption procedures
   An exemption may only be granted for a requirement that has been enacted by a state.
Subpart C: Listing of specific state and local exemptions
   See CFR Section 808.53 for specific exemptions for different states.

Part 809: *In Vitro* Diagnostic Products for Human Use

Subpart A: General provision
   1. *In vitro* diagnostic products are the reagents, instruments, and systems intended for use in the diagnosis of disease or other conditions.
   2. Product class relates to all products intended for use for a particular determination with common or related use.
Subpart B: Labeling
   1. Labels shall in general state proprietary name and intended use, name and place of business or manufacture, and a warning statement: "For *in vitro* diagnostic use."

2. Labels for reagents shall also state quantity, concentration of reactive ingredients, source for biological material, date of manufacture and required storage conditions, expiration date, lot number, and statement of an observable alteration or degradation of the product.
3. For additional required label information, see CFR 809.10.

Subpart C: Requirements for manufacturers and producers
1. *In vitro* diagnostic products shall be manufactured in accordance with the good manufacturing practice requirements found in the section on Part 820 in this chapter.
2. Analyzed specific reagents (ASRs) are restricted to be sold to:
- *In vitro* diagnostic manufacturers
- Clinical laboratories
    - Facilities where sample testing is performed in a laboratory, using screening tests recognized by the Food and Drug Administration

Part 810: Medical Device Recall Authority

Subpart A: General provisions (definitions)
1. **Cease distribution and notification strategy or mandatory recall strategy**: A planned, specific course of action to be taken by the person named in a cease distribution and notification order or in a mandatory recall order.
2. **Consignee**: Any person or firm that has received, purchased, or used a device that is subject to a cease distribution.
3. **Correction**: Repair, modification, adjustment, relabeling, destruction, or inspection (including patient monitoring) of a device, without its physical removal from its point of use to some other location.
4. **Device user facility**: A hospital, ambulatory surgical facility, nursing home, or outpatient treatment or diagnostic facility that is not a physician's office.
5. **Health professionals**: Practitioners that have a role in using a device for human use.
6. **Reasonable probability**: That it is more likely than not that an event will occur.
7. **Serious, adverse health consequence**: Any significant adverse experience.
8. **Recall**: The correction or removal of a device for human use where the FDA finds that there is a reasonable probability that

the device would cause serious, adverse health consequences or death.
9. **Removal**: The physical removal of a device from its point of use to some other location.

Subpart B: Mandatory medical device recall procedures

Cease distribution and notification order

If, after providing the appropriate person with an opportunity to consult with the agency, the FDA finds that there is a reasonable probability that a device intended for human use would cause serious adverse health consequences or death, the agency may issue a cease distribution and notification order.

Regulatory hearing

1. Any request for a regulatory hearing shall be submitted in writing to the agency employee identified in the order within the time frame specified by the FDA.
2. In lieu of requesting a regulatory hearing under 810.11, the person named in a cease distribution and notification order may submit a written request to the FDA asking that the order be modified or vacated.
3. If a person named in a cease distribution and notification order does not request a regulatory hearing or submit a request for agency review of the order, the FDA shall amend the order to require such a recall.

Cease distribution notification or mandatory recall strategy

The person named in a cease distribution and notification order issued under paragraph 810.10 CFR shall comply with the order and develop a recall strategy that meets all requirements of this section.

Communications concerning a cease distribution and notification or mandatory recall order

1. The person named in a cease distribution and notification order may request termination of the order by submitting a written request to the FDA.
2. The agency will make available to the public in the weekly *FDA Enforcement Report* a descriptive listing of each new mandatory recall.

Part 812: Investigational Device Exemptions

Subpart A: General provisions
1. The purpose of this part is to encourage the discovery and development of useful devices intended for human use.

2. This part applies to all clinical investigations of a device to determine safety and effectiveness.
3. An investigation of a device, other than a significant risk device, may be started by obtaining institutional review board (IRB) approval.
4. A brief explanation of why the device is not a significant risk device must be presented to the IRB.

Definitions
1. **Custom device**: A device that necessarily deviates from devices generally available or from an applicable performance standard or premarket approval requirement and is not offered for commercial distribution through labeling or advertising.
2. **Implant**: A device that is placed into a surgically or naturally formed cavity of the human body.
3. **Institution**: A person, other than an individual, who engages in the conduct of research on subjects or in the delivery of medical services.
4. **Institutional review board** (IRB): Any board, committee, or other group formally designated by an institution to review biomedical research involving subjects and established, operated, and functioning in conformance with CFR 56.
5. **Investigator**: An individual who actually conducts a clinical investigation, i.e., under whose immediate direction the test article is administered or dispensed.
6. **Principal investigator**: An individual who is responsible for designing and coordinating all studies conducted by investigators.
7. **Monitor**: An individual designated by a sponsor or contract research organization to oversee the progress of an investigation.
8. **Noninvasive**: One that does not by design or intention penetrate or pierce the skin, mucous membranes, or body.
9. **Significant risk device**: Investigational device that is intended as an implant, is purported or represented to be for use in supporting or sustaining human life, or presents a potential for serious risk to the health, safety, or welfare of a subject.
10. **Sponsor**: A person who initiates a study, but who does not actually conduct the investigation.
11. **Sponsor-investigator**: An individual who both initiates and actually conducts an investigation.
12. **Transitional device**: A device subject to Section 520(1) of the act, that is, a device that the FDA considered to be a new drug or an antibiotic drug before May 28, 1976.

13. **Unanticipated adverse device effect**: Any serious adverse effect on health or safety, or any life-threatening problem or death caused by, or associated with, a device, or a death that was not previously identified in nature, severity, or degree of incidence in the investigational plan.

Labeling and promotion
1. An investigational device or its immediate package shall bear a label with the following information: the name and place of business and "CAUTION: Investigational device. Limited by Federal (or United States) law to investigational use."
2. Devices for animal research shall bear the label "CAUTION: Device for investigational use in laboratory animals or other tests that do not involve human subjects."
3. A sponsor, investigator, or any person acting for or on behalf of a sponsor or investigator shall not:
    - Promote or test market an investigational device until after the FDA has approved the device for commercial distribution
    - Commercialize an investigational device by charging the subjects or investigators for a device a price larger than that necessary to recover costs of manufacture, research, development, and handling

Address for IDE correspondence
On the outside wrapper of each submission, the purpose of the submission must be stated. For example, an "IDE application," a "supplemental IDE application," or a "correspondence concerning an IDE (or an IDE application)."

Subpart B: Application and Administrative Action
1. A sponsor shall submit an application to the FDA if the sponsor intends to use a significant risk device in an investigation.
2. A sponsor shall not begin an investigation until the FDA has approved the application.

Investigational plan
The investigational plan shall include, in the following order:
- Protocol
- Risk analysis
- Description of device
- Monitoring procedures
- Consent materials
- IRB information
- Other institutions
- Additional records and reports

Report of prior investigations
  1. The report of prior investigations shall include reports of all prior clinical, animal, and laboratory testing of the device and shall be comprehensive and adequate to justify the proposed investigation.
  2. The FDA will notify the sponsor in writing of the date it receives an application. An investigation may not begin until 30 days after the FDA receives the application and approves it.

Supplemental applications
  1. A sponsor must obtain approval of a supplemental application.
  2. A device under clinical investigation may be used in the treatment of patients not in the trial under the provision of a treatment IDE for desperately ill patients.
  3. The FDA will not disclose the existence of an IDE unless its existence has previously been publicly disclosed or acknowledged.

Subpart C: Responsibilities of sponsors
  1. A sponsor is responsible for selecting qualified investigators and providing them with the information they need to conduct the investigation properly, ensuring proper monitoring of the investigation, ensuring that IRB review and approval are obtained, submitting an IDE application to FDA, and ensuring that any reviewing IRB and the FDA are promptly informed of significant new information.
  2. A sponsor shall not begin an investigation or part of an investigation until both an IRB and the FDA have approved the application or supplemental application relating to the investigation or part of an investigation.
  3. A sponsor shall select investigators qualified by training or experience to investigate the device.
  4. A sponsor shall ship investigational devices only to qualified investigators participating in the investigation.
  5. A sponsor shall obtain a signed agreement from each participating investigator.

Subpart D: IRB review and approval
  An IRB shall review and have authority to approve, require modification (to secure approval), or disapprove all investigations.

Subpart E: Responsibilities of investigators
  1. An investigator is responsible for ensuring that an investigation is conducted according to the signed agreement, the investigational plan, and applicable FDA regulations, for protecting the rights, safety, and welfare, and for the control of devices under investigation.

2. If the FDA has information indicating that an investigator has repeatedly or deliberately failed to comply with the requirements of this part, it will furnish the investigator written notice of the matter.

Subpart F: Reserved

Subpart G: Records and Reports

Records

A participating investigator shall maintain accurate, complete, and current records relating to the investigator's participation in an investigation.

Inspections

A sponsor or an investigator who has authority to grant access to a facility shall permit authorized FDA employees to inspect any establishment.

Reports

An investigator shall prepare and submit any of the following applicable reports in a complete, accurate, and timely manner:

Unanticipated adverse device effects

Withdrawal of IRB approval

Progress

Deviations from the investigation

Informed consent from patient

Final report

This part applies to any Class III medical device whether it is new and has not been classified (automatically Class III) or has been designated Class III by the FDA.

Definitions

1. **Master file**: A reference source that a person submits to the FDA. A master file may contain detailed information on a specific manufacturing facility, process, methodology, or component used in the manufacture, processing, or packaging of a medical device.
2. **PMA**: Any premarket approval application for a Class III medical device, including all information submitted with or incorporated by reference therein.
3. **PMA amendment**: Information an applicant submits to the FDA to modify a pending PMA or a pending PMA supplement.
4. **PMA supplement**: A supplemental application to an approved PMA.
5. **Thirty-day PMA supplement**: A supplemental application to an approved PMA in accordance with paragraph 814 39(e).

6. **Serious, adverse health consequences**: Any significant adverse experience, including those that may be either life threatening or involve permanent or long-term injuries.
7. **HDE**: A humane device exemption to a premarket approval.

Confidentiality of data and information in a PMA file

A PMA file includes all data and information submitted with the PMA, any IDE incorporated into the PMA, any PMA supplement, any report, any master file, or any other PMA-related submission and is considered confidential.

Research conducted outside the U.S.

A study conducted outside the U.S. submitted in support of a PMA and conducted under an IDE shall comply with Part 812 (IDE requirements).

Product development protocol (PDP)

A Class III device for which the FDA has declared a product development protocol completed under this chapter will be considered to have an approved PMA. (*Note*: PDP was discussed in the "Special Considerations" section of this chapter.)

Subpart B: Premarket approval application (PMA)

Note: This list contains only important items and is not intended to be exhaustive. Additional information may be obtained from the web address at the end of the section.

1. The applicant or an authorized representative shall sign the PMA.
2. A table of contents that specifies the volume and page number for each item referred to in the table.
3. A summary in sufficient detail that the reader may gain a general understanding of the data and information in the application.
4. A general description of the disease or condition the device will diagnose, treat, prevent, cure, or mitigate, including a description of the patient population for which the device is intended.
5. An explanation of how the device functions and the basic scientific concepts that form the basis for the device.
6. A description of existing alternative practices or procedures for diagnosing, treating, preventing, curing, or mitigating the disease or condition.
7. A brief description of the foreign and U.S. marketing history of the device, if any.
8. An abstract of any information or report described in the PMA.
9. A summary of the nonclinical laboratory studies submitted in the application.
10. A summary of the clinical investigation.
11. Conclusions drawn from the studies.

12. A complete description of:
    - The device
    - Each of the functional components
    - The properties of the device
    - The principles of operation
    - The method used
    - Reference to any performance standard
    - Adequate information to demonstrate how the device meets, or justification of any deviation from any performance standards
    - Any deviation from a voluntary standard
    - A section containing results of the nonclinical laboratory studies with the device, including microbiological, toxicological, immunological, and biocompatibility tests
    - A section containing results of the clinical investigations involving human subjects with the device, including clinical protocols, number of investigators, and subjects per investigator
    - A statement with respect to each study that it was conducted in compliance with the institutional review board regulations
    - A statement that each study was conducted in compliance with Part 812 (IDE section) or Part 814 (PMA section) concerning sponsors of clinical investigations and clinical investigators
    - For a PMA supported solely by data from one investigation, a justification showing that data and other information from a single investigator are sufficient
    - A bibliography of all published reports, whether adverse or supportive, known to the applicant
    - One or more samples of the device and its components
    - Copies of all proposed labeling for the device
    - An environmental assessment
    - A financial certification or disclosure statement
    - Periodical updates of the device's its pending application

The FDA has issued a PMA guidance document to assist the applicant in the arrangement and content of a PMA. This guidance document is available at http://www.fda.gov/cdrh/dsma/pmaman/front.html.

PMA amendments and resubmitted PMAs
- An applicant may amend a pending PMA or PMA supplement to revise existing information or provide additional information.
- After the FDA's approval of a PMA, an applicant shall submit a PMA supplement for review and approval by the FDA before making a change affecting the safety or effectiveness of the device for which the applicant has an approved PMA.

Subpart C: FDA action on a PMA
   Time frames for reviewing a PMA
      Within 180 days of receipt of an application that is accepted for filing, the FDA will review the PMA and, after receiving appropriate FDA advisory committee input, send the applicant a reply.
Subpart D: Administrative review (reserved)
Subpart E: Postapproval requirements
   The FDA may require postapproval requirements as part of the PMA approval.
Subpart F: Reserved
Subpart G: Reserved
Subpart H: HDE amendment and resubmitted HDEs
   If the FDA requests an HDE applicant to submit an HDE amendment and a written response to the FDA's request is not received within 75 days of the date of the request, the FDA will consider the pending HDE or HDE supplement to be withdrawn voluntarily by the applicant.

Part 820: Quality System Regulation

Subpart A: General provision
   1. Current good manufacturing practice (cGMP): Requirements are set forth in this Quality System Regulation (QSR). The requirements in this part govern the methods, facilities, and controls used for the design, manufacture, packaging, labeling, storage, installation and servicing of all finished devices intended for human use.
   2. **Foreign manufacturers**: If a manufacturer who offers devices for import into the U.S. refuses to permit or allow the completion of an FDA inspection of the foreign facility for the purpose of determining compliance with cGMP, then the devices manufactured at that facility are considered adulterated under Section 501(h) of the act.
   3. **Quality system**: Each manufacturer shall establish and maintain a quality system.
Subpart B: Quality system requirements
   Management responsibility
      1. Quality policy: Management with executive responsibility shall establish its policy, objectives, and commitments to quality. Management with executive responsibility shall ensure that the quality policy is understood, implemented, and maintained at all levels of the organization. Specifically, the management shall describe:

- Quality policy
- Organization
- Responsibility and authority
- Resources
- Management representative
- Management review
- Quality planning
- Quality system procedures

2. Each manufacturer shall establish a quality audit procedure and perform audits.
3. Each manufacturer shall have sufficient personnel with necessary education to operate the facility.

Subpart C: Design controls
Design controls must include:
- Design and development planning
- Design input
- Design review
- Design output
- Design verification
- Design validation
- Design transfer
- Design changes
- Design history file

Subpart D: Document controls
Each manufacturer shall establish and maintain a document control function.

Subpart E: Purchasing controls
Each manufacturer shall establish and maintain a purchasing control function.

Subpart F: Identification and traceability
Each manufacturer shall establish and maintain manufacturing traceability.

Subpart G: Production and process controls
The following information must be in place:
- Instruction documents
- Monitoring and process control
- Compliance with specified reference standards or codes
- The qualification of process and process equipment
- Criteria for workmanship that shall be expressed in documented standards
- Production and process changes
- Environmental control
- Personnel records

- Building records
- Equipment records
- Maintenance schedule
- Inspection records
- Adjustment records
- Manufacturing material description
- Automated processes description
- Control of inspection, measuring, and test equipment
- Process validation records

Subpart H: Acceptance activities
- Receiving, in-process, and finished device acceptance logs must be available.
- Acceptance status records must be complete.

Subpart I: Nonconforming product (NCP)
An NCP shall be controlled and isolated.

Subpart J: Corrective and preventive action (CPA)
CPA procedure records must be up-to-date.

Subpart K: Labeling and packaging control
Control must include:
- Label integrity
- Labeling inspection
- Labeling storage
- Labeling operations
- Control number

Subpart L: Handling, storage, distribution, and installation
A procedure must be in place before manufacturing begins.

Subpart M: Records
- Design history file
- Device master record
- Device history record
- Quality system record
- Complaint files

Subpart N: Servicing
If servicing is specified, procedures must be in place.

Subpart O: Statistical techniques
Applicable statistical techniques must be in place to cover:
- Statistical process control
- Sampling plans

Part 821: Medical Device Tracking Requirements

Subpart A: General provisions
- Manufacturer must have a tracking system.

- Manufacturing must define exemptions and variances.
- Serious adverse health consequences must be tracked.
- Life-supporting or life-sustaining device used outside a device user facility must be traceable.

Subpart B: Tracking requirements

A manufacturer of any Class II or III device must track that device in accordance with this part.

A manufacturer of a tracked device shall adopt a method of tracking that allows information to be provided to the FDA within 3 days, with the name, address, and telephone number of the distributor, multiple distributors, or final distributor holding the device for distribution and the location of the device.

Furthermore, within 10 days of a request from the FDA for tracked devices that are intended for use by a single patient over the life of the device, after distribution to or implantation in a patient, the following is required:

1. The lot number, batch number, model number, or serial number of the device
2. The date the device was shipped by the manufacturer
3. The name, address, telephone number, and social security number (if available) of the patient receiving the device
4. The date the device was provided to the patient

Also, a manufacturer of a tracked device shall establish a written standard operating procedure for the collection, maintenance, and auditing of the data.

Subpart C: Additional requirements and responsibilities

A distributor must promptly provide the manufacturer tracking the device with the following information:
- Name and address of the distributor
- Lot number, batch number, model number, or serial number of the device
- Date the device was received
- Person from whom the device was received
- Final distributor, upon sale or other distribution of a tracked device

Subpart D: Records and inspection

Manufacturers, distributors, multiple distributors, and final distributors shall, upon the presentation by an FDA representative of official credentials and the issuance of Form 482, make all records and information required to be collected and maintained under this part, and all records and information related to the events and persons identified in such records, available to FDA personnel. Records under this part shall be maintained for the useful life of each tracked device that is manufactured or distributed.

Part 822: Postmarket Surveillance

Subpart A: General provisions
This part provides procedures and requirements for postmarket surveillance of Class II and III devices that meet any of the following criteria:
1. Failure of the device would be reasonably likely to have serious adverse consequences.
2. The device is intended to be implanted in the human body for more than 1 year.
3. The device is intended to be used outside a user facility to support or sustain life.

Subpart B: Notification
- The FDA will notify in writing the company that is required to conduct postmarketing surveillance.
- If the company does not agree with the surveillance requirements, a review of the order may be requested.

Subpart C: Postmarket surveillance plan
A plan must be submitted within 30 days of the date you receive the postmarket surveillance order. The submission must include the following:
1. Organizational/administrative information
2. Your name and address
3. Generic and trade names of your device
4. Name and address of the contact person for the submission
5. Table of contents identifying the page numbers for each section of the submission
6. Subscription of the device
7. Product codes and a list of all relevant model numbers
8. Indications for use and claims for the device
9. Postmarket surveillance plan

If the company stops marketing the device subject to postmarket surveillance, it must continue to conduct postmarket surveillance in accordance with its approved plan even if it no longer markets the device.

Subpart D: FDA review and action
The FDA will determine whether the surveillance report is complete and notify the company.

Subpart E: Responsibilities of manufacturers
1. If the company changes ownership, the new owners must continue the surveillance plan.

2. If the company goes out of business, the FDA must be notified within 30 days, and the method by which the surveillance is continued should be discussed with the FDA.
3. If the company stops marketing the device subject to postmarket surveillance, it must continue surveillance in accordance with an approved plan.

Subpart F: Waivers and exemptions

Waivers may be requested for any specific requirement.

Subpart G: Records and reports

All correspondence with your investigators or the FDA must be kept for a minimum of 2 years, including:
1. Signed agreements from each of your investigators
2. Your approved postmarket surveillance plan
3. All data collected and analyses conducted in support of your postmarket surveillance plan
4. Any other records that the FDA requires to be maintained by regulation or by order

Part 860: Medical Device Classification Procedures

Subpart A: General
1. **Class I**: The class of devices that are subject to only the general controls.
2. **Class II**: The class of devices that are or eventually will be subject to special controls.
3. **Class III**: The class of devices for which premarket approval is or will be required. A device is in Class III if insufficient information exists to determine that general controls are sufficient to provide reasonable assurance of its safety and effectiveness.

The classification panels, in reviewing evidence concerning the safety and effectiveness of a device, will consider:
- The persons for whose use the device is represented or intended
- The conditions of use for the device
- The probable benefit to health
- The reliability of the device

Subpart B: Classification
1. This subpart sets forth the procedures for the original classification of distribution before May 28, 1976, or is substantially equivalent to a device that was in commercial distribution before that date. Such a device will be Class I (general controls), Class II (special controls), or Class III (premarket approval), depending

upon the level of reasonable assurance of the safety and effectiveness of the device.
2. The commissioner refers the device to the appropriate classification panel.
3. In order to make recommendations to the commissioner on the class of regulatory control (Class I, II, or III) appropriate for the device, the panel reviews the device for safety and effectiveness.
4. Based upon its review of evidence of the safety and effectiveness of the device, and applying the definition of each class, the panel submits to the commissioner a recommendation regarding the classification of the device.
5. The commissioner publishes the panel's recommendation in the *Federal Register*.
6. The classification panel will recommend classification into Class III of any implant or life-supporting or life-sustaining device.

Subpart C: Reclassification
Any petition for reclassification of a device shall include the following:
1. A specification of the type of device
2. A statement of the action requested by the petitioner
3. A completed supplemental data sheet applicable to the device
4. A completed classification questionnaire applicable to the device
5. A statement of the basis for disagreement with the present classification
6. A full statement of the reasons why the device should not be classified into its present classification
7. Representative data and information known by the petitioner that are unfavorable to the petitioner's position
8. If the petition is based upon new information, a summary of the new information

Note: Consultation with the panel is allowed.

Part 861: Procedures for Performance Standards Development

Subpart A: General
1. This part describes the establishment, amendment, and revocation of performance standards applicable to devices intended for human use.
2. The Food and Drub Administration may determine that a performance standard is necessary to provide effectiveness of the device.

In carrying out its duties under this section, the Food and Drug Administration will, to the maximum extent practical:

1. Use personnel, facilities, and other technical support available in other federal agencies
2. Consult with other federal agencies concerned with a standard setting and other nationally or internationally recognized standard-setting entities
3. Invite participation, through conferences, workshops, or other means, by representatives of scientific, professional, industry, or consumer organizations that can make as significant contribution

Any performance standard established under this part will include:
1. Performance characteristics of the device
2. The design, construction, components, ingredients, and properties of the device
3. The manufacturing processes
4. Testing of the device
5. The publication of the results of each test
6. Manufacturer's certification to purchasers that the device conforms to the applicable performance standard.

Subpart B: Procedures for Performance Standards Development and Publication
1. The Food and Drug Administration may accept an existing standard, a proposed standard, or a draft standard.
2. The Food and Drug Administration will establish advisory committees to which the proposed regulations may be referred.

Parts 862 to 1050

These parts describe special requirements for the following devices:

862 Clinical chemistry and clinical toxicology devices
864 Hematology and pathology devices
866 Immunology and microbiology devices
868 Anesthesiology devices
870 Cardiovascular devices
872 Dental devices
874 Ear, nose, and throat devices
876 Gastroenterology–urology devices
878 General and plastic surgery devices
880 General hospital and personal use devices
882 Neurological devices
884 Obstetrical and gynecological devices
886 Orthopedic devices
888 Physical medicine devices

890 Radiology devices
892 Banned devices
898 Performance standard for electrode lead wires and patient cables
900 Mammography
1004 Repurchase, repairs, or replacement of electronic products
1005 Importation of electronic products
1010 Performance standards for electronic products: general
1020 Performance standards for ionizing radiation-emitting products
1030 Performance standards for microwave- and radio frequency-emitting products
1040 Performance standards for light-emitting products
1050 Performance standards for sonic, infrasonic, and ultrasonic radiation-emitting products

ABBREVIATIONS

International and National Standard Abbreviations

AAMI	Association for the Advancement of Medical Instrumentation
ANSI	American National Standards Institute
ASTM	American Society for Testing and Materials
CB	Certified body
IEC	International Electrotechnical Commission
ISO	International Organization of Standardization
NBMed	Notified bodies medical devices

Regulatory Abbreviations

510(k)	Premarket notification
CADx	Computer-aided diagnosis
CAPA	Corrective action/preventative action
CBER	Center for Biologics Evaluation and Research
CDRH	Center for Devices and Radiological Health
CFR	*Code of Federal Regulations*
cGMP	Current good manufacturing practice
CLIA	Clinical laboratory improvement amendments
CMS	Centers for Medicare and Medicaid Services
DEN	Device experience network
DHF	Design history file
DMR	Device master record
DSMICA	Division of Small Manufacturers, International and Consumer Assistance

FDA	Food and Drug Administration
FOI	Freedom of Information Act
GAO	General Accounting Office
GCP	Good clinical practice
GLP	Good laboratory practice
GMP	Good manufacturing practice
GPO	Government Printing Office
HCFA	Health Care Financing Administration
HDE	Humanitarian device exemption
HUD	Humanitarian use device
ID	Intended use
IDE	Investigational Device Exemption
IFU	Instruction for use
IRB	Investigative review board
IVD	*In vitro* diagnostics
MAUDE	Manufacturer and user facility device experience
MDR	Medical device report
NSR	Nonsignificant risk
OCER	Office of Communication, Education, and Radiation Programs
ODE	Office of Device Evaluation
OIVD	Office of *In Vitro* Diagnostic Device Evaluation and Safety
OSEL	Office of Science and Engineering Laboratories (formerly OST)
PDP	Product development protocol
PMA	Premarket approval
QSIT	Guide to Inspections of Quality Systems
QSR	Quality System Regulation
SE	Substantial equivalence
SMDA	Safe Medical Devices Act
SR	Significant risk

11

INTRODUCTION TO BIOCOMPATIBILITY TESTING

Northview Laboratories

CONTENTS

What Is Device Biocompatibility?.. 268
What Are the FDA and EU/ISO Requirements for Biocompatibility
  Testing?... 268
Do I Need Biocompatibility Data? 269
How Do I Determine Which Tests I Need? 270
Should I Test Device Materials, or Only a Composite of the Finished
  Device?... 270
Is GLP Treatment Required for Biocompatibility Testing? 271
Designing Your Biocompatibility Program 271
All About Extracts 272
Sample Preparation 274
Noncontact Devices 277
Biological Tests Methods 280
  Cytotoxicity (Tissue Culture) 280
  Sensitization Assays 284
  Irritation Tests 284
  Acute Systemic Toxicity 285
  Subchronic Toxicity 285
  Genotoxicity 286
  Implantation Tests 286
  Hemocompatibility 287
  Carcinogenesis Bioassay 288
  Reproductive and Developmental Toxicity 288
  Pharmacokinetics 289

Preclinical Safety Testing 289
Histopathology Services 290
Analytical Testing of Biomaterials 290
Material Characterization 291
Extractable Material Characterization 291
Tests on Extracting Media 292
Bulk Material Characterization 292
Surface Characterization 292
References 293
About This Chapter 294
Acknowledgments 294

WHAT IS DEVICE BIOCOMPATIBILITY?

The word *biocompatibility* refers to the interaction between a medical device and the tissues and physiological systems of the patient treated with the device. An evaluation of biocompatibility is one part of the overall safety assessment of a device. Biocompatibility of devices is investigated using analytical chemistry, *in vitro* tests, and animal models. The biocompatibility of a device depends on several factors, including:

- The chemical and physical nature of its component materials
- The types of patient tissue that will be exposed to the device
- The duration of that exposure.

Of course, the primary purpose of a device biocompatibility assessment is to protect patient safety. Manufacturers will also want to consider corporate regulatory goals and compliance risks in planning a biocompatibility testing program. Inevitably, evaluating the biocompatibility of a device is a risk assessment exercise. There is no risk-free device or device material. The goal of device designers is to minimize risk while maximizing benefit to patients.

WHAT ARE THE FDA AND EU/ISO REQUIREMENTS FOR BIOCOMPATIBILITY TESTING?

The best starting point for understanding biocompatibility requirements is ISO 10993, *Biological Evaluation of Medical Devices*. Part 1 of the standard is the "Guidance on Selection of Tests," Part 2 covers animal welfare requirements, and Parts 3 through 19 are guidelines for specific test procedures or other testing-related issues. (A list of the individual sections of ISO 10993 can be found on p. 4.)

Testing strategies that comply with the ISO 10993 family of documents are acceptable in Europe and Asia. In 1995, the Food and Drug Administration (FDA) issued a *Blue Book Memorandum G95-1*, which replaced the Tripartite Guidance (the previous biocompatibility testing standard). The FDA substantially adopted the International Organization of Standardization (ISO) guideline, although in some areas FDA's testing requirements go beyond those of ISO.

The specific ISO test procedures vary slightly from the U.S. Pharmacoepia (USP) procedures historically used for FDA submissions. The ISO procedures tend to be more stringent, so companies planning to register their product in both Europe and the U.S. should follow ISO test methods. FDA requirements should be verified since additional testing may be needed. Japanese procedures for sample preparation and testing are slightly different from either USP or ISO tests.

Northview highly recommends discussing your proposed biocompatibility testing plan with an FDA reviewer before initiating testing.

DO I NEED BIOCOMPATIBILITY DATA?

Biocompatibility data of one kind or another is almost always required for devices that have significant tissue contact. Refer to the flowchart from ISO 10993-1 to help determine if your device needs biocompatibility testing.

Most commonly, companies arrange for their own biocompatibility studies. You may be able to reduce the amount of testing you will need on a specific device if you have some or all of the following types of biocompatibility data:

1. **Data from previous submissions**: If data are available from a previous submission, consider the following points as you apply the data to your current device. You will need to perform confirmatory testing if there are significant changes in any of these areas:
   a. Materials selection
   b. Manufacturing processes
   c. Chemical composition of materials
   d. Nature of patient contact
   e. Sterilization methods
2. **Data from suppliers of materials or components**: If vendor data are used, manufacturers should obtain copies of the original study reports. It is important that the laboratory that generated the reports has an experienced staff, a strong track record of current good manufacturing practice (cGMP) and good laboratory practices (GLP) compliance, and an AAALAC (Association for Assessment and Accreditation of Laboratory Animal Care, www.aaalac.org)

accredited animal science program. Usually manufacturers will want to conduct at least some confirmatory testing of their own (e.g., cytotoxicity and hemocompatibility studies).
3. **Analytical data**: Manufacturers may use analytical data to help demonstrate that a device has a low overall risk or a low risk of producing a given biological effect. Section 18 of ISO 10993, *Chemical Characterization of Materials*, gives some guidance on this process.
4. **Clinical data**: Clinical data can be used to satisfy some biological effects categories from the ISO 10993-1 test selection matrix. The data may come from clinical trials of the device in question, or from clinical experience with predicate devices or devices containing similar components or materials.

HOW DO I DETERMINE WHICH TESTS I NEED?

The core of the ISO standard is confirmation of the fitness of the device for its intended use. The first step in this process is chemical characterization of device components. See page 13 for specifics of such a program.

Biological testing is probably the most critical step in a biocompatibility evaluation. The ISO materials biocompatibility matrix (p. 5) categorizes devices based on the type and duration of body contact. It also presents a list of potential biological effects. For each device category, certain effects must be considered and addressed in the regulatory submission for that device. ISO 10993-1 does not prescribe a specific battery of tests for any particular medical device. Rather, it provides a framework that can be used to design a biocompatibility testing program.

Device designers should generally consult with an experienced device toxicologist and their clinical investigators to determine how best to meet the requirements of the materials biocompatibility matrix. For each biological effect category, the rationale for the testing strategy should be documented. This is especially true when a manufacturer decides not to perform testing for an effect specified by the matrix for the category of devices.

SHOULD I TEST DEVICE MATERIALS, OR ONLY A COMPOSITE OF THE FINISHED DEVICE?

Each component of a device that contacts the patient should be tested according to the ISO standard. In addition, you should definitely conduct testing on the finished device as specified by ISO 10993-1. Generally, the best approach is to:

1. Assemble vendor data on candidate materials.
2. Conduct analytical and *in vitro* screening of materials.

3. Conduct confirmatory testing on a weighted composite sample from the finished device.

There is a risk in testing the finished device without developing data on component materials. If an adverse result occurs, it can be difficult to track down the component that is causing the problem. You may end delaying your regulatory submission while you repeat testing on the individual components.

Screening device materials minimizes this risk. The initial chemical characterization should detect leachable materials that could compromise device safety. Inexpensive nonanimal studies (such as cytotoxicity and hemocompatibility tests) provide an additional screen for material safety. Material screening tests also help ensure that you will not be forced to redesign your device due to biocompatibility test failures. Many manufacturers assemble data on a library of qualified materials used in their products.

Some test procedures do not lend themselves to testing of composite samples. Due to physical limitations, agar overlay or direct contact cytotoxicity tests and implant studies require separate testing of each device component. *For all biocompatibility studies, test samples should be sterilized using the same method as will be used for the finished device.*

IS GLP TREATMENT REQUIRED FOR BIOCOMPATIBILITY TESTING?

All biocompatibility testing should be performed in compliance with good laboratory practice (GLP) regulations (FDA or OECD).

GLP regulations apply to biological safety studies conducted in support of regulatory submissions. They govern all phases of testing, including preparation and approval of study protocols, monitoring tests in progress, and issuance of final reports, as well as facility and study management and the role of the quality assurance unit. GLP treatment is explicitly required for IDE and PMA submissions. FDA reviewers say they strongly prefer GLP treatment for studies supporting 510(k)s.

For European submissions, ISO 10993-1 seems to require GLP treatment, but the wording is somewhat ambiguous. In practice, studies are usually not rejected for lack of GLP treatment. Manufacturers of device components and materials should have their biocompatibility studies done per GLPs so that their clients can use the data in any type of regulatory submission.

DESIGNING YOUR BIOCOMPATIBILITY PROGRAM

Selecting and qualifying materials to be used in medical devices is a complicated and at times overwhelming task. Good judgment is necessary to determine the extent of safety testing required for a given device or material. The more extensive the use of a material, the larger the database necessary to ensure the safety of the patient population. Likewise, the nature and duration of human contact with the device help to determine the type and degree of testing that is needed.

The following sections of this booklet are dedicated to making your testing decisions easier. The flowchart below (Figure 11.1) gives a step-by-step approach aimed at helping you design a biocompatibility testing program that will satisfy FDA or international regulatory agency requirements.

ALL ABOUT EXTRACTS

Medical device biocompatibility problems are most often caused by toxins that leach out of the device into the surrounding tissues or body fluids. So in the laboratory, extracts of device materials are often used in assessing biocompatibility. These extracts are generally prepared using exaggerated conditions of time and temperature to allow a margin of safety over normal physiological conditions.

Analytical extraction studies allow the chemist to identify and quantitate specific leachable moieties. These data can in turn help the device toxicologist or risk assessor determine the worst-case scenario for patient exposure and the risk to patient health.

Extracts are also used in many of the biological tests specified by ISO 10993. Table 11.1 lists the most commonly used extracting media. *For most devices, only saline and vegetable oil extracts are needed.*

Extracts are selected on the basis of the biological environment in which the test material is to be used. A saline extract approximates the aqueous, hydrophilic fluids in the body. It also permits the use of extreme temperatures in preparing the extracts, thus simulating certain sterilization conditions. Tissue culture media may even more closely approximate aqueous body fluids, but cannot be used for high-temperature extractions. Vegetable oils are nonpolar, hydrophobic solvents and simulate the lipid fluids in the body. For technical reasons, dimethyl sulfide (DMSO) extracts are often used in certain genotoxicity and sensitization tests. Alcohol in sodium chloride for injection, USP (SCI) and polyethylene glycol (PEG) should be used only if they approximate the solvent properties of drugs or other materials that will contact the device during its normal use. SCI is a polar or hydrophilic solvent that simulates the aqueous fluids found in the body.

Extraction conditions (temperature and time) should be at least as extreme as any conditions the device or material will encounter during sterilization or clinical use. Generally, you will want to choose the highest extraction temperature that does not melt or fuse the material or cause

Introduction to Biocompatibility Testing ■ 273

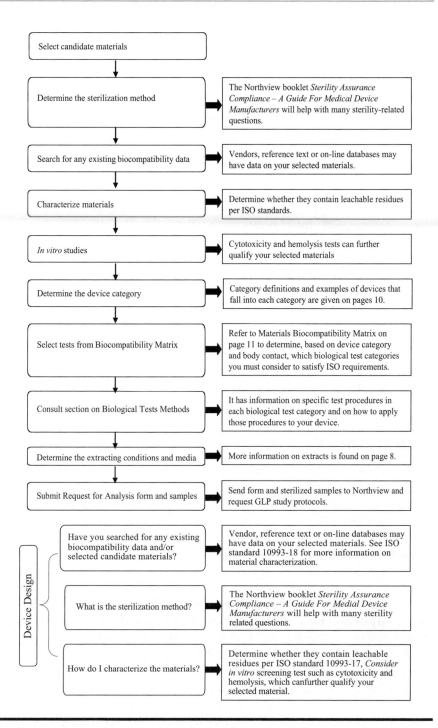

Figure 11.1   Designing your biocompatibility program.

Table 11.1 Extracting Media

Sodium chloride for injection, USP (SCI)
Vegetable oil
1:20 alcohol in SCI
Polyethylene glycol 400 (PEG)
DMSO
Clinically relevant solvents

Table 11.2 Extraction Conditions

37°C for 24 hours
37°C for 72 hours
50°C for 72 hours
70°C for 24 hours
121°C for 1 hour
Other conditions (justification required)

chemical changes. To provide some margin of safety for use conditions, Northview recommends an extraction condition of at least 50°C for 72 hours. For devices that are susceptible to heat, an extraction condition of 37°C for 72 hours may be acceptable. Table 11.2 lists common extraction conditions.

SAMPLE PREPARATION

The simplest method for determining the surface area of a device is usually to use the computer-aided design (CAD) program from the design engineering group. Typically, the surface area can be calculated with a just a few keystrokes. Alternatively, you can calculate the surface area using the equations below. Or you can submit a sample device or engineering drawing to Northview, and our staff will perform the calculations.

Typically, the standard surface area of your device is used to determine the volume of extract needed for each test performed. This area includes the combined area of both sides of the device, but excludes indeterminate surface irregularities. If the surface area cannot be determined due to the configuration of the device, a mass/volume of extracting fluid can be used. In either case, the device is cut into small pieces before extraction to enhance exposure to the extracting media. In some cases, it is not appropriate to cut the device; such devices are tested intact.

The table on page 12 lists the amount of sample required for many procedures. Generally, we recommend using the ratio of sample to extracting media specified in ISO 19993-12 (i.e., 6 or 3 cm^2/ml, depending on the thickness of the test material, or by weight). For some types of materials, the ratio used for USP elastomeric closures for injections (1.25 cm^2/ml) is preferred.

Formulas for Surface Area Calculation

Device Shape	Formula	Device Shape	Formula
Square or rectangle	A = L × W	Solid cylinder (including ends)	A = (OD × π × L) + (2πr^2)
Hollow cylinder	A = (ID + OD) π × L	Triangle	A = (b × h)/2
Disk	A (one side) = πr^2	Sphere	A = 4 × π × r^2
Ellipse	A = (π × X × Y)/4	Trapezoid	A = (h × [p + q])/2
Regular polygon	A = (b × h × n)/2	Circular ring	4π^{2}R$_r$r$_c$

Note: A = surface area; ID = inner diameter; OD = outer diameter; L = length; W = width; R = radius; R$_R$ = ring radius (circular ring); r$_c$ = cross section radius (circular ring); X, Y = longest and shortest distances through the center of an ellipse; π = 3.14; h = height; b = base length; p, q = length of the parallel sides of a trapezoid; n = number of sides of a polygon; r$_o$ = 1/2 OD; r$_i$ = 1/2 ID.

ISO 10993: Biological Evaluation of Medical Devices

Part	Topic
	Listing of Individual Parts
1	Evaluation and Testing
2	Animal Welfare Requirements
3	Tests for Genotoxicty, Carcinogenicity, and Reproductive Toxicity
4	Selection of Tests for Interactions with Blood
5	Tests for Cytotoxicity: *In Vitro* Methods
6	Tests for Local Effects after Implantation
7	Ethylene Oxide Sterilization Residuals
8	Selection and Qualification of Reference Materials for Biological Test
9	Framework for Identification and Quantification of Potential Degradation Products
10	Test for Irritation and Sensitization
11	Test for Systemic Toxicity
12	Sample Preparation and Reference Materials
13	Identification and Quantification of Degradation Products from Polymers

Continued

ISO 10993: Biological Evaluation of Medical Devices (Continued)

Part	Topic
	Listing of Individual Parts
14	Identification and Quantification of Degradation Products from Ceramics
15	Identification and Quantification of Degradation Products from Coated and Uncoated Metals and Alloys
16	Toxicokinetic Study Design for Degradation Products and Leachables
17	Establishment of Allowable Limits for Leachable Substances

Device Categories: Definitions and Examples

Device Categories		Examples
Surface device	Skin	Devices that contact intact skin surfaces only. Examples include electrodes, external prostheses, fixation tapes, compression bandages, and monitors of various types.
	Mucous membrane	Devices communicating with intact mucosal membranes. Examples include contact lenses, urinary catheters, intravaginal and intraintestinal devices (stomach tubes, sigmoidoscopes, colonoscopes, gastroscopes), endotracheal tubes, bronchoscopes, dental prostheses, orthodontic devices, and IUDs.
	Breached or compromised surfaces	Devices that contact breached or otherwise compromised external body surfaces. Examples include ulcer, burn and granulation tissue dressings or healing devices, and occlusive patches.
External communicating device	Blood path, indirect	Devices that contact the blood path at one point and serve as a conduit for entry into the vascular system. Examples include solution administration sets, extension sets, transfer sets, and blood administration sets.

Continued

Device Categories: Definitions and Examples (Continued)

Device Categories		Examples
	Tissue/bone/ dentin communicating	Devices communicating with tissue, bone, and pulp/dentin system. Examples include laparoscopes, arthroscopes, draining systems, dental cements, dental filling materials, and skin staples. Devices that contact internal tissues (rather than blood contact devices). Examples include many surgical instruments and accessories.
	Circulating blood	Devices that contact circulating blood. Examples include intravascular catheters, temporary pacemaker electrodes, oxygenators, extracorporeal oxygenator tubing and accessories, hemoadsorbents, and immunoadsorbents.
Implant device	Tissue/bone	Devices principally contacting bone. Examples include orthopedic pins, plates, replacement joints, bone prostheses, cements, and intraosseous devices. Devices principally contacting tissue and tissues fluid. Examples include pacemakers, drug supply devices, neuromuscular sensors and stimulators, replacement tendons, breast implants, artificial larynxes, subperiosteal implants, and ligation clips.
	Blood	Devices principally contacting blood. Examples include pacemaker electrodes, artificial arteriovenous fistulae, heart valves, vascular grafts and stents, internal drug delivery catheters, and ventricular assist devices.

NONCONTACT DEVICES

These are devices that do not contact the patient's body directly or indirectly. Examples include *in vitro* diagnostic devices. Regulatory agencies rarely require biocompatibility testing for such devices.

278 ■ The Medical Device R&D Handbook

ISO Materials Biocompatibility Matrix

Medical Device Categorization by			Biological Effect												
Nature of Body Contact			Initial Evaluation Tests								Supplementary Evaluation Tests				
Category	Contact	Contact Duration*	Cytotoxicity	Sensitization	Irritation or Intracutaneous Reactivity	Systemic Toxicity (Acute)	Subacute and Subchronic Toxicity	Genotoxicity	Implantation	Hemocompatibility	Chronic Toxicity	Carcinogenicity	Reproductive/ Developmental	Biodegradation[c]
Surface Device	Skin	A	•	•	•									
		B	•	•	•									
		C	•	•	•									
	Mucosal membrane	A	•	•	•									
		B	•	•	•	F	F	•	F					
		C	•	•	•	F	F	•	F		F			
	Breached or compromised surface	A	•	•	•	F								
		B	•	•	•	F	F	•	F					
		C	•	•	•	F	F	•	F		F			

External communicating device	Blood path, indirect	A	•	•	•	•	•					
		B	•	•	F	•	•	F		•	•	
		C	•	•	•	•	•	•	F	•	•	
	Tissue/bone/dentin[a]	A	•	•	F	•	•	F				
		B	•	•	•	•	•	•	•	•		
		C	•	•	•	•	•	•	•	•	F	
	Circulating blood	A	•	•	•	•	•	•	F[b]	•	•	
		B	•	•	•	•	•	•	•	•	•	
		C	•	•	•	•	•	•	•	•	•	
Implant device	Tissue/bone	A	•	•	F	F	•					
		B	•	•	•	•	•	•	•			
		C	•	•	•	•	•	•	•			
	Blood	A	•	•	•	•	•	•	•	•	•	
		B	•	•	•	•	•	•	•	•	•	
		C	•		•	•	•	•	•	•	•	

Note: This table is only a framework for the development of an assessment program for your device and is not a checklist. Bullet = ISO evaluation tests for consideration. F = additional tests that may be required for U.S. submissions.

* A = Limited (≤24 hours), B = Prolonged (24 hours–30 days), and C = Permanent (> 30 days).
[a] Tissue includes tissue fluids and subcutaneous spaces.
[b] For all devices used in extracorporeal circuits.
[c] Depends on specific nature of the device and its component materials.

Consult with the FDA before performing any biocompatibility testing if you are submitting an IDE or you have a device/drug combination.

BIOLOGICAL TESTS METHODS

The following sections describe some of the specific procedures recommended for biocompatibility testing. This listing does not imply that all procedures are necessary for any given device, nor does it indicate that these are the only available tests.

Cytotoxicity (Tissue Culture)

Cell culture assays are used to assess the biocompatibility of a material or extract through the use of isolated cells *in vitro*. These techniques are useful in evaluating the toxicity or irritancy potential of materials and chemicals. They provide an excellent way to screen materials prior to *in vivo* tests.

There are three cytotoxicity tests commonly used for medical devices. The *direct contact* procedure is recommended for low-density materials, such as contact lens polymers. In this method, a piece of test material is placed directly onto cells growing on culture medium. The cells are then incubated. During incubation, leachable chemicals in the test material can diffuse into the culture medium and contact the cell layer. Reactivity of the test sample is indicated by malformation, degeneration, and lysis of cells around the test material.

The *agar diffusion* assay is appropriate for high-density materials, such as elastomeric closures. In this method, a thin layer of nutrient-supplemented agar is placed over the cultured cells. The test material (or an extract of the test material dried on filter paper) is placed on top of the agar layer and the cells are incubated. A zone of malformed, degenerative, or lysed cells under and around the test material indicates cytotoxicity.

The *MEM elution* assay uses different extracting media and extraction conditions to test devices according to actual use conditions or to exaggerate those conditions. Extracts can be titrated to yield a semiquantitative measurement of cytotoxicity. After preparation, the extracts are transferred onto a layer of cells and incubated. Following incubation, the cells are examined microscopically for malformation, degeneration, and lysis of the cells. (See p. 3 for more information on the selection of extracting media and conditions.) At least one type of cytotoxicity test should be performed on each component of any device.

Test Turnaround Time and Sample Requirements

Requirement	Test Name	Sample Amount[a]			Turnaround (weeks)
		Surface Area (cm²)	Weight (g or ml)		
Cytotoxicity	USP agar overlay	1 cm² × 2 pieces	2		1–3
	USP MEM elution	1 cm² × 2 pieces			
	USP direct contact	60[b]			
	ISO agar overlay	1 cm² × 3 pieces			
	ISO MEM elution	1 cm² × 3 pieces			
	ISO direct contact	60[b]			
Sensitization	Murine local lymph node assay (LLNA)	120 cm²			4–5
	Maximization test	240[b]	16		6–8
	Closed-patch test	NA	50		8–10
Irritation	USP intracutaneous test	60[b]	4		2–3
	ISO intracutaneous test	60[b]	4		
	ISO dermal irritation	60[b]	10		2–4
	FHSA primary skin irritation	NA	10		
	ISO ocular irritation	60[b]	10		4–10
	FHSA primary eye irritation	NA	10		
	Mucous membrane irritation	60[b]	Varies		Varies
	Human skin irritation	NA	0.2 g or 0.4 ml		2–4
Systemic toxicity	USP systemic injection test	60[b]	4		3
	Material-mediated pyrogen test	10 devices	4		2–3

Continued

Test Turnaround Time and Sample Requirements (Continued)

Requirement	Test Name	Sample Amount[a]			Turnaround (weeks)
		Surface Area (cm^2)	Weight (g or ml)		
Subchronic (14–180 days)	Intraperitoneal test	12 devices	55		6–7
	Intravenous test	12 devices			Varies
	Implant tests	d			Varies
	Other procedures	Varies	Varies		Varies
Genotoxicity	Ames test	120[b]	8		5
	Mouse lymphoma assay	900[b]	60		10
	Mouse micronucleus assay	120[b]	8		11
	Chromosomal aberration test	120[b]	8		15
Implantation	Implantation test	15 strips, 1 × 10 mm			
	Acute, 7 days				3
	Subchronic, 14–180 days				4–26
	Chronic, >180 days				54
	Histopathology	NA			3–4
Hemocompatibility	Hemolysis, direct contact (duplicate)	NA	2		2
	Hemolysis, direct contact (triplicate)	3 devices	6		2
	Hemolysis, sample extract (duplicate)	120[b]	NA		2
	Hemolysis, sample extract (triplicate)	3 devices	NA		2

		6- to 2 1/2-inch-long pieces	10–12
	In vivo thrombogenicity		
	In vitro platelet aggregation assay	150[b]	10	4–6
	In vitro hemocompatibility assay	150[b]	10	4–6
	PTT, PT	60[b]	4	4–6
	Complement activation	60[b]	2	4–6
Chronic	Long-term implant	Inquire		Inquire
	Lifetime toxicity	Inquire		Inquire
Carcinogenesis	Lifetime toxicity	Inquire		Inquire
Analytical tests	USP physicochemical tests	720	NA	2
	Infrared scan	5 × 1 cm (minutes)	NA	2
	Other procedures	Inquire		Inquire

FHSA = Federal Hazardous Substances Act, MEM = mammalian cell culture medium, PT = prothrombin time, PTT = partial thromboplastin time.

[a] Sample requirements based on surface area calculations. The weight of the device may be used if the surface area cannot be calculated.
[b] Double these amounts for materials <0.5 mm in thickness.
[c] Depends on duration of implant.
[d] Fifteen strips per time point, each strip 1 × 10 mm; sample should be supplied by sponsor in specified size, separately packaged and sterilized, and ends should be smooth and rounded.

Sensitization Assays

Sensitization studies help to determine whether a material contains chemicals that cause adverse local or systemic effects after repeated or prolonged exposure. These allergic or hypersensitivity reactions involve immunologic mechanisms. Studies to determine sensitization potential may be performed using either specific chemicals from the test material, the test material itself, or, most often, extracts of the test material. The materials biocompatibility matrix recommends sensitization testing for all classes of medical devices.

The *guinea pig maximization test* (Magnusson–Kligman method) is recommended for devices that will have externally communicating or internal contact with the body or body fluids. In this study the test material is mixed with complete Freund's adjuvant (CFA) to enhance the skin sensitization response.

The *closed-patch test* involves multiple topical doses and is recommended only for devices that will contact unbroken skin only.

The *murine local lymph node assay* (LLNA) determines the quantitative increase in lymphocytes in response to a sensitizer. If a molecule acts as a skin sensitizer, it will induce the epidermal Langherhans cells to transport the allergen to the draining lymph nodes, which in turn causes T-lymphocytes to proliferate and differentiate. *From an animal welfare perspective, this test is preferable to the guinea pig maximization test or the closed-patch test.*

Irritation Tests

These tests estimate the local irritation potential of devices, materials, or extracts using sites such as skin or mucous membranes, usually in an animal model. The route of exposure (skin, eye, mucosa) and duration of contact should be analogous to the anticipated clinical use of the device, but it is often prudent to exaggerate exposure conditions somewhat to establish a margin of safety for patients.

In the *intracutaneous test*, extracts of the test material and blanks are injected intradermally. The injection sites are scored for erythema and edema (redness and swelling). This procedure is recommended for devices that will have externally communicating or internal contact with the body or body fluids. It reliably detects the potential for local irritation due to chemicals that may be extracted from a biomaterial.

The *primary skin irritation* test should be considered for topical devices that have external contact with intact or breached skin. In this procedure, the test material or an extract is applied directly to intact and abraded sites on the skin of a rabbit. After a 24-hour exposure, the material is removed and the sites are scored for erythema and edema.

Mucous membrane irritation tests are recommended for devices that will have externally communicating contact with intact natural channels or tissues. These studies often use extracts rather than the material itself. Some common procedures include vaginal, cheek pouch, and eye irritation studies. (See p. 3 for more information on extracts.)

Acute Systemic Toxicity

By using extracts of the device or device material, the *acute systemic toxicity* test detects leachables that produce systemic (as opposed to local) toxic effects. The extracts of the test material and negative control blanks are injected into mice (intravenously or intraperitoneally, depending on the extracting media). The mice are observed for toxic signs just after injection and at four other time points. The materials biocompatibility matrix recommends this test for all blood contact devices. It may also be appropriate for any other device that contacts internal tissues.

The *material-mediated pyrogen* test evaluates the potential of a material to cause a pyrogenic response, or fever, when introduced into the blood. Lot release testing for pyrogenicity is done *in vitro* using the *bacterial endotoxin* (limulus amebocyte lystate [LAL]) test. It must be validated for each device or material. However, for assessing biocompatibility, the rabbit pyrogen test is preferred. The rabbit test, in addition to detecting bacterial endotoxins, is sensitive to material-mediated pyrogens that may be found in test materials or extracts.

Subchronic Toxicity

Tests for *subchronic toxicity* are used to determine potentially harmful effects from longer-term or multiple exposures to test materials or extracts during a period of up to 10% of the total lifespan of the test animal (e.g., up to 90 days in rats). Actual use conditions of a medical device need to be taken into account when selecting an animal model for subchronic toxicity. Appropriate animal models are determined on a case-by-case basis.

Northview offers two standard protocols for subchronic testing that are appropriate for many devices. Both are done in mice. One uses *intraperitoneal* administration of an extract of the device or device material. The other uses an *intravenous* route of administration. Implant tests are often performed at different durations appropriate to assess subchronic toxicity of devices and device materials.

Subchronic tests are required for all permanent devices and should be considered for those with prolonged contact with internal tissues.

Genotoxicity

Genotoxicity evaluations use a set of *in vitro* and *in vivo* tests to detect mutagens, substances that can directly or indirectly induce genetic damage directly through a variety of mechanisms. This damage can occur in either somatic or germline cells, increasing the risk of cancer or inheritable defects. A strong correlation exists between mutagenicity and carcinogenicity.

Genotoxic effects fall into one of three categories: point mutations along a strand of DNA, damage to the overall structure of the DNA, or damage to the structure of the chromosome (which contains the DNA). A variety of tests have been developed to determine if damage has occurred at any of these levels. These assays complement one another and are performed as a battery.

The most common test for mutagenicity, the *Ames test*, detects point mutations by employing several strains of the bacteria *Salmonella typhimurium*, which have been selected for their sensitivity to mutagens. The mouse lymphoma and hypoxanthine guanine phosphoribosyl transferase (HGPRT) assays are common procedures using mammalian cells to detect point mutations. The *mouse lymphoma* assay is also able to detect clastogenic lesions in genes (chromosome damage). Assays for DNA damage and repair include both *in vitro* and *in vivo* unscheduled DNA synthesis (UDS). Cytogenetic assays allow direct observation of chromosome damage. There are both *in vitro* and *in vivo* methods, including the *chromosomal aberration* and the *mouse micronucleus* assays. ISO/ANSI 10993-1 specifies an assessment of genotoxic potential for permanent devices and for those with prolonged contact (>24 hours) with internal tissues and blood. Extracorporeal devices with limited contact (<24 hours) may require a genotoxicity evaluation. Generally, devices with long-term exposure require an Ames test and two *in vivo* methods, usually the chromosomal aberration and mouse micronucleus tests. Devices with less critical body contact may be able to be tested using only the Ames test.

When selecting a battery of genotoxicity tests, you should consider the requirements of the specific regulatory agency where your submission will be made. Because of the high cost of genotoxicity testing, Northview strongly recommends that you consult your FDA reviewer *before* you authorize testing.

Implantation Tests

Implant studies are used to determine the biocompatibility of medical devices or biomaterials that directly contact living tissue other than skin (e.g., sutures, surgical ligating clips, implantable devices, etc.). These tests can evaluate devices that, in clinical use, are intended to be implanted for either short-term or long-term periods. Implantation techniques may be used to evaluate both absorbable and nonabsorbable materials. To provide a reasonable assessment of safety, the implant study should closely approximate the intended clinical use.

The dynamics of biochemical exchange and cellular and immunologic responses may be assessed in implantation studies, especially through the use of histopathology. Histopathological analysis of implant sites greatly increases the amount of information obtained from these studies. More information on histopathology service is available on page 11.

Hemocompatibility

Materials used in blood contacting devices (e.g., intravenous catheters, hemodialysis sets, blood transfusion sets, vascular prostheses) must be characterized for blood compatibility to establish their safety. In practice, all materials are to some degree incompatible with blood because they can either disrupt the blood cells (hemolysis) or activate the coagulation pathways (thrombogenicity) or the complement system.

The *hemolysis assay* is recommended for all devices or device materials except those that contact only intact skin or mucous membranes. This test measures the damage to red blood cells when they are exposed to materials or their extracts, and compares it to positive and negative controls.

Coagulation assays measure the effect of the test article on human blood coagulation time. They are recommended for all devices with blood contact. The *prothrombin time assay* (PT) is a general screening test for the detection of coagulation abnormalities in the extrinsic pathway. The most common test *for thrombogenicity* is the *in vivo* method. For devices unsuitable to this test method, ISO 10993-4 requires tests in each of four categories: coagulation, platelets, hematology, and the complement system.

Complement activation testing is recommended for implant devices with contact with circulatory blood. This *in vitro* assay measures complement activation in human plasma as a result of exposure of the plasma to the test article or an extract. The measure of complement actuation indicates whether a test article is capable of inducing a complement-induced inflammatory immune response in humans.

Other blood compatibility tests and specific *in vivo* studies may be required to complete the assessment of material–blood interactions, especially to meet ISO requirements.

Devices or Device Components That Contact Circulating Blood and the Categories of Appropriate Testing: External Communicating Devices

Device Examples	Test Category				
	Thrombosis	Coagulation	Platelets	Hematology	Complement System
Atherectomy devices				x[a]	
Blood monitors	x			x[a]	
Blood storage and administration equipment, blood collection devices, extension sets		x	x	x[a]	
Extracorporeal membrane oxygenator systems, hemodialysis/hemofiltration equipment, percutaneous circulatory support devices	x	x	x	x	x
Catheters, guidewires, intravascular endoscopes, intravascular ultrasound, laser systems, retrograde coronary perfusion catheters	x	x		x[a]	
Cell savers		x	x	x[a]	
Devices for absorption of specific substances from blood		x	x	x	x
Donor and therapeutic apheresis equipment		x	x	x	x

[a] Hemolysis testing only.

Carcinogenesis Bioassay

These assays are used to determine the tumorigenic potential of test materials or extracts from either a single or multiple exposures over a period consisting of the total lifespan of the test system (e.g., 2 years for rat, 18 months for mouse, or 7 years for dog). Carcinogenicity testing of devices is expensive, highly problematic, and controversial. Manufacturers can almost always negotiate an alternative to full-scale carcinogenicity testing of their devices.

Reproductive and Developmental Toxicity

These studies evaluate the potential effects of test materials or extracts on fertility, reproductive function, and prenatal and early postnatal development. They are often required for devices with permanent contact with internal tissue.

Devices or Device Components That Contact Circulating Blood and the Categories of Appropriate Testing: Implant Devices

Device Examples	Thrombosis	Coagulation	Platelets	Hematology	Complement System
Annuloplasty rings, mechanical heart valves	x			x[a]	
Intra-aortic balloon pumps	x	x	x	x	x
Total artificial hearts, ventricular-assist devices	x			x	
Embolization devices				x[a]	
Endovascular grafts	x			x[a]	
Implantable defibrillators and cardioverters	x			x[a]	
Pacemaker leads	x			x[a]	
Leukocyte removal filter		x	x	x[a]	
Prosthetic (synthetic) vascular grafts and patches, including arteriovenous shunts	x			x[a]	
Stents	x			x[a]	
Tissue heart valves	x			x[a]	
Tissue vascular grafts and patches, including arteriovenous shunts	x			x[a]	
Vena cava filters	x			x[a]	

[a] Hemolysis testing only.

Pharmacokinetics

Pharmacokinetic (PK) or ADME (absorption/distribution/metabolism/excretion) studies are used to investigate the metabolic processes of absorption, distribution, biotransformation, and elimination of toxic leachables and potential degradation products from test materials or extracts. They are especially appropriate for bioabsorbable materials. Our teams of dedicated toxicologists are happy to work with you in setting up the appropriate PK or ADME study for your compound.

Preclinical Safety Testing

The objectives of preclinical safety studies are to define pharmacological and toxicological effects not only prior to initiation of human studies, but throughout clinical development. Both *in vitro* and *in vivo* studies can contribute to this characterization.

Histopathology Services

Implant studies are often the most meaningful evaluation of device biocompatibility. The test material is placed in direct contact with living tissue. After an appropriate period, the implant site is recovered and examined microscopically for tissue reactions. The histopathologist can detect and describe many types of tissue and immune system reactions.

Similarly, in subchronic and chronic studies, various organs and tissues are harvested at necropsy and evaluated microscopically for toxic effects. Many of these studies also call for clinical chemistry analysis of specimens or serum samples from the test animals.

ANALYTICAL TESTING OF BIOMATERIALS

Analytical procedures provide another means to investigate the biocompatibility of medical device materials. Studies of extractables will help manufacturers assess the risks of *in vivo* reactivity. Accurate characterization of device materials and their extractable components helps preclude subsequent toxicology problems with finished devices. Increasingly, the FDA has been asking for analytical characterization of device materials and potential leachables (per ISO 10993-17). Many firms also use analytical procedures for routine quality control (QC) of raw materials or finished products.

The steps below can be used to plan a program for analytical testing of a device or device material:

1. List all raw materials, known impurities, and processing agents. Consider unreacted monomers, oligomers, coloring agents, antioxidants, plasticizers, slip agents, and inhibitors.
2. List possible leachables, including reaction and degradation products.
3. Calculate theoretical upper limits for patient exposure to these chemicals.
4. Conduct a literature search on potential toxic effects of leachables.
5. Design extraction protocols based on worst-case exposure assumptions. Exhaustive extraction or long-term extraction at physiological conditions is recommended.
6. Plan analytical strategy and choose analytical methods. Check to be sure that detection limits are appropriate.

MATERIAL CHARACTERIZATION

In the very near future the use of chemical characterization of materials to establish biocompatibility will become essential with the goal to identify and quantify the chemical constituents of a material to help establish its biocompatibility.

Testing of medical devices is a risk assessment exercise beginning with the identification and quantification of chemicals in your device.

Consideration of the chemical characterization of the materials from which medical devices are made is a necessary first step in assessing the biological safety of the device. It is also important in judging equivalence of a proposed material to a clinically established material and a prototype device to a final device.

The degree of chemical characterization required should reflect the nature and duration of the clinical exposure and should be determined based on the data necessary to evaluate the biological safety of the device. It will also depend on the nature of the materials used, e.g., liquids, gels, polymers, metals, ceramics, composites, or biologically sourced material.

The information generated from chemical characterization can be used for a range of important applications, some of which are listed below:

1. As part of an assessment of the overall biological safety of a medical device
2. Measurement of the level of any leachable substance in a medical device in order to allow the assessment of compliance with the allowable limit derived for that substance from health-based risk assessment
3. Judging equivalence of a proposed material to a clinically established material
4. Judging equivalence of a final device to a prototype device to check the relevance of data on the latter to be used to support the assessment of the former
5. Screening of potential new materials for suitability in a medical device for a proposed clinical application.

Extractable Material Characterization

- USP physicochemical tests: plastics
- USP physicochemical test panel for elastomeric closures for injections
- USP polyethylene containers tests: heavy metals and nonvolatile residues

- Indirect food additives and polymers extractables (21 CFR 177)
- Sterilant residues: ethylene oxide, ethylene chlorohydrin, ethylene glycol
- Metals determination by atomic absorption spectroscopy
  - Extractable metals
  - Total metal content
- Nonroutine characterization of organic extractable material
  - Ultraviolet/visible spectroscopy
  - Gas chromatography
  - Liquid chromatography
  - Gravimetry
  - Protein assay
  - Infrared spectroscopy

Tests on Extracting Media

- Total organic carbon (TOC)
- Organic solvent residues
- Nonvolatile residues

Bulk Material Characterization

- Infrared spectroscopy analysis for identity and estimation of gross composition
- Transmission spectroscopy
- Differential scanning calorimetry
- Thermogravimetric analysis (TGA)

Surface Characterization

- Infrared (IR) reflectance spectroscopy
- Scanning electron microscopy (SEM)
- Energy-dispersive x-ray analysis (EDX)

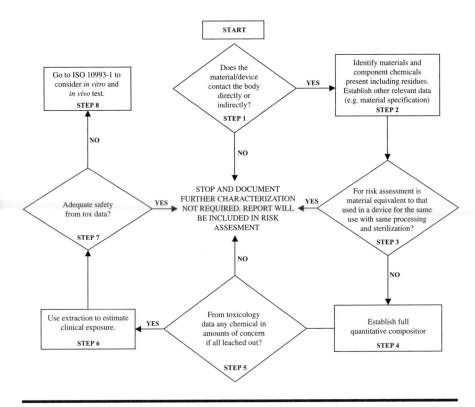

Figure 11.2 Flowchart summarizing the stepwise generation and use of chemical characterization data in risk assessment.

REFERENCES

AAMI Standards and Recommended Practices, Vol. 4, *Biological Evaluation of Medical Devices*, which includes AAMI/ANSI/ISO 10993. (Annex B of 10993-1 is an extensive bibliography of U.S. and international reference documents.)

ASTM F-748-98, *Practice for Selecting Generic Biological Test Methods for Materials and Devices*.

Stark, Nancy J., *Biocompatibility Testing and Management*, Clinical Design Group, Chicago, 1994.

ISO Standard 10993, *Biological Evaluation of Medical Devices*, Parts 1–19.

Guidelines for the Intraarticular Prosthetic Knee Ligament (FDA).

PTCA Catheter System Testing Guideline (FDA).

Cox Gad, Shayne, *Safety Evaluation of Medical Devices*, Marcel Dekker, New York, 1977.

USP 1031, *The Biocompatibility of Materials Used in Drug Containers, Medical Devices, and Implants*.

ABOUT THIS CHAPTER

This chapter was adapted from the Northview Laboratories publication *Assessing Biocompatibility* booklet. The regulatory requirements for biocompatibility are changing, and the information in this chapter was current at the time of writing.

Northview may have an updated version available that contains additional and up-to-date information on this subject. Please contact Northview (see below) for the most current version of the booklet, and with questions regarding your specific requirements. The complete version of this booklet includes a number of helpful charts and checklists to help design your biocompatibility testing.

Northview Atlantic
106 Venture Blvd.
Spartanburg, SC 29306
Phone: 864-574-7728

Northview Laboratories
1880 Holste Rd.
Northbrook, IL 60062
Phone: 847-564-8181

Northview Pacific
551 Linus Pauling D.
Hercules, CA 94547
Phone: 510-964-9000
www.northviewlabs.com

ACKNOWLEDGMENTS

The assistance of Tom Spauding, president of Northview Laboratories, and the staff of Northview is gratefully acknowledged for making this chapter available and helping to prepare and edit it.

INTERVIEW WITH THOMAS FOGARTY, M.D.

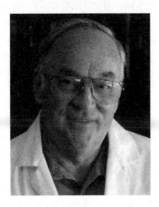

Thomas J. Fogarty, M.D., is a legend in the medical device community. He is a retired vascular surgeon, a highly regarded winemaker,[1] a venture capitalist, and a leading medical technology innovator. He has founded or co-founded more than 30 companies in the medical device or services field, holds more than 100 patents, and is author of more than 170 scientific and medical articles. Dr. Fogarty invented the Fogarty embolectomy catheter while still a medical student and also developed the stent graft that replaced highly invasive open AAA (abdominal aortic aneurysm) surgery.[2] Dr. Fogarty is one of the most successful medical device innovators of all time. He is a recipient of the Laufman-Greatbatch Prize[3] for advances in medical instrumentation and received the MIT-Lemelson Prize for Innovation in 2000.[4] He was inducted into the Inventor's Hall of Fame in December, 2001.[5]

MDR&D: You have been a successful practicing physician as well as a pioneering medical device innovator. Could you tell me about some of the innovations and the companies you've founded?

---

[1] http://www.fogartywinery.com/
[2] http://wwwp.medtronic.com/Newsroom/NewsReleaseDetails.do?itemId=1095281449245&lang=en_US
[3] http://new.aami.org/awards/greatbatch.html
[4] http://web.mit.edu/invent/a-winners/a-fogarty.html
[5] http://www.invent.org/hall_of_fame/162.html

TJF: Yes, I can tell you about a few, but I can't tell you about all. The initial ones were essentially licensing patents. The first was to a company called Edwards, which licensed the first therapeutic balloon catheter. I also licensed a few of the Fogarty clamps, which were the first truly atraumatic vascular clamps. Edwards also had an option to buy a tissue heart valve and had the right to exercise that option in a 6-month period. They chose not to, so I started a company called Hancock Laboratories, where the first successful tissue heart valve reached the marketplace. I became involved with Bentley Laboratories by serving on the board and as a consultant. After that, I got involved in early stage companies.[6]

MDR&D: You often mention the term "clinical utility" as something that should drive a medical innovation. Could you describe the concept of clinical utility?

TJF: I have people interpret clinical utility as something that helps a physician, but more importantly, it should help the patient. Physicians don't always hear the perspective of a patient, but in order for something to have clinical utility, it has to satisfy both patient and doctor.

MDR&D: You have said that an invention and an innovation are not the same thing — that there's a difference between the two.

TJF: Yes, there is. An invention can be an innovation, and an innovation can be an invention. However, you could innovate a service, but not invent it. In other words, you may come up with a different type of service to benefit the patient, but not invent anything. Or you may come up with a technique and an instrument, which is closer to invention than innovation.

MDR&D: So, if somebody says, "I have a great idea."

TJF: It is an idea and nothing else.

MDR&D: And, it doesn't have a lot of value…

TJF: It has zero, unless the idea is implemented.

MDR&D: You have described some of the critical factors to producing medical device innovation such as having an idea of the market, the people, sales and distribution and clinical utility.

TJF: Well that's part of it, but the first thing is recognizing a need. There are certain technologies and inventions to which a physician will say, "Well I don't need that." One has to accept the fact, which is difficult for physicians to do, that they are lacking

---

[6] For more information on these companies see: In Vivo: The Business & Medicine Report, February 2003, http://www.windhover.com/contents/monthly/exex/e_2003800031.htm

because they are intelligent and have been taught to stay out of trouble by doing things the same way to take care of the patient. A lot of doctors have never recognized the need because they are not willing to admit that they are not doing the best job. The same is true of technicians. If you come up with a technology that replaces a technician or replaces a nurse, you're going to have a hard time.

MDR&D: You have also mentioned that it takes different types of people to generate a marketable innovation, such as those who are good at concepts and those who can finish "the last ten percent."

TJF: Yes, the finishers are actually the hardest to find, since engineers are all perfectionists. So there comes a time in an engineer's life where somebody has to stop them because they will go on forever. It's a natural tendency of engineers; the enemy of good is better. So there's a fine balance between when to stop and when not to stop. They have to recognize that even when they put it into the marketplace and it gets clinical use, they're going to have additional work. You cannot anticipate everything; you have to acknowledge that. But, if you're going in the wrong direction, you have to make sure you're going in the wrong direction.

MDR&D: What management techniques do you use to keep up a high pace of innovation?

TJF: I think it's a balance of interfering, but not interfering. You have to intercede at the right time with more encouragement than criticism. Innovation surrounding new companies is not a 9 to 5 job, period. Commitment is critically important and leaders have to create that environment of commitment.

MDR&D: You have described Fogarty Engineering is a "percolator" rather than an "incubator." What is the difference?

TJF: An incubator implies that there's a certain time frame. For a human, it's 9 months. Innovation cannot be scheduled because you cannot create consistently in a time frame. When you say incubate, that means incubate. You cannot do that with innovation. You may work and get there quicker or get there later. With an incubator no matter how you work, it's going to come out in 9 months. That's why I call it a "percolator." You can't always tell when the water is going to boil. There are a lot of things that influence the process.

MDR&D: What does "You have to cannibalize yourself to innovate" mean?

TJF: You have to replace it yourself. If the technology is going to replace something, it's better that you do it yourself. It's kind of like you're in a trap, a steel trap. To get out you have to chew your way out. Unless you do it fast, you aren't going to get there. If you have enough vision and have an interest in it, you can. It's hard to cannibalize yourself, but you have to do it. If you don't do it, somebody else will.

MDR&D: One of the characteristics of your innovations is simplicity. Could you speak to the need for simplicity in medical device design?

TJF: That's because that's the way it is. You usually go through a stage of complexity and then return to simplicity. What helps that is when you prototype, you see the issues with making it yourself. And if you start thinking if I make it this way, will it work? And if I make it simple, will it be accepted by more people?

MDR&D: The person doing the design work should be the one doing the prototyping?

TJF: It doesn't have to be, but that has always worked well for me. If I can't do the prototyping myself, the engineers will and then I'll ask, "Let me see you make that." Then I'll say, "Well maybe I can make it this way." If I change the deployment, the engineer will understand, but he won't understand how a surgeon can use a different technique and achieve the same thing. The first thing that physicians will do, if something doesn't work, is blame the engineer. Then he will immediately want to go back and have the engineer change it. You don't need to always do that; you can change the technique.

MDR&D: Then it's not just the device itself; it's how the physician interacts with the device?

TJF: That's correct.

MDR&D: Are there differences between technology driven products and clinical needs driven products?

TJF: There is a difference. If you have a technology that's complicated, then the manufacturing process is going to be too expensive. If you have something that's complicated in terms of physician use, it's going to be difficult. In other words, if he finds it hard to use, he would rather just do what he always did. Then there are clinical needs. Clinical needs should be first from the patient's perspective, not the specialist's perspective. It may help him do something. It may help him make more money. It may help him take one procedure from another specialty.

MDR&D: I understand that when you first came up with catheter interventions, putting balloons on catheters and putting them in blood vessels, you had a tremendous uphill battle.

TJF: Absolutely. The concept was if you manipulated the inside of a vessel with anything, much less scrape it with a balloon, it was totally inappropriate. When I was a medical student at the University of Cincinnati, the professor of surgery said, "Only one so uninformed and inexperienced would dare do such a thing."

MDR&D: You proved the conventional wisdom was not right.

TJF: Right. The golden rule ain't so golden.

MDR&D: What does the statement "First do no harm" really mean?

TJF: It means that's the obligation of a physician. And you do no harm by doing what you were taught to do and always did. That's why physicians aren't so venturesome.

MDR&D: You have said what doctors say they need, and what they want, and what they'll pay for are three different things.

TJF: They are. Absolutely.

MDR&D: Does "First do no harm" mean "do what you've always done?"

TJF: It doesn't mean that. All physicians interpret that as doing what they've always done and not venturing out into what they haven't done or what is not properly documented by someone's criteria. That someone is usually an academic. And what it does for the patient is a fourth different thing. You should look at what's best for the patient.

MDR&D: That's the way to find a real clinical need and find real clinical utility?

TJF: Hopefully the needs match, but sometimes they don't. In other words what's best for the patient and best for the doctor. If they can be therapeutically better and economically better for both the doctor and the patient, that is a good match.

MDR&D: At a medical technology conference, you talked about the different set of priorities between a university teaching hospital and a community-based hospital.

TJF: Most physicians residing in an academic center are focusing close on what they call science and teaching. And, "oh by the way" we do occasionally take care of real patients representing real pathology. There's a difference between science and technology. Science is the explanation of a theory to prove or disprove the validity of the theory explored. Technology is the application of science that is already proven. You may use the scientific method in documenting the technology and you may use the science of epidemiology and the science of statistics to prove the efficacy of a technology.

MDR&D: You have said that the physician–entrepreneur sometimes gets caught in a trap of conflict of interest.

TJF: It's not sometimes, it's always.

MDR&D: Do doctors have difficulty participating in the clinical evaluation of their own technology due to conflict of interest problems?

TJF: Depending upon the institution. At most academic centers it remains an unresolved problem.

MDR&D: How did the Three Arch Partners venture capital fund start?

TJF: I have always been involved in medical technology. When I say always, by that I mean, I have had exposure to the hospital environment and physicians since age 12. With this familiarity, I became interested in it. I then became an inventor in the field of medical technology and then finished my training in medical technology. I continued to develop devices over these years. Twelve years ago, I took a year off for the purpose of further developing Fogarty Engineering. In that process some venture groups asked me to be a partner. I looked at the opportunity and felt that most venture firms mostly graded theses. I do not want to spend my life grading theses so I started to explore the possibility of creating what I call an entrepreneurial venture group. This in fact had been done in other areas besides medical technology. I had exposure to two young venture capitalists who were members of the same boards of companies I had founded. I asked if they wanted to start a "different" venture group, which they agreed to. They named the partnership Three Arch Partners.

MDR&D: Are there any particular red flags that would keep you from investing in a company?

TJF: If it's offshore or part of it is. Or if the physician/founder/inventor insists on being a CEO. The fourth thing is obvious unawareness of the regulatory and reimbursement issues. There are probably many, many others.

MDR&D: What's more important when you look at a company to invest in? The people or the technology?

TJF: Both.

MDR&D: How do you overcome reimbursement challenges?

TJF: It depends upon the product. And whether or not it's FDA approved, or whether it's in clinical trials. Those sort of challenges aren't consistent. You can actually have a CPT code but have no reimbursement either by a governmental agency, a state, or a national approval or acceptance of payment. Payment and coverage are different. So you could have coverage but no payment.

MDR&D: So there can be a CPT code to cover it but getting the reimbursement from the insurance company is other matter?

TJF: That is correct. FDA approval is not correlated with CMS (Center for Medicare and Medicaid Services). It's quite possible that the whole process will take 8 years at a minimum. The rapid pace of technology will exceed the ability of the regulatory agencies that currently exist to keep up.

MDR&D: Do you see the packaging of products and services together as important to the future of medical device technology?

TJF: It's essential. Not important. It's more than important.

MDR&D: How has the medical device field changed over the last 10 years?

TJF: In 10 years, what has really changed back and forth and what has been inconsistent is the regulatory, the reimbursement, social economics, lifestyle, considerations of safety, and who is considering that — the patient, the consumer, the company, the producer of drugs, and the makers of technology by the way of large device companies. And that's only a small sample. They have changed for worse or for better. It is a serious problem. There has been no semblance of consistency.

MDR&D: What advice would you give to someone who is just getting started in this field?

TJF: If you don't have the capacity to listen to others, including the janitor and your secretary, get out.

MDR&D: What are some of the important clinical needs that you see now that don't have good solutions?

TJF: Sleep apnea, obesity, and all areas of preventive medicine are in critical need of being addressed.

MDR&D: You are unique in the sense that you have four successful careers in parallel, a practicing surgeon, medical device entrepreneur, venture capitalist and winemaker. How do you get them all to work together?

TJF: They're all related. Wine drinking is an extremely valuable preventative medicine. Venture capital is absolutely critical to the progress of technology. Innovation and invention go hand in hand.

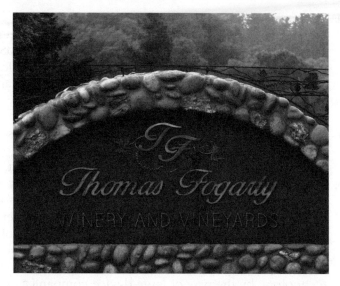

Fogarty Winery is nestled in the Santa Cruz Mountains. (Photo: Ted Kucklick.)

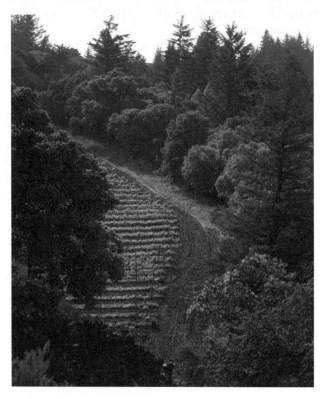

A spectaculular view of the vineyard. (Photo: Ted Kucklick.)

OTHER INTERVIEWS WITH DR. FOGARTY:

Doctors of Invention, *Modern Physician,* July 2004.
Five Questions, *Endovascular Today,* March 2003.
Berlin, Linda, Stanford Doctor to be Honored for Inventions, *San Francisco Chronicle,* October 5, 2001.
Bestard, Nicole, Finding a Better Way, *Gentry,* June, 2003.
Cassack, David, The Inventor's Inventor, *In Vivo,* February 2003.
Fogarty, Thomas J., Physicians as Entrepreneurs, *IEEE Grid,* December 1994 .
Frost, Bob, Leading Questions, *San Jose Mercury News,* October 18, 1998.
Hiltzik, Michael, Medicine's Own Thomas Edison, *Los Angeles Times,* June 5, 2003.
Quinn, Jim, Failure is the Preamble to Success, *American Heritage of Invention and Technology Magazine* Winter 2004.
Roggins, Christine, Transforming Ideas into Products, *Stanford Medicine,* Fall, 2000.
Romano, Michael, *Venture Reporter,* October 15, 2003.
The Stanford Innovators Workbench interview with Thomas J. Fogarty is available on DVD from the Stanford Biodesign Program website at: http://innovatorsworkbench.stanford.edu/store/index.html.

INTERVIEW WITH PAUL YOCK, M.D.

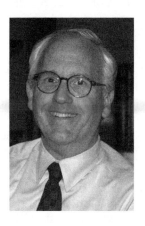

Paul G. Yock, M.D., is the Martha Meier Weiland professor of medicine and professor of mechanical engineering. Dr. Yock is cochair of Stanford's new Department of Bioengineering and director of the Stanford Program in Biodesign. Dr. Yock is a Stanford cardiologist internationally known for his work in inventing, developing, and testing new devices, including the Rapid Exchange™ balloon angioplasty system, which is the dominant angioplasty system in use worldwide. Yock also invented a Doppler-guided hypodermic needle system, the Smart Needle™, and P-D Access™. Dr. Yock is director of the Center for Research in Cardiovascular Interventions, a Stanford facility that develops and tests new technologies in cardiovascular medicine. The focus of Dr. Yock's research program is the field of intravascular ultrasound. He authored the fundamental patents for intravascular ultrasound imaging and founded Cardiovascular Imaging Systems, now a division of Boston Scientific. In 1998 Dr. Yock developed a new interdepartmental and interschool program at Stanford, the Medical Device Network (MDN). Recently MDN has been expanded under Dr. Yock's leadership into a broader research and educational initiative, the Stanford Program in Biodesign. MDN is now BDN, the Biodesign Network. The primary mission of Biodesign is to promote the invention and implementation of new health technologies through interdisciplinary research and education at the frontiers of engineering and the biomedical sciences.[1]

MDR&D: I understand that you are an inventor on least 36 patents.
PGY: I think that's true. I think there are 40-some now.
MDR&D: Some of the inventions are the rapid exchange catheter and intervascular ultrasound. And you're a practicing cardiologist?
PGY: Yes.
MDR&D: Also, professor of medicine, and cochair of the Stanford Bioengineering Department, as well as cofounder with Dr. Peter Fitzgerald of the Center for Research and Cardiovascular intervention, as well as director of the Stanford Biodesign Program.
PGY: Typical academic list of 47 things.
MDR&D: What first inspired you to go into medicine?
PGY: That's a great question. I hadn't thought about that in a long time. My dad was a dentist. And we grew up appreciating the fact that he got great satisfaction from taking care of his patients. But he also told us that medicine had a lot more potential, and he kind of nudged us in that direction. I think it was a combination of those influences with the fact that I love the sciences and I loved the biological sciences in high school and college that pointed me in that direction.
MDR&D: Where did you go to school?
PGY: I went to a public high school in Minnesota. Then I went to Amherst College for undergraduate. And then I spent a couple years at Oxford, mainly studying philosophy, actually. And got a master's there. Then med school at Harvard.
MDR&D: And so from this master's in philosophy, what inspired you to combine an interest in medicine and an interest in philosophy with an interest in engineering and invention?
PGY: From reasonably early on, I just liked design itself. If I had the talent, I think I would've been an architect because I loved designing things as a kid. Not building things so much, but just sort of solving problems, design problems. And as I got into medicine, I just kept doing those things. I remember when I was in college I did a summer research project, and it involved an animal technique that was called *ganztierenfrieren*, which basically means you drop a rat in a vat of liquid nitrogen and they get frozen like that. The reason for doing that was to get a snapshot of a metabolic process, knowing when you anesthetize

---

[1] From http://innovation.stanford.edu/jsp/global/template2.jsp?id=15.

an animal and then sacrifice it, the metabolism changes a lot. So to get a metabolic snapshot, you need to do something quickly.

I designed a device, a little biopsy sucker so that — we were working on kidneys at the time — it froze a section of the kidney rather than freezing the whole animal, and it delivered it in a little vial of liquid nitrogen.

I always had the inclination to design things like that and just kept doing so through college and medical school, internship and residency. Most of the ideas were terrible.

MDR&D: You probably met a lot of people, especially the people you worked with, that you consider to be particularly great innovators and inventors and people who inspired you. Who were some of the most interesting and inspiring people in your opinion in the medical device field?

PGY: I'd start with the people I had the benefit of working with. I did my fellowship in angioplasty with Dr. John Simpson. That was a marvelous opportunity to have mentoring from one of the great people in the field. John actually helped me to get CVIS, Inc., going, which was the first company I was involved with. It was an intervascular ultrasound company. And I've actually thought a lot about what made him so effective as a mentor, because that's something that we're trying to do now with the Biodesign Program at Stanford. And it turns out that it's not easy to be as good a mentor as he is. And I think the thing that makes him so unique is he has a way of making you feel like it's possible to do big things. Just something about being around him makes you believe that you can do it, too. And I think it's partly that he's a folksy sort of guy and a very friendly guy. Lots of people around him have gone on to start companies. I think he just has this aura that causes people to have the motivation and the gumption to do these things.

Tom Fogarty was another big influence for me. Tom actually also helped start CVIS, invested in it, was a director. And I think Tom is the best needs finder that I've ever met in my life. He understands. He has some kind of sixth sense about identifying important clinical needs and needs that have a market attached to them, too. He does that better, faster, clearer than anybody I've ever met. He's brilliant that way.

MDR&D: What are some of the major problems and opportunities you see in medicine?

PGY: A detection of massive events that are about to occur, like stroke, myocardial infarction, early treatment sensing other metabolic processes. Sensing that the early stage of an inflammatory or infectious condition. For example, you've just been seeded with a rhinovirus and can see that you're just starting up that curve, and those technologies will give us some warning about what's happening. That will drive the development of therapies that will hit at the early stage of these diseases. There are huge untapped areas in cardiovascular. We've made minimal progress in congestive heart failure. It is a major epidemiologic problem. Certainly stroke. I mean stroke is appalling the way we treat it now. Atrial fibrillation. Huge problem. We haven't begun to sort it out. Those are some of the areas I would say in cardiology that are worth looking at.

MDR&D: So you see some of those as maybe some of the grand problems in the field?

PGY: Yes. Absolutely. And then I think the other big problem, the biggest of all, the grand-daddy, epidemiologic problem is the whole obesity, metabolic, insulin resistance area — it's enormous. And that's upstream a little bit from heart disease and cerebrovascular disease, but it is in some sense the biggest epidemic that we'll deal with in the next 20 years.

MDR&D: How has the medical device development field changed since you first became involved?

PGY: That's a great question, too. I think in my area, cardiovascular, when I first got involved we were at the early stages of catheter interventions, and there were relatively easy solutions to making procedures better, easier, faster. Those mechanical solutions, the gizmo solutions, are a little harder to come by right now. I'm convinced that they're still out there, they're just not as easy to have. One thing I really want to say is that biologic device convergence is really important. But there are still simple device strategies out there that haven't been thought of that are elegant, simple, and important. And there will always be those things. And you see something come along like vascular closure, for example, that just took characterizing the problem, understanding the problem, and solving it. There are several mechanical solutions to that, which are not terribly difficult to come up with. I think those are all still out there ahead of us; it's just again a question of appreciating the need.

MDR&D: How do you identify and develop a new product idea? One thing that you were saying is understanding the problem better.

PGY: You have to start with a need. And the successful, the effective people in medical technology invention start with a clinical need, and they have the ability to find that need and to characterize it and to understand how important it is. That is more than half of the secret to successful inventing.

MDR&D: Another invention that you're known for is the rapid exchange catheter. Could you describe what this is and how it was developed?

PGY: It is a way that a catheter and a guidewire work together that allows a single operator to perform angioplasty and a single operator to change in and out a catheter over a guidewire. I was a fellow with John Simpson when I was learning angioplasty. At that time we were using over-the-wire angioplasty equipment. What that meant was that you had a catheter that was approximately 3 feet long. In order to keep the place in the coronary artery, you had to have a guidewire that was 10 feet long, 5 or 6 feet of which stuck out of the patient, and there had to be two operators. The guy with the skill and experience was up front moving the catheter up and down, and the flunky, which was me, was at the foot of the bed trying to hold the guidewire in place while the other guy was moving the catheter. You've got a 10-foot-long guidewire, and you're trying to hold it in place where a quarter of an inch matters. You've got a problem with that system, the guy holding the guidewire is always at fault. So I kept being the guy who was screwing up the case. And I couldn't stand that. I said there's got to be a better way to do this that doesn't have this dumb 10-foot-long guidewire. That was my needs statement — I didn't want to be the goat in the procedure anymore. It just occurred to me that there was nothing written that said we had to use an over-the-wire system for the whole length of the catheter. That all we cared about was that it was over the wire inside the artery, and the rest of it didn't have to be over the wire. That was the way that system started. The way I characterize it is that the part of the catheter outside of the guiding catheter in the artery is exactly like an over-the-wire catheter. But back in the guiding catheter, the guidewire exits the catheter so that it functions with a single-operator system with a much shorter guidewire length.

MDR&D: A lot less sterile field problem also.

PGY: Exactly right.

MDR&D: Another intervention you're noted for is intervascular ultrasound. How did this come about and why?

PGY: So that came about because I was around in the early days of atherectomy. And I had just been studying for my cardiology boards, and I happened to know from studying that most plaques in arteries develop on one side of the artery only. The other side is pretty normal. And yet on the angiogram when you get a narrowing it looks like the plaque is all the way around. I got real worried when I saw the directional atherectomy device, the first prototypes, and I said, "Wait a minute. The angiogram is going to teach us to cut around the clock 360°." But for part of that clock we're going to be cutting a normal wall with the atherectomy device. I said, "There's got to be some way of understanding where the plaque is that's better than angiography." I started thinking about techniques that would allow us to look below the surface of the vessel. I had some ultrasound background. It occurred to me that if we could pull it off, ultrasound would be a good way to do that.

MDR&D: I heard that when you went to a certain large company and told them what you wanted, they told you it was impossible.

PGY: It's true that everyone was worried about the fact that we would not be able to make good images, especially when the catheters serve as antennas for noise in the cath lab environment. All the engineers who looked at that problem said there's no way you'll be able to make a clean image with that little tiny transducer at the end of a catheter, the whole catheter serving as an antenna for noise. The cath lab being one of the noisiest electronic environments you can possibly imagine. You've got an unsolvable problem there.

MDR&D: But you did it?

PGY: No, I correct you. The engineers did it. I had the naivete to think that it should be doable and was lucky enough to partner up with some really good engineers who figured out how to do it.

MDR&D: What advice would you give to somebody starting out in the medical device field? What training should they have? What kind of experience? What kind of education? What would make somebody entering the field successful?

PGY: Well, one important thing is that there is a huge breadth of knowledge in medical technology. It spans medicine and areas of engineering. One trap is to educate yourself real broadly but not have an area of deep expertise. My one piece of advice would be as you get your education in preparation for going into medical technology, make sure there is one area, and it can be an area of engineering or it can be an area of medicine, where you are really expert — where you can put yourself up against anybody coming out at the same level of training and hold your own. If that's mechanical engineering, you should really understand the fundamentals of mechanical engineering well, and then have the vocabulary of some medical specialties and so on. But don't trade off that deep expertise in one area because both from a standpoint of companies hiring you and also from the standpoint of your own discipline, and focus, and effectiveness, you need to be an expert. The only way to be a deep expert is to have one area of focus.

MDR&D: What are some of the most common mistakes medical device designers and entrepreneurs make?

PGY: The most common mistake I think by far is to try to develop too complicated a technology. The older I get, the more I appreciate this. At least for procedural technologies, it has to be very simple. It has to be very clean. It has to be easy to learn. Devices that are complicated, demanding, require significant operator training are severely disadvantaged compared to something that's simple. Keep it simple is in my lexicon as rule number one. Another mistake that has nothing to do with technology but is maybe the most common mistake I'm seeing now is not taking into account the regulatory and reimbursement pathways in designing a device. It absolutely doesn't matter anymore if you have the best device in the world if you can't get that paid for. It will not succeed. You need to understand that at the early stages of your design process you need to know what the reimbursement parameters are and what the FDA parameters are. Of those two, reimbursement is actually the more important and the more difficult.

INTERVIEW WITH DANE MILLER, PH.D.

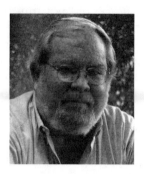

Dane Miller, Ph.D., is president and CEO of Biomet, Inc., a major force in the orthopedics marketplace. From humble beginnings in 1977, Biomet has grown into one of the most respected names in the orthopedics and medical device industries, delivering consistent year-in and year-out double-digit growth. I met with Dr. Miller for this interview at the headquarters of Biomet in Warsaw, IN.

MDR&D: Thank you again, Dane, for this interview. Could you describe how Biomet was founded?

DM: Well, I guess the very starting point was a conversation that Jerry Ferguson and I had in late 1975 when I had made a decision to leave my current employer and Jerry's employer Zimmer, and move to California to join Cutter Biomedical. We talked somewhat facetiously about the prospects of starting a company. By the time we thought about it, I think we realized it was probably impossible. Jerry then called me again in early '77 and said, "Well I think it's time." So we began the planning with a group of people. Ultimately Jerry and I were the only surviving partners and we added Niles Noblet and Ray Harroff and incorporated the company in November of '77, which became our official start date, but began operations in January of '78. Our original plans were to found a company that could utilize the manufacturing support industry here in Warsaw, IN, and we would simply develop and distribute products to the orthopedic market.

MDR&D: Tell me what Biomet has grown into today from those beginnings in 1975 to '77.

DM: At the end of fiscal year 2004, we finished with revenues of about $1.6 billion. That's from first-year sales in 1978 of $17,000.

MDR&D: I understand that you did not run in the black that first year.

DM: No, we operated probably our first 2 or 3 years in the red, expecting as we got our feet planted, got a product line launched, or a series of product lines launched, that we wouldn't be making money. It was probably not until fiscal '81 or '82 that we had much black ink on the bottom line.

MDR&D: What was the founding team's vision when they started as far as the values that you had and the commitment to innovation and service?

DM: Well, we were strong believers that it all starts with people and the way you treat your people; whether they be customers, distributors, or in-house team members. If you treat people with respect and give them the flexibility to sign on to their own job and make their own decisions, ultimately a company can be successful.

MDR&D: You mentioned in Biomet's corporate history book, *From Warsaw to the World*, that one of the things you learned at big companies is how not to do things. What were some of the things that you didn't want to duplicate at your company?

DM: Most importantly, we didn't want to get in the way of creative people doing their jobs. What often happens with bigger companies, and I should point out that I don't think big is necessarily defined by revenues or the number of square feet a company occupies or number of employees or team members. It's more than that. It's a state of mind. We at Biomet work very hard to create an environment and harbor an environment where people can do their best work. For example, I think with some companies when something goes wrong, the political engines begin to run and people start pointing fingers and trying to find blame. The important thing when something goes wrong is what can be learned from it, not a concerted effort to see to it that it never happens again. We look at what was not predicted at the front end that led to the unfortunate outcome and what can be put in the books as a lesson. Too often when something goes wrong, companies write a new policy that prevents that and lots of other things from happening again, instead of learning from it.

MDR&D: So you don't have a policy manual a foot thick at Biomet?

DM: No, we don't. Certainly there are certain things that have to be documented in the form of policies, such as personnel interactions and so forth. But we try to avoid writing a policy every time something happens.

MDR&D: What are Biomet's principles and approach to medical device research and development?

DM: Because of the technical orientation of Biomet's senior management, I think we take a little more of a technical approach than some companies in healthcare medical devices. We don't let the market drive technical decisions, I think, because a number of us have backgrounds in science and engineering. We tend to take a somewhat more disciplined scientific approach to issues.

MDR&D: What do you look for in a product development associate at Biomet? Somebody, say, who comes in as an engineer.

DM: Independence and self-motivation. We don't believe in strong day-to-day or hour-to-hour management. We feel that creative people have to be given the flexibility to take possession of their jobs and do them well. And we look for a self-starter, I guess, as much as anything.

MDR&D: Biomet has had a steady march of double-digit growth each year. How has Biomet been able to maintain this growth?

DM: By retaining the founding principles of the company to maintain an entrepreneurial environment, one where you're continuing to make progress with new products and new technologies. And we also happen to be fortunate that we're in a market that's growing nicely, as well.

MDR&D: There have been some growth stages in the history of Biomet from entrepreneurial start-up; then you've had a middle stage at about the $300 million revenue mark. And then today you're over $1 billion in sales and a worldwide market presence and a worldwide manufacturing presence. What did you need to do at each stage to move the company up to the next level?

DM: I'm not sure they are clearly separable stages. I think the important thing is we looked at what worked yesterday and do more of it today. And we look at what didn't work quite so well yesterday, and do less of it. We have a 26- to 27-year history of operating our business in that way.

MDR&D: Describe how Biomet sees opportunity where others see problems?

DM: I think the challenges are not to get consumed by problems. Not to let a negative approach to dealing with problems get in your way. When things aren't going the way you hoped, the key is to redouble your effort and get by it and move on and not get hung up with your problems.

MDR&D: You've had one situation — when you acquired Lorenz Surgical — in which you actually turned what could have been a real problem into a great opportunity. Could you describe how that happened and what you did to turn that into an opportunity and salvage it from a problem?

DM: Well that was certainly a challenging time. Just a little history of the Lorenz acquisition. We acquired Lorenz, which included a relationship with a German manufacturer, which products made up the vast majority of the Lorenz revenue stream. Not too long after acquiring them we were informed after working very hard to protect and deal carefully with the relationship that they would no longer supply product to us. We did everything humanly possible to harbor a good relationship with the German manufacturer and did not begin manufacturing our own product in-house, such as to create rift in that relationship, only to find the German manufacturer had chosen not to continue shipping us product. As I recollect, we were informed in early November that at the end of that particular calendar year no more orders would be accepted or shipments made to us. And that probably amounted to 80% of our product line or revenue stream at the time from Lorenz. And only a few days later we found that, in fact, the three senior principals at Lorenz were leaving the company to form a new company to distribute those manufacturers' products. So not only did we lose access to the principal supplier for the company, but also we lost senior management at that point. So, we cranked up our ability to manufacture the product back here in Indiana. They're much smaller products than we produced. It required different tooling and different capital equipment, but we unleashed our engineering and manufacturing teams on making sure that there weren't any blanks in product availability, and I think did a pretty good job of showing the sales force, who had been preconditioned to the thought that if Lorenz lost its supplier, the company was in big trouble. In fact, we proved that was not going to be the case.

MDR&D: And you proved it, actually, in a very convincing way at a sales meeting where you showed them an example of what you could pull off.

DM: Yes, we provided them a couple of competitive catalogs and asked the sales force to pick a product, a particular plate design that we had never manufactured, that Lorenz had never man ufactured, and we would unleash our engineering team from late morning to early afternoon and see if they could reverse engineer and produce a product, and do all the design work, all the CNC machining, and CNC programming necessary to make it. By the end of that day we handed the Lorenz sales force a prototype of the product.

MDR&D: How has Biomet dealt with the continuing squeeze in reimbursements for innovative medical technologies in the managed care environment?

DM: We have for many years focused on reimbursement and total cost of treatment in our product development activities. After all, if we can provide a total hip or a total knee that costs an additional $500, but help the hospital deliver that treatment for a thousand dollars less, we've all come out ahead. And that's been the focus of I think most medical device product development in the healthcare field.

MDR&D: So you do start with reimbursement strategy up front?

DM: Absolutely.

MDR&D: And what about the way that the environment has changed under managed care? Ten to 15 years ago the doctors had a lot more leverage and say so over what they could provide. And now much more is being dictated by insurance companies.

DM: I think doctors are signed on to the concept of saving money in ultimate care and treatment of patients. After all, our big challenge going forward is how we're going to provide this expanding group of baby boomers the increased healthcare demands that they're going to place on the system for less money. That is, less money on a per unit basis.

MDR&D: So that's an area where you're seeking out new clinical needs, in that aging baby boomer population?

DM: Absolutely. As the wave of baby boomers reach their retirement and orthopedic care age, which is somewhere in the 55 to 65 age category, we're going to need to figure out more economical and efficient means of treating them.

MDR&D: How does Biomet maintain such a rapid pace of new product introduction?

DM: We don't have the largest R&D group in the industry, but I would have to say I think we have the most efficient R&D team anywhere in the industry. Each of our major divisions funds an R&D operation. And I think they're all as efficient as anybody in those markets.

MDR&D: Your company has a motto: "Driven by Engineering." What does this motto mean?

DM: If you look at the rest of the orthopedic industry, much of senior management comes from either finance and accounting or marketing and sales ranks. Here at Biomet most of our senior management comes from science and engineering ranks. And we think its science and engineering that's driving Biomet's decision making, and not marketing.

MDR&D: I've talked to a number of sales reps, and Biomet is known as one of the best companies in orthopedics to sell for. How have you developed and maintained that reputation and that relationship?

DM: First, we have a very talented distribution system. And we just work hard to deliver what they need, what their customers need. And don't treat them like just a sales force. They're part of the team.

MDR&D: You and your fellow founders seem to be driven by strong principles. What are the sources for these principles and ideals?

DM: Oh, I think it's upbringing as much as anything. I think it's unusual today to look at a group of people in their 50s and 60s who are married to their first wives The company began 27 years ago and we're still married to our first wives.

MDR&D: And maybe a few more toys.

DM: We all have a few more toys and they're a little bigger toys, but we're still the same people we were 27 years ago.

MDR&D: How do you see the development of the combination of biologics and devices? This seems to be an area that Biomet is pioneering in. How do you see the future of biomaterials in orthopedics?

DM: Somewhat oversimplified, I see biomaterials assisting the orthopedic surgeon in doing procedures through needles instead of 6-inch incisions. I think the real advent of minimally invasive surgery, minimally invasive treatment techniques will come through the assistance of biomaterials technology.

MDR&D: And you personally got involved in biomaterials testing early on. Tell me how you personally tested titanium for implants?

DM: I was involved in some preclinical research involving a particular titanium alloy and particular surface treatment. And one afternoon a couple of tornadoes blew through the area, taking out the entire power grid in this county. I couldn't go into my office at work because there wasn't any light. So I called a friend in Fort Wayne and took a small bar of titanium that was designed for animal tests and asked if he would implant it in my arm.

MDR&D: And you kept that in your arm for quite a while?

DM: About 10 years.

MDR&D: So you have firsthand experience with biomaterials testing and trying out titanium. It's like the old story, you didn't just contribute, you got involved.

DM: Yes, as a matter of fact, that piece of titanium came out about 10 years later. We did the histology work, and it looked precisely the way it did when it was implanted 10 years prior. And the tissue response was absolutely minimal. The tissue had grown right up to the implant surface.

MDR&D: If you were a new Ph.D. today or an engineer and you wanted to build the next Biomet, or build a successful innovative medical technology company, how would you go about it, starting today? You just graduated from school.

DM: Well, first make sure you put your formal education behind you and be prepared to start to learn all over again. And second, make sure you never hide behind your education as a shield. Get out there and learn what it takes. Educate yourself beyond what your formal education could ever have provided you. When I started I knew absolutely nothing about stock options or finance, for example. I had to learn all of that.

MDR&D: If you think that your formal education did everything that it needed to do, then that would be a mistake?

DM: Absolutely. Your formal education is only the footing. The rest of it, the rest of the structure, comes through experience.

For more information on the history of Biomet, see Richard Hubbard and Jerry Rodengen's *Biomet: From Warsaw to the World* (Write Stuff Enterprises, Ft. Lauderdale, FL, 2002). This is the official corporate history of Biomet and is available from Biomet.

OTHER INTERVIEWS WITH DANE MILLER

Executive Interview, Knowledge Enterprises *OrthoKnow*, July 2004, www.orthoworld.com.

CEO Says Total Joint Replacement Is the Biggest Growth for Biomet, *The Wall Street Transcript*, January 15, 2004, http://www.twst.com/notes/articles/waj608.html.

Herper, Matthew, Dane Miller: CEO Value to the Bone, Forbes.com, May 8, 2001.

INTERVIEW WITH INGEMAR LUNDQUIST

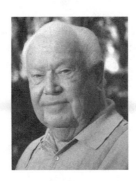

Ingemar Lundquist is a prolific inventor and was one of the early developers of catheters and manufacturing equipment for Advanced Cardiovascular Systems. He developed the indeflator, the standard device for inflating and deflating an angioplasty balloon, and helped develop over-the-wire angioplasty. One of his first successful designs was an automatic postal meter for Friden (now Friden-Alcatel) He was also a pioneer in the design of steerable catheters for EPT, and a cofounder of Vidamed, Inc. His wife, Linda Lundquist, also participated in this interview.

MDR&D: You came here from Sweden with $200 in your pocket. What year was that?

LL: It was 1948 or '49.

MDR&D: You worked on postal meters and you worked on taxi meters and different mechanical things. How did you make the jump from that to medical devices?

IL: My father died of a heart attack. He asked me to develop devices for the medical field at that time. But he was thinking mostly of some means of moving a patient from one bed to another and stuff like that because the nurses had such a hard time moving people within the hospital from one bed to the other.

MDR&D: From your background going from postage meters to catheters and medical devices, what are the practical skills you used, the

	most useful skills that you found translated into developing medical devices.
IL:	My skills as a machinist, basically. And my know-how about the machines used to develop things, like lathes, milling machines, and so forth.
MDR&D:	Did you ever get something right the first time, or did you have to do it several times?
IL:	Well you develop something, you usually don't get it right the first time. You step one little piece at a time to get it eventually the way you want it. You usually don't get that in one shot. It's more than one try.
MDR&D:	So this goes back to your machine shop school that seeing the real thing and holding it in your hands is something that's an essential part of doing product development.
IL:	Definitely. I don't think I could've developed products just on paper. I had to develop them by actually making the products. I could not convince myself on a piece of paper that it worked. So I had to develop it and see how it functioned physically.
MDR&D:	Have you found that using a computer was something that helped you?
IL:	It helped a little bit. The thing that really helped me was developing the prototype so I could see with my own hands and eyes if it worked the way I expected it to.
MDR&D:	What was a typical workday or a workweek like for you, if there was such a thing?
IL:	I don't know if I had a typical workweek. I worked; when I had a project going, I just worked on it all the time usually. I would go to bed and dream about it, so to speak, and wake up the next morning and just continue.
LL:	That's true. You stayed down in the basement working and working and working until he got it finished to another step.
MDR&D:	Would you work on several projects at one time or would you focus on one thing?
IL:	I usually focused on one thing. I didn't spread myself too thin in that respect.
MDR&D:	Do you actually consider yourself an inventor, or do you consider yourself more of an engineer or designer or problem solver?
IL:	I think I would say for myself as an inventor, and a product development engineer.
LL:	Very seldom would he ever mention it to anybody that he had invented.

MDR&D: If you were to, say, define what an invention is, what would you say?
IL: An invention must be something that is different than anybody has developed. An invention is basically a product or a device that is unique and you think you can patent it.
MDR&D: What do you think about the patent process? Is it more difficult to do now than it used to be, or is it easier?
IL: I think it is probably more difficult now because there are more inventions to sort out. It used to be easier. It is quicker now to sort through them because there are more tools available to help you as far as computers and databases.

INTERVIEW WITH
J. CASEY MCGLYNN

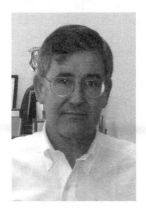

J. Casey McGlynn is one the most experienced attorneys in the medical device industry. Mr. McGlynn is chairman of the Life Sciences Group at Wilson Sonsini Goodrich and Rosati (WSGR) and a nationally recognized leader in the representation of startup and emerging growth companies in the life sciences field. The Life Sciences Group at WSGR offers focused resources and capabilities to meet the most critical needs of startup and emerging growth companies including private and venture capital financings; public offerings; university licensing, strategic collaborations and strategic patent counseling. Mr. McGlynn is a frequent speaker and contributor to magazines and newsletters on issues relating to the life sciences industry, and moderates the annual WSGR Medical Device Conference.[1]

MDR&D: How did you decide to go into law originally and what led you to specialize in the life science area?

JCM: Getting into law was just something I was interested in even as a young kid. It was a goal that I set very early on in my life. But with regard to getting into healthcare law, I knew I was interested in business, and when I interviewed, I interviewed at a number of firms. It turned out that Wilson Sonsini

---

[1] For more information see: http://www.wsgr.com

was in this fantastic place called Silicon Valley. As I interviewed here, I realized it was a unique place, so different from the rest of the world. It was only as I began the practice here that I realized how unique it was. One of the first companies that I incorporated was a company in the healthcare area, and that's really how I began to do things in the life sciences. The first company was called Advanced Cardiovascular Systems. It was incorporated originally as Advanced Catheter Systems, and it became the vascular division of Guidant Corporation. It was first started with angel capital, later funded by venture capitalists and eventually sold to Eli Lilly to form a piece of their medical device business. Eli Lilly spun off its device business and ACS was spun out as part of Guidant Corporation about 10 years ago.

MDR&D: How is practicing corporate law in the life science area different than other areas, for example high-tech electronics?

JCM: The fundamentals of being a good lawyer are much the same. The issues related to financing and public offerings and mergers and acquisitions are similar. What's different is specific market knowledge about the industry and about what goes on in the industry. Concerns that might be different would be: who is interested in investing in this sector, or what percentage should officers and directors get of companies, or how have other companies in similar situations dealt with particular issues? When you come to a fork in the road you may have two choices, both of which might actually be logical choices. If you have a long history in the life sciences area, you'll know what roads other people have taken and in many cases which ones worked out and which ones didn't. Industry specific knowledge is very valuable in the life sciences area. It has allowed me to help clients sort out the business issues they face day to day.

MDR&D: According to a 1997 interview in *Business Week*, Larry Sonsini challenged WSGR to branch out from a concentration in electronics to develop a dominating position in the life science area. According to the article, you took on this challenge and built the WSGR life science practice. Could you tell me about this?

JCM: The firm had a very large practice in life sciences before the life sciences group was formed, but it was a very disparate group. We had several hundred attorneys at that time and everybody had some life science clients. I might have had a bigger practice in the life sciences area at the firm, but there were a number of other attorneys also practicing in the area. One person didn't really know what the others were doing. So the first goal was to figure out what companies WSGR represented. How many of them were there? The next thing was to get people together to begin talking about life sciences. We ran educational programs internally on both the device side and on the biopharmaceutical side. Finally, we began to run an educational program for the industry, aimed at teaching best practices in collaboration, financing, M&A (mergers and acquisitions) regulatory law, and reimbursement.

MDR&D: You took what already existed and organized it?

JCM: That's correct. We did a study. I think we collected 100 key people in the life sciences industry. We hired somebody to go out and interview those people. What came out of that study was that people in the life sciences area really wanted people who were focused on their industry. They didn't want generalists, they wanted specialists that were focused, understood the science, understood some of the quirks in that particular area. That's the feedback we were responding to. We formed an independent group that was just focused on the life sciences.

MDR&D: You were responding to what you saw as a demand and also seeing that the industry had grown large enough to support that sort of an activity?

JCM: We knew it was an important industry, and we had enough clients to form an independent group

MDR&D: Each year Wilson Sonsini produces the WSGR Medical Device Conference. Could you tell me how this conference came to be and how it has grown over the years?

JCM: We run a lot of different conferences. Probably the largest every year is the WSGR Medical Device Conference. It was actually the first industry-specific conference that WSGR organized. It started off to help entrepreneurs understand the critical issues they would face in starting a new business. It was intended as a workshop to help entrepreneurs understand the nuts and bolts in getting a company organized, funded, public, sold, etc. There were probably 100 people, maybe a little bit less the first time we did the event. I think this last year we probably had about 450 people. We've done it for about 12 years now. It has become an annual event where people get together, when they may not have seen each other for a long time, and have an opportunity to talk about what they're doing and what's new in their lives. We feel that a number of really great companies have had their spark or beginnings at that meeting. So we feel that it's been a very useful thing in terms of entrepreneurs and getting new businesses started.

MDR&D: You mentioned before about how Silicon Valley was an exciting place to be and this is where you wanted to be. What do you think makes Silicon Valley tick? What makes it different?

JCM: What I like about Silicon Valley, what I am amazed at, is that I meet a lot of very technically talented people very early in their careers and they are very driven by their vision of how they want to change the world. They are not focused on creating great wealth for themselves but in changing the world. And in many cases obviously they become wealthy. But wealth is not the real driver. And honestly in my early days, when I had a big plate full of electronics companies, I found the people in those industries to be really interesting people with incredible drive. I find there's one additional element in the life sciences area that for me is one of the reasons that I'm still practicing law. It's great to have a great idea, to be passionate about that idea, to create it and to transform the world with it. But the thing about healthcare that's so fantastic is that in the process you are not just transforming the world. You are actually helping save lives, making the world a much better place than it was before you got there. And to me, that is the one thing about the medical device industry, and the biopharmaceutical industry, that is just fantastic. It just makes me feel really great about a lot of the companies that I've had an opportunity in my career to be a part of and help because I know I've indirectly helped a lot of people live longer and healthier lives.

MDR&D: Do you think that Wilson Sonsini as a firm has helped to shape Silicon Valley corporate culture?

JCM: To say we shaped corporate culture would be too egotistical on our part. But we've been a part of the valley from the very beginning. And our goal has always been to service companies from start up through the large multi-national company. Our model is to provide all the services those companies need. Companies need different services at different times. Start-ups need things that are really radically different than a large company like Hewlett Packard might need. The key is to know when to bring those services to bear to help clients move forward and be as successful as they possibly can be. I don't know whether we transformed the valley. That's probably too egotistical, too. But I would say we've definitely been a part of the valley from the very beginning.

MDR&D: How does a life science start up lay a foundation for growth and success?

JCM: I'd say for me when I look at a new opportunity it's about the people and it's about the idea. And those are the two key pieces. It doesn't mean that you have a complete management team on hand on day one. But it means that there is a special person in that organization. It might be an engineer, it might be a scientist, or it might be a doctor that really, really understands the field that he's moving into and really has a vision of what needs to be changed. It's that one change maker, if you will, that's absolutely critical on the people side. And then again it's this product concept. What I have found interesting on the product concept side is that many of the entrepreneurs that have an idea may not have fully crystallized that idea. It's only through networking with a lot of other very talented people in this industry that they're able to really crystallize the right application. So I guess it's really people first. But it has to be an idea that makes some sense, even though it may not be the final crystallized idea.

MDR&D: How does a company change over time from a small entrepreneurial seed stage company through its growth stages and ultimate exit?

JCM: It changes obviously by hiring people. Each person a startup hires has such a profound influence on the culture of that company and also on the company's capabilities. And it's a very expensive process. Every employee is a very expensive addition to an enterprise early on in a company's life. So you really have to pick those people very carefully. For me the companies that turn out to be the best are the ones whose founder or CEO has the passion for real excellence and is very, very focused on making sure he gets the best and the brightest into his organization because those are the people that can really transform a good idea into a great idea or can make a company that has potential to really sing. To me the hiring process is really critical in terms of creating a great organization. When I say people, it's not just the people that the companies hire. It is also the investor that they select. Everybody that you bring into your organization, whether it be service providers like lawyers or accountants, whether it be venture capitalists, whether it be your scientific advisory board, all those people tell about who you are and what kind of company you want to become. So I say, focus on the best and the brightest and make sure that you set a very high standard for yourself because people will judge you by the decisions that you make in terms of creating that organization.

MDR&D: What are some of the biggest mistakes start up companies make?
JCM: It's so interesting because there are so many ways to fail and there's probably only one path to success in a particular given company. In other words, you can make a big mistake by hiring the wrong CEO. You can make a big mistake by raising too much money. You can make a big mistake by getting the wrong venture capitalist associated with your business. You can make a big mistake a lot of other ways. The problem is that every one of these mistakes has a lasting impact on the organization. It's something we can't get rid of for the next 4 or 5 years. There are a lot of different mistakes that entrepreneurs can make that can turn out to be very serious. I'd say some of the biggest problems people have run into were when people underestimated the clinical challenges with regard to products. They thought that they could build it and the product would just be fine. And they weren't rigorous enough with regard to clinical development. We had a lot of failures in the late 1980s and early 1990s because of that kind of problem. I don't think today that clinical failure is nearly as likely as it was 10 or 15 years ago. Today I'd say one of the areas where people can continue to under-appreciate the seriousness of the problem is in reimbursement. This is not an area I would have been talking about 10 or 15 years ago but today it's a very serious issue. It's one of those things that the best companies focus on early. In many cases, though, a company will move forward through development, clinical trials, regulatory approval, and release of the product, and it's only after the product gets into the marketplace that management realizes what a huge problem reimbursement is. So again, I think today reimbursement is one of the biggest challenges for the industry as a whole.
MDR&D: You're saying reimbursement issues could kill a company?
JCM: That's right.
MDR&D: Do you see any solutions to the problems with reimbursements any time in the future?
JCM: Companies need to become more sophisticated about reimbursement. It's really a question of understanding what it takes to get reimbursement and putting that process in place. Maybe collecting additional data in early clinicals and getting peer-reviewed articles published. There's a whole litany of things that can be done to make sure that you'll be able to be reimbursed earlier, but you've got to work on it ahead of time. I think that's the process that we're going through right now. The best managers are more sophisticated and are working on reimbursement

MDR&D: One of the things that is essential for a start up is capital, and it's been said that a good venture capitalist provides more than just money. What else does a good angel or VC provide?

JCM: Today it's almost impossible in my mind to finance a company without venture capital. You have to start with the premise that sooner or later you're going to have venture capitalists in your company. The question is really when do you want to have them? I do think that they bring a lot of experience and a lot of connections. There are a lot of companies out there. When it comes time for people to make decisions, when it comes time for investment bankers to decide which companies they want to take public, or when it comes time for some of the big healthcare companies to decide who they want to acquire, there are a whole bunch of companies in almost every one of the areas. The question is which one are they going to pick? All I can say is you create sign posts with every action you take. One of the signposts is to have a great group of venture capitalists associated with your business. They're going to know the investment bankers and have relationships with them. They're going to know the major healthcare companies and have relationships with them. They're going to be able to make introductions and help you. Those are signposts for both the investment banker and the healthcare company. It makes them look a little bit more closely at your company than they would otherwise look. That allows you to create a company that has a better chance of being successful. I do think that their contacts and relationships are very useful for companies and can increase the probability of success. I'd say the best and the brightest venture capitalists can be very useful and can be very helpful in terms of helping you make decisions, thinking about what actions you want to take based on the things that failed for them in the past and the things that were successful for them in the past. As I always tell my CEOs, it's ultimately up to the CEO to make these decisions. You have to call on the venture folk to get their comments and thoughts, but every fact pattern is different. It's up to the CEOs to evaluate what they are hearing from their venture friends and figure out the right course of action. It's never black and white. It's never "It was this way the last time and therefore it has to be this way." I think the VCs have a lot of good advice and a lot of good connections that could be very useful for CEOs.

earlier. I do think we're getting better at it but it's still one of those issues on which we have a lot of work to do.

MDR&D: You said before that choosing the wrong VC partner can be harmful to a company. How can it be harmful to a company to have a mismatch between a company and a VC?

JCM: I've sat on a lot of boards where the management and the VCs did not get along at all. And it wasn't a question of the company not doing the right things or not trying to build the business, or the CEO not being competent. But it was a situation where it was just incredibly adversarial at the board level. That is a very destructive thing. It's very disheartening for management to try and create value. It's not about being challenged, but it's about being directed or crushed. There are a whole bunch of words we could use. But it can be a very destructive process if the management of an organization and the venture capitalists are really at odds. The venture capitalist can say, "We can change management." as they can, and they can put more money into the company. But these are all sad stories because it takes a long time to fire a CEO and to find a replacement. And it costs a lot of money. And it's just a huge amount of lost time and energy. A lot of the companies that fail, fail because they've got complex personalities inside their organization that are just at loggerheads with each other. So for the CEOs or founders, you have to choose your investors really wisely. And that means you need to really understand who these people are by doing some background checks. If you don't know your investors before the financing, you risk relationships that are destructive.

MDR&D: How does a new company find venture capital? How do you get the partners' attention, and how do you get in front of them to make your pitch?

JCM: Palo Alto and Menlo Park, for example, have a huge number of venture capitalists. So the question really is finding the ones that are interested in your business. If you're a healthcare company, you don't want to go to a fund that's primarily focused on electronics. If you're interested in medical devices, you don't want to end up at a venture capital firm that's primarily focused on doing biotechnology. You need to find somebody that can help you identify who the key players are in your sector. If you happen to have a CEO that's already done it once before, that CEO is probably going to be very knowledgeable and there is not going to be an issue. But if you are a first-time founder of a company, it's going to be important to find somebody who has a huge network of relationships and really knows who these people are, what kinds of deals they've done in the past, and what focus they have so that you can get an idea about who you should go see. So that's the first thing. Now, getting in to see the right people is simple if you work with somebody who has a relationship with them. The venture capitalists are interested in meeting entrepreneurs and seeing new ideas but they've got so many things crossing their desks. The entrepreneur must find some way to help the VC know this is a project they should spend some time on. The key variable is making sure that somebody who has a relationship with that venture fund is the one that's contacting them for you. You can't send an e-mail or a business plan to them without some prior introduction from some third party that actually knows them. The introduction can come from lawyers, from other CEOs, or from other venture capitalists. The network is pretty broad and it's just a question of identifying some people who can help you make those introductions. The next piece, obviously, is getting in there and having a great story to tell. That story involves your background and who you are and why you're unique and why you're a person that somebody should give millions of dollars to, and why your idea is unique and important and something that's going to transform the world. Assume you've got about 30 to 40 minutes in your first meeting in order to convince them that the founders and the ideas are special, not run of the mill. So you need to spend a lot of time on the presentation thinking about what it is you want to cover in that short meeting. You're not going to get a second chance unless you capture their imagination at the first meeting.

MDR&D: Describe the amount of effort it can take for companies that get that first meeting with a VC to finally get to a term sheet?

JCM: It could be as immediate as your first meeting, if you happen to hit the sweet spot for that venture capitalist, if your project is something that the VCs are already interested in, and if you look like the absolute right person to execute on this particular opportunity. And it could be literally less than a month before you have a term sheet from the venture fund. On the other hand it can take a long time. I think at the last WSGR Medical Device Conference Karen Talmadge, the founder of Kyphon, said it took several years during which time she had over 100 meetings before she found a firm that wanted to invest in her company. So it can take a long time, too. Tenacity is a very important attribute of the great entrepreneurs because not everybody is going to see your vision. In the case of Kyphon, obviously, a lot of people said no. And yet today the company is worth over a billion dollars. Fundamentally the product that they're selling today is exactly the product that the founder of Kyphon was talking about at each one of those initial meetings with venture capitalists. The VCs just didn't see the opportunity because it wasn't quite in their sweet spot.

MDR&D: What are some of the elements of a good term sheet?

JCM: First you'd want to be dealing with a first class venture fund that you feel is going to be a real team player and not an adversary in the company building process. And then you want to get the highest valuation reasonable. And after that you need to look at the stylized terms that financings typically have. One of the provisions that we typically see is dividends. Dividends could be cumulative or non-cumulative. We'd like to see them non-cumulative, which means that they are only paid if declared, and these dividends will never be declared for start up companies. So it becomes a benign provision. But if it turns out to be cumulative dividends, then of course that's like having a promissory note with an interest rate. It's going to grow every year. If it has a 9 or 10% dividend rate, you know that in 7 or 8 years they're going to double the value of their investment. It can be a very expensive provision to give in on and something that we wouldn't want to have in a deal.

The next provision and perhaps the most important provision and the most discussed provision is liquidation preference. I'd say today there's going to be a liquidation preference. You're going to be selling preferred stock. The goal would be to just have a 1X liquidation preference without what is called participating preferred. The goal is to make the investor choose between either getting his money back or getting what the founders and other shareholders, the common shareholders, would be getting for a share of the company. Today the venture capitalists are pushing for participating preferred. It may be a full participating preferred, or it may be a participating preferred that's capped at some maximum number. But participating preferred means that investors get their money back before the other common shareholders get anything, and then they participate along with the common shareholders on a share-for-share basis so that in addition to the liquidation preference they get the same thing that the common shareholders would get. So that at the end of the day if the common shareholders got a dollar back, the preferred investor would have gotten that dollar back on his share plus he would have gotten back his initial investment.

There are a lot of other kinds of provisions. There are voting provisions. There are redemption provisions. And I think with each provision, I could go into a lot of detail, but suffice it to say the way I look at term sheets is I ask myself: "Which things are going to cap the wealth creation opportunity for the entrepreneur?" And: "Which things are really there to help minimize the risk for the investor?" I like to look at those things separately. In my mind the more important issues are those that avoid limiting the upside in the wealth creation process for the entrepreneur as opposed to focusing on some of the fears that the venture capitalist might have. To me if things don't go well, there's probably not going to be anything for anybody. But if things do go well, we're going to be dividing up a pie and we want to make sure that we get as fair a deal as possible for the entrepreneur. Those are some of my thoughts with regard to term sheets.

MDR&D: What percentage of ownership can founders expect to retain after seed rounds and VC rounds?

JCM: It's hard to say. And it's all over the place. I would say there is a lot of dilution in companies. So you have to be real smart about building a financing strategy with regard to your company and also making sure that you use capital really efficiently. It's funny, sometimes people brag about how much money they have raised or how much money they raised in this particular round of financing. But it's not about how much money you raise, it's about how far you get on the least amount of money possible with the lowest amount of dilution possible because that's how we create wealth for entrepreneurs. It really has to be a mind set from the very beginning that we're going to try to do this as frugally as possible. That being said, the difference in burn rates between companies is radically different. I mean it's absolutely amazing, if you looked at how lean and mean some companies were and what percent of the company they ended up with. There's a company called Cutera that went public. I think that the founders owned over 50% of the company when it went public last year. They did two rounds of financing before the public offering. Just to give you a sense of how capital efficient they were, they never even dipped into the second round of financing. On the other hand, there are companies that have raised over 100 million dollars privately before they got ready for their public offering. In those cases the founders have obviously been decimated by the dilution that they've suffered and own at most two percent of the company.

So again I think capital efficiency is probably the most important factor once you've gotten your company financed.

MDR&D: On the subject of legal representation strategy, what should a medical device start-up look for when shopping for good legal representation?

JCM: I'd say a couple of things. One, you would like somebody that's very experienced in terms of representing your industry. So in the life sciences area he or she understands the industry, understands who the players are in the industry, has lots and lots of contacts and relationships so that you can use those relationships and contacts for your benefit. I think next you want a law firm that has the capability of solving your problems now and in the future so you don't feel obligated to move later on. When you are a very young company, you are very capital focused. So you want a firm with lots of experience with private financing, corporate partnering, and licensing, as well as patent prosecution. As you get larger there are other problems that you'll face, so you want a firm with public finance, employment law, tax, M&A, FDA, and litigation. Finally I think you want a firm that is responsive and that is very motivated to help you succeed.

MDR&D: Going back to your other statement about capital conservation, how does a company conserve capital with respect to its legal costs? How does it get the best representation and the best services while still conserving capital and preserving its capital efficiency?

JCM: I think that's a great question. The way we typically work with our clients is try to build a team. Because lawyers are very expensive, we have a partner, and an associate, and a paralegal on that team so that the most serious strategic issues can be worked on by somebody who has worked on lots of deals, has lots of great experience, and can help get to the right decision. So that's the first level. The second level is implementation of what might be a term sheet, a letter of intent or whatever. And there I think being able to move it down to a lot less expensive person with adequate supervision will save a huge amount of money for the client. And then finally there are those things that have to get done but are of a mundane nature like preparation of stock certificates or stock option agreements. These can be done by paralegals again at a much lower rate. So the goal is really to find a way to do it as inexpensively as possible. One other way to save money is to work with people who have lots of experience with the work you need done. If you hire experienced people, you're going to get people that don't need to reinvent the wheel when it comes to the next transaction. Those are ways to minimize the cost with regard to lawyers.

MDR&D: How has the financing and business model for the life science company changed since the "class of 1996?"

JCM: In 1996 most of the medtech companies that went public were development stage without an approved product or sales. They projected when they thought they would get regulatory approval and when they would be able to launch their product, and what the product launch would look like. The analysts carefully wrote down all of those promises and worked it into a model, valued the companies and then took them public. The problem was that the performance after that public offering in most cases was pretty dismal. When the companies missed their projections their valuations were slammed. But the companies that we see going public today are companies with real muscle mass. They are companies that have approved products, that have a predictable revenue ramp, and that are approaching profitability. It's a much better place to be if you're going to be public to have products that are in the marketplace, already approved and where you're able to predict with increased accuracy the growth rate with regard to your company. I think those are important variables that have really changed since the "Class of 1996."

MDR&D: How is going public different today with regulations such as Sarbanes-Oxley?

JCM: The actual IPO process has not changed that much, but the liabilities are much more in people's minds today. It's not that there was not significant exposure in the past for management and the board of directors with regard to misstatements of fact in a registration statement. But recently enacted laws, the focus of the SEC on management, and the increases in lawsuits from plaintiffs' attorneys make us all a lot more cautious. We see people being much more concerned, and cautious, with regard to the preparation of the registration statement. Because many of the rules in Sarbanes-Oxley focus on reporting after the public offering, we see companies that have gone public need larger accounting staffs, and a lot more work is being done on verification of the financial information that's being reported to the CFO and then finally to the board of directors and the public. The responsibility of management has really increased. The Ken Lay defense of: "I didn't know it was happening" is no longer available. Because of that there is a lot more emphasis on due diligence and making sure of the accuracy of financial statements in order to avoid liability. So it is a period of increased scrutiny, and, therefore, I think increased anxiety for the management of a public company.

MDR&D: Following up on that, describe the relative advantages of a company being acquired versus going public?

JCM: Selling a company allows management to take the money off the table, walk away, and start a new enterprise a short time later. For the CEO and management it's a great opportunity to cash in and to begin again. In the IPO situation it's not going to be possible for management to cash in and walk away because the world is going to be looking at management to meet the promises it made to the public. And the public is going to be watching all of management's filings so that if you are an active seller into the marketplace, the public is going to wonder why it should be holding your stock. So it is much more difficult for management to find a way to diversify by selling the stock in its company. I will say, however, that some of the biggest and best stories in the medical device industry have been companies that have gone public, have continued as a public entity for 2 or 3 years, built real muscle mass and then sold the company to a large medical device manufacturer. These are some of the largest deals in the industry as opposed to oftentimes smaller deals that get done in a merger and acquisition context prior to a public offering. So it is a complex equation trying to figure out whether or not you want to take your company public, or whether you want to sell it. I would say you need to be opportunistic because you owe your fiduciary duty to your shareholders. And it may be that, for example, you would love to do a merger but that because of the market environment the IPO is really the right thing for you to do for your shareholders.

MDR&D: You have worked with a number of "serial entrepreneurs." What are the qualities of the ones that are really successful, the really great ones?

JCM: I would say they tend to be technically very astute, with vast knowledge about their area of expertise. There's a second category of entrepreneur who is not as technically astute but is a manager as opposed to an engineer, or scientist, or doctor. The manager entrepreneur understands people and markets, and his expertise can supercharge the company.

MDR&D: What advice would you have for someone who is a company founder who has had a great idea, worked hard, executed properly, and has really done well? What do you do after you've "made it?"

JCM: Hopefully, the really successful entrepreneurs will find a way to give back something to the industry. There are a lot of very experienced people interested in helping young entrepreneurs, and I think that's great for our industry and it can be very satisfying for those who do the executive mentoring of the young entrepreneur.

MDR&D: What are some of the exciting medtech areas that you see on the horizon?

JCM: There is a lot going on in orthopedics and in congestive heart failure. There's always a lot going on in the cardiovascular area, and I am also very excited about women's health. It's an area that 10 years ago the first companies with which I was associated turned out not to be that successful. But we've had some incredible successes since then. I also like the aesthetics field. These products are private-pay and don't have reimbursement issues. The aging population has created a real demand for these products.

INDEX

A

AALAC, *see* Association for Assessment and Accreditation of Laboratory Animal Care
Abbreviated 510(k), 238
Abrams' needle, 105
ABS, *see* Acrylonitrile–butadine–styrene
AC, *see* Alternating current
Accredited Persons Program, purpose of, 233
Acetal, 34
ACM, *see* Association for Computing Machinery
ACM Siggraph, 191
Acorn tip catheter, 79
Acrylic, 31, 40
Acrylonitrile–butadine–styrene (ABS), 23, 31, 39
  Magnum®, 38
  medical-grade, 40
  PC/ABS, 40
  stereolithography and, 122
ACS, *see* Advanced Cardiovascular Systems, Inc.
Acuity, 105
Acute systemic toxicity test, 285
Additive object modelers, 116
ADME studies, *see* Adsorption/distribution/metabolism/excretion studies
Adobe Photoshop®, 173, 204, 206
Adsorption/distribution/metabolism/excretion (ADME) studies, 289
Advanced Cardiovascular Systems, Inc. (ACS), 59
Advanced Polymer Corporation, 58
Advanced Polymers, 76, 86

Advanced Surgical Planning Interactive Research Environment (ASPIRE) system, 186
Agar
  cutting needle, 105
  diffusion assay, 280
Albinus, 7, 198
Alias, 138, 189
Alternating current (AC), 13, 14
American Helicopter Association, 133
AMI, *see* Association of Medical Illustrators
Amplatz catheter, 79
Analytical extraction studies, 272
Anatomical atlases, 194
Anatomical Chart Company, 210, 214
Anatomical reconstruction for visualization, 168
Anatomy
  digital reconstruction from, 202
  erroneous understanding of, 198
  first textbooks of, 196
Aneurysm needle, 105
Angiography catheter, 79
Angioplasty industry, plastic balloon catheters for, 59
Angle of rotation, 105
Animal models, 218
Animal Welfare Act, 218
Animation, three-dimensional, 212
Anneal, 106
Anticoring heel blast, 106
Apec®, 41
Aptic Superbones, 189
Arcam AB, 131
Arm probe scanners, 184, 185
Art(s)
  -based industrial design field, 9
  definition of, 6, 9

341

internal conflict, 8
scientific information communicated via, 7
skill applied to aesthetics, 7
ultimate goal of, 8–9
Art for art's sake, 8
Arthroscopy and Medical Equipment International, 188
Artistic anatomy, 215
Aspirating needle, 106
ASPIRE system, see Advanced Surgical Planning Interactive Research Environment system
Association for Assessment and Accreditation of Laboratory Animal Care (AAALAC), 269–270
Association for Computing Machinery (ACM), 191
Association of Medical Illustrators (AMI), 202, 216
Association of Medical Illustrators Sourcebook, 216
ASTM A 967-96, 106
Atherectomy catheter, 79
Atomic absorption spectroscopy, 292
Autocad, 138, 173
Automated fabrication, 116
Automated Fabrication, 156
Automated touch probe scanners, 183
Avid Medical, 110

B

Back bevels, 106
Bacterial endotoxin test, 285
Balloon
  bonding, 77
  catheter, 79
  dip molds, 63
  inflation, hole punching for, 73
Balloon angioplasty
  market for, 10
  pioneering figure in, 83
Balloon blowing
  airflow for, 56
  equipment, 57
  molds, 58
Barex®, 47
Baydur®, 42
Bayer Plastics, 40, 41

B Braun, 75
Beahm Designs, 57, 65, 86
Beckton-Dickinson, co founder of, 108
Bench-top testing, 217
Bentham, Jeremy, 200
Bevel length, 106
BG Sulzle, 110
Bias, 106
Bierce, Ambrose, 3
Biocompatibility
  program, design of, 271, 273
  relative, 21
  test matrix, 27, 28–29
Biocompatibility testing, 22, 267–294
  analytical testing of biomaterials, 290
  biocompatibility data, 269–270
  biological tests methods, 280–290
    acute systemic toxicity, 285
    carcinogenesis bioassay, 288
    cytotoxicity, 280
    genotoxicity, 286
    hemocompatibility, 287
    histopathology services, 290
    implantation tests, 286–287
    irritation tests, 284–285
    pharmacokinetics, 289
    preclinical safety testing, 289–290
    reproductive and developmental toxicity, 288
    sensitization assays, 284
    subchronic toxicity, 285
  design of biocompatibility program, 271–272
  determination of tests needed, 270
  device biocompatibility, 268
  extracts, 272–274
  FDA and EU/ISO requirements, 268–269
  GLP treatment, 271
  material characterization, 291–292
    bulk material characterization, 292
    extractable material characterization, 291–292
    surface characterization, 292
    tests on extracting media, 292
  noncontact devices, 277–280
  sample preparation, 274–277
  testing of device materials or composite of finished device, 270–271
Biomaterials, analytical testing of, 290
Biomaterials Access Assurance Act, 22
Biomedical Modeling, Inc, 190–191

Biopsy needle track placement, 184
Bitmap editing program, 206
Black-and-white cartooning techniques, 206
Blood-borne pathogens, 179
Blood compatibility tests, 287
Blunt dilators, 103
Blunt end, 106
Blunt needles, 99
Body Phantoms, 211
Boedeker Plastics, 30
Bohr, Niels, 6
Bonding (heat), 79
Bone models, 42, 188
The Bone Room, 188–189
Boston Scientific, 68
Bougie tip, 80
Bozeman–Fritsch, 80
Braasch catheter, 80
Braid, 80
BrainLab system, 184
Brevet, 75
Bricolage, 165
Bricoleur, 165
Bridgeport-type knee mills, 134
Brockenbrough needle, 106
Broedel, Max, 201
Bronchoscope, cannibalizing of, 174
Brush catheter, 80
Bulk material characterization, 292
Burke, James, 12
Burr, 106

C

CAD, see Computer-aided design
Cadaver(s)
  history of procurement of in Britain, 200
  tissue, 195
CADCAM Net, 157
CAD/CAM Zone, 157
Calibration Phantoms, 211
Calibre®, 41
CAM systems, see Computer-aided manufacturing systems
Cannuflow® ClearVu™, 176
Cannula, 106
Capture tubes, 59
Carbothane®, 42
Carcinogenesis bioassay, 288
Cardiac device project, 176
Cardiac pacemaker, inventor of, 16
Cardiotech Inc., 42
CARS, see Computer-aided radiology and surgery
CARS Society, see Computer Aided Radiology and Surgery Society
Casting materials, shrinking of, 142
Castle Island Company, 156, 191
Cast nylon, 35
Cataract needle, 106
Catheter, 80
  attaching proximal luer fitting, 74
  -based interventional radiology, father of, 52
  basic accessory in forming, 56
  bonding, 52
  definition of, 67
  design, opportunities for innovative, 68
  drill, punch, 80
  expanding, 52
  flaring, 52
  free blowing, 52
  illustration, 208
  in vitro prototype, 71, 72
  laminating, 52
  necking, 52
  prototypes, 75
  proximal luer fitting, 69
  pull wire, 72
  relay, 69
  steerable, 68, 70
  tipping, 52
  tubes, examples of punched, 64
Catheter assembly, basics of, 67–87
  assembly of proximal steering hub, 77–79
  attaching of balloon to catheter shaft assembly, 76
  attaching of proximal luer fitting, 74–76
  formation of distal tip assembly, 71
  glossary of catheter terms, 79–86
  how catheter is built, 68–70
  joining distal tip assembly and proximal shift, 73
  other ways to tip catheter, 71–72
  punching of air hole for balloon inflation, 73–74
  resources, 86–87
Catheter-forming equipment and operations, 51–65
  automated hole punching, 62–63

balloon dip molds, 63–64
basic forming operations, 52–53, 56–59
    balloon blowing, 57–59
    glass molds, 57
    mandrels, 56–57
    features and user controls, 55–56
        airflow control and airflow gauge, 55–56
        cooling air nozzle, 56
        temperature gauge, 55
        thermal nozzle, 56
    history of development of glass catheter molds, 59–60
    hole punching, 61
    hot-air station, 53–54
    moisture filters, 54–55
    particle filters, 54
    resources, 65
    safety, 55
    slug ejection, 61–62
    types of compressors, 54
CavLab, 191
CBA, see Center for Bits and Atoms
CDRH, see Center for Devices and Radiological Health
Center for Bits and Atoms (CBA), 155
Center for Devices and Radiological Health (CDRH), 241
Centerline Precision, 86
Central venous catheter, 80
Cerebral spinal fluid (CSF), 108
CerLAM™, 128
Certificate for foreign government (CFG), 235
CFA, see Complete Freund's adjuvant
CFG, see Certificate for foreign government
CFR, see Code of Federal Regulations
CGI Corporation, 186
cGMP, see Current good manufacturing practice
Charnley, John, 37
Charrière gauge scale, 92
Chemical characterization, 291, 293
Chemical Inkjet Printer (ChIP), 154
Chevron-Phillips Chemical, 42
Chiba needle, 106
ChIP, see Chemical Inkjet Printer
Chromosomal aberration assay, 286
Chronoflex®, 42
Ciba-Geigy Corporation, 201–202
CIRS, Inc., 211

Clamshell mold, 76, 77
Classical sculptors, 197
ClearVu™ flexible arthroscopic cannula, 175, 177
Clemente Anatomy: A Regional Atlas of the Human Body, 213
Clemente's Anatomy Dissector, 213
Closed-patch test, 284
CMM, see Coordinate measuring machine
CNC machining, see Computer numeric-controlled machining
Coagulation assays, 287
Code of Federal Regulations (CFR), 228, 241–242
    establishment registration, 246
    exemptions from federal preemption, 248
    general requirements, 243
    investigational device exemptions, 250
    in vitro diagnostic products, 248
    labeling, 243
    medical device classification procedures, 262
    medical device recall authority, 249
    medical device reporting, 244
    medical device tracking requirements, 259
    postmarket surveillance, 261
    procedures for performance standards development, 263
    Quality System Regulation, 257
    reports of corrections and removals, 246
    special requirements for devices, 264
Color Atlas of Anatomy, 213
Commodity plastics, 39
Competitive product analysis, 168
Compleat RPML Archives, 157
Complement activation testing, 287
Complete Freund's adjuvant (CFA), 284
Compliance, 80
Compressors, types of, 54
Computed tomography (CT), 128, 166, 211
    reconstruction, 190
    scans, 185
Computer-aided design (CAD), 115
    data, generation of, 115
    model(s)
        surgical approach planning illustration with, 205
        three-dimensional, 167
        orthopedic implant design in, 126

programs, accessory realistic rendering program in, 204
reverse engineering and, 166
sample preparation and, 274
software, 138
systems, digital exchange of information among, 139
Computer-aided manufacturing (CAM) systems, 116
Computer-aided radiology and surgery (CARS), 202
Computer Aided Radiology and Surgery (CARS) Society, 157, 191
Computer numeric-controlled (CNC) machining, 115, 133
 fabricated prototypes, 31
 full-size VMC, 135
 in-house, 134
 milling machines, three-axis, 120
 Roland, 135
 SLA and, 122
 subtractive rapid prototyping and, 116
Computer programs, copyrighted, 166
Connecticut Hypodermics, 110
Continuity, types of, 182
Cooling air nozzle, 56
Coordinate measuring machine (CMM), 185, 186
Cope's needle, 106
Corel Draw®, 173
Corel Painter™, 206
Corrective and preventive action (CPA), 259
Cosmetic laser system, Nd:YAG, 131
CPA, see Corrective and preventive action
Create, definition of, 2
CSA International, 164
CSF, see Cerebral spinal fluid
CT, see Computed tomography
Current good manufacturing practice (cGMP), 257, 269
Curve analysis tools, 181
CYA, see Cyanoacrylate adhesive
Cyanoacrylate adhesive (CYA), 33, 80
Cyberware, Inc., 183, 190
Cycolac®, 40
Cyrex®, 40
Cyro Corporation, 32, 40
Cyrolite®, 40
Cytotoxicity, 280
Czech Technical University department of Cybernetics, 140

D

Danforth Biomedical, 60
DARPA, see Defense Advanced Research Projects Agency
DaVinci, 7
DC, see Direct current
Defense Advanced Research Projects Agency (DARPA), 158
DEHP, see Diethylhexyl phthalate
Delrin, 34, 136
De novo classification, 238
dePezzer, 80
Depth-seeking needle, 99
Dermilaon™, 103
Deschamps' needle, 106
Design
 art and, 6
 definition of, 6
 history record (DHR), 205
 iterative process of, 4
Desktop
 milling machines, makers of, 135
 replacement laptops, 115
DesktopNC.com, 134, 157
Device
 biocompatibility, 268
 master record (DMR), 238
DHR, see Design history record
DICOM, see Digital Imaging and Communications in Medicine
Diethylhexyl phthalate (DEHP), 43
Differential scanning calorimetry, 292
Digital ear impression product, 183
Digital Imaging and Communications in Medicine (DICOM), 181
Digital impression, 146
Digital light processing (DLP), 130
Digitally controlled additive fabrication, 116
Digital Millennium Copyright Act (DMCA), 166
Digitizing, 169
Dilators, 103
Dimethyl sulfide (DMSO), 272
Dip molds, 64
Direct current (DC), 13
Direct manufacturing freedom of creation, 154
Discovery, science and, 4
Disposable Instrument Company, 110–111
Dissections, recording of by Hippocratic Greek physicians, 196

Division of Small Manufacturers, International and Consumer Assistance (DSMICA), 227
DLP, see Digital light processing
DMCA, see Digital Millennium Copyright Act
DMR, see Device master record
DMSO, see Dimethyl sulfide
DNA
  damage, assays for, 286
  model, 145
Dotter, Charles, 52, 80
Dow Chemical, 38, 40, 41, 42
Drainage catheter, 81
Drawing interchange file (DXF), 140, 180
Drew–Smythe catheter, 81
Drucker, Peter, 10–11
Drug-eluting stents, 85
DSMICA, see Division of Small Manufacturers, International and Consumer Assistance
DSM Somos, 122
Dumb objects, 179
DuPont, 34
DXF, see Drawing interchange file
Dymax, Inc., 75, 86
Dyson, Freeman, 17

E

Eagle Stainless, 111
Ear on a mouse, 149
EBM, see Electron Beam Melting
Echotip, 106
Eden PolyJet™ system, 125, 126
Eden™ RP machines, 129–130
Edison, Thomas, 1, 3, 9, 12
EDX, see Energy-dispersive x-ray analysis
Elastomeric plastics, 41
Electron Beam Melting (EBM), 131
Electron Microscopy Services, 111
Emerson, Ralph Waldo, 163
Emulsifying needle, 106
Energy-dispersive x-ray analysis (EDX), 292
English Birmingham wire gauge, 91
Envisiontec GmbH
  Bioplotter®, 150
  Perfactory, 130
EOS, EOSINT machines, 131
EP catheter, 81
EPTFE, see Expanded PTFE
Equilasers, 131

Ergonomic studies, models for, 118
Ethibond™/T i-cron™, 103
Ethilon™, 103
Ethylene vinyl acetate (EVA), 44
Eureka! moment, 4
European suture, 102
EVA, see Ethylene vinyl acetate
Ex-One Corporation ProMetal™ process, 131
Expanded PTFE (EPTFE), 46
Extractable material characterization, 291
Extracting media, 274, 292
Extraction
  conditions, 272, 274
  protocols, 290
Extrusion, 81
Extrusioneering, Inc., 86
Eyeglass lenses, programmable printer for, 153
Eye movements, analysis of, 184

F

Fabbers.com, 157
Fallopio, Gabriello, 198
Faraday, Michael, 5
Farleigh Dickinson, 84
Farlow's Scientific Glassblowing, Inc. (FSG), 57, 59, 65, 86, 211, 212
Faro and Immersion Corporation, 170
FDA, see Food and Drug Administration
FDAMA, see FDA Modernization Act
FDB mission, see Food and Drug Branch mission
FD &C, see Federal Food, Drug and Cosmetics Act
FDM, see Fused deposition modeling
Federal Food, Drug and Cosmetics Act (FD & C), 227, 233, 235
Fenestrations, 81
FEP, see Fluorinated ethylene propylene
File exchange map, 207
Flame retardant (FR), 33
Flared end, 106
Flaring, 81
Flatbed scanner, use of for three-dimensional reconstruction, 173
Fluorinated ethylene propylene (FEP), 35, 38, 73
Fluoropolymers, 37, 52
Foam sheet material, 48

FOC, *see* Freedom of Creation
Fogarty, Thomas, 4, 11
Fogarty catheter, 81
Foley catheter, 82
Food and Drug Administration (FDA), 15, 206, 217
    additional regulations by different states, 235
    authority, 226
    Blue Book Memorandum G95-1, 269
    Center for Biologics Evaluation and Research, 226
    Center for Devices and Radiological Health, 226
    Center for Drug Evaluation and Research, 226
    Center for Food Safety and Applied Nutrition, 226
    Center for Veterinary Medicine, 226
    -compliant materials, 25
    device classification, 229
    device functional classification, 230
    device listing, 228
    Division of Small Manufacturers, International and Consumer Assistance, 227
    establishment registration, 228
    exporting devices, 234
    Export Reform and Enhancement Act, 227
    Federal Food, Drug and Cosmetics Act, 227, 235
    510(k) premarket notification, 230
    importing into U.S., 234
    international regulations, 227
    investigational device exemption, 232
    Medical Device Amendments, 227, 230
    Medical Device User Fee Modernization Act, 227
    Modernization Act (FDAMA), 227
    monitoring of device problem data, 240
    Office of the Commissioner, 226
    Office of Regulatory Affairs, 226, 241
    premarket approval submission, 232
    Quality System Regulation, 225
    reorganization, 227
    requirements for biocompatibility testing, 268
    Safe Medical Devices Act, 227
    Substantial equivalence, 230, 231
    tests for regulation of medical devices, 26
    third-party submission review by accredited parties, 233
Food and Drug Branch (FDB) mission, 235
Food, Drug, and Cosmetic Act, 233
Forensic engineering, 192
Forssmann, Werner, 82
FR, *see* Flame retardant
Freedom of Creation (FOC), 154
Free length, 107
Freeman Manufacturing and Supply, 136, 137
Free-market capitalism, 9
French scale, 82, 90, 92
FSG, *see* Farlow's Scientific Glassblowing, Inc.
Functional freeform fabrication, 158
Fused deposition modeling (FDM), 124, 125

G

Gastroscopes, four-way steering of, 70
Gauge, 107
GCP, *see* Good clinical practice
GE, 40
Gehr Plastics, 32
General Dynamics, 133
Genotoxicity tests, 286
GEO™ Structure Vertebral Body Replacement implants, 127, 146
German Industrial Designers Association, 163
Gibbs CAM, 135
Glass
    molds, catheter tubing formed using, 57
    transition temperature, 55
Glendo Corporation, 95, 96
GLP, *see* Good laboratory practices
Glutaraldehyde sterilant, 179
GMP, *see* Good manufacturing practice
The Golem Project, 158
Good clinical practice (GCP), 241
Good laboratory practices (GLP), 218, 220, 242, 271
Good manufacturing practice (GMP), 57, 96, 227, 235, 240
Gouley's catheter, 82
Graphical Representation and Analysis of Structure Server (GRASS), 144

GRASS, see Graphical Representation and Analysis of Structure Server
Gray's Anatomy, 201
Gray's Anatomy for Students, 214
Greatbach, Wilson, 16
Grit blast, 107
Gruentzig, Andreas, 83
Guidant, 68
Guidewire, 83
Guiding catheter, 83
Guinea pig maximization test, 284
Gutenberg printing press, 3

H

Hagedorn's needles, 107
Hardware store materials, 21
Harvey, William, 198
Hasson cannula, 107
Hasson trocar, 107
Hazlitt, William, 8
HDE, see Humanitarian device exemption
HDPE, see High-density polyethylene
Heat shrink tubing, 41
Helisys Corporation, 127
Hemolysin molecule, 129
Hemolysis assay, 287
Hemostasis valve, 83
HGPRT assay, see Hypoxanthine guanine phosphoribosyl transferase assay
High-density polyethylene (HDPE), 41
High-performance engineering plastics, 23, 30, 35, 46
Histopathology services, 290
Hole forming, types of, 61
Hole punching, automated, 62
Hook burr, 107
Hot-air box, 68
Hot-air station
    airflow control knob, 55
    prototype development, 53
    temperature gauge, 55
Hub, 83, 107
HUD, see Humanitarian use device
Humanitarian device exemption (HDE), 239
Humanitarian use device (HUD), 240
Huntsman Advanced Materials, 122–123
Hydlar®, 35
Hydrophillic, 83
Hydrophobic, 83

Hypodermic needle features, 95
Hypodermic tube vendors, 110
Hypodermic tubing, 91, 94
Hypoxanthine guanine phosphoribosyl transferase (HGPRT) assay, 286

I

IACUC, see Institutional Animal Care and Use Committee
IBM, 133
ID, see Inner diameter
IDE, see Investigational device exemption
IDEO, 165
IFUs, see Instructions for use
IGES, see Initial Graphics Exchange Specification
Image reconstruction, 185
Imaging Phantoms, 211
Immersion Corporation, 190
Implantation tests, 286, 290
Index of CARS Resources, 157
Indexed Visuals (IV), 216
Indwelling catheter, 84
Infrared reflectance spectroscopy, 292
Initial Graphics Exchange Specification (IGES), 139, 180
Initial importer, definition of, 234
Injection molding, 25, 35, 38
Inkjet-style modelers, 116
In-line water trap, 55
Inner diameter (ID), 91, 92
Innovate, definition of, 2
Innovation(s)
    capital and, 15
    definition of, 11
    essential ingredient, 4
Innovation vs. Imitation, 163
Innovator, key skill of, 5
Innovmetric, PolyWorks™, 170–173
Institutional Animal Care and Use Committee (IACUC), 219
Institutional review board (IRB), 233
Instructions for use (IFUs), 209
Insurance reimbursement, 16
Intellectual property, 5, 162, 163
    development, 206
    patents and, 12
International Anti-Counterfeiting Coalition, 164

International Organization of
  Standardization (ISO), 25, 269
  device testing approach, 270
  flowchart, 269
  ISO 9626, 107
  ISO 10993, 275
  materials biocompatibility matrix, 270,
    278–279
International Polymer Engineering, 46
International quality systems, 226
International Society for Computer Aided
  Surgery, 157
International Society for Computer Assisted
  Orthopaedic Surgery, 157, 191
Internet, RP service bureau and, 140
Interpore Cross, 127, 145
Intracutaneous test, 284
Introducer, 84
Intuition, 8
Invent, definition of, 2
Invention
  discovery and, 2
  Edison's rules for, 13
  human clinical need and, 11
Invention, innovation, and creativity, 1–17
  art and design, 6–9
  finding the need, 9–17
  science and discovery, 4–6
Investigational device exemption (IDE),
    220, 227, 232, 239
Investment cast orthopedic implants, 145
Investor presentations, 209
InVision™ multijet modeling, 120
In vitro diagnostic devices, 277
In vivo study, 217, 218, 219
  data collection, 220
  good laboratory practices, 220
  team, 220
IRB, *see* Institutional review board
Irritation tests, 284
ISO, *see* International Organization of
  Standardization
IV, *see* Indexed Visuals

J

Javelin 3D, 128, 185, 190
Jewelry industry, Solidscape systems in, 127
Johnson & Johnson, Ethicon division of, 164
.JPEG file, 204
Judkins catheter, 84

K

Kevlar fiber, 35
Kewanee Oil v. Bicron, 163
Kilgore International, 211
Klöckner Pentaplast, 47
Knife needle, 107
Knowledge for knowledge's sake, 8
Konica Minolta, 183
Kraton®, 42
K-Resin®, 42
Kroemer, Herbert, 17
K-Tube, 111

L

Lab notebook illustrations, 206, 208
Laerdal Corporation, 211
LAL test, *see* Limulus amebocyte lystate
Laminated object modeling (LOM), 127
Lancets, 95, 107
Laserform® material, 137
Laser sintering, 131
Latex, 45
Law of hysteresis, discovery of, 14
LDPE, *see* Low-density polyethylene
LED-based curing wands, 75
Leonardo da Vinci, 197, 199
Lexan®, 32, 41
Ligature needle, 107
Light beam scanners, 183
Limulus amebocyte lystate (LAL) test, 285
Liquid latex, 45
LLNA, *see* Local lymph node assay
Local lymph node assay (LLNA), 284
Locke, John, 2
Loctite, Inc., 33, 75, 86
LOM, *see* Laminated object modeling
Lost-wax casting, 127
Low Cost Eyeglasses, 153
Low-density polyethylene (LDPE), 41
Luer fittings, 84, 87, 108
Lumen, 108
Lustran®, 40

M

Magnetic permeability, 108
Magnetic resonance imaging (MRI), 10, 95,
    134, 166, 185, 190, 211

Magnum®, 38, 40
Malleable, 108
Managed care, 16
Mandrels, 56, 94
Manifold, 84
Marconi, Guglielmo, 14
Marketers, buying decisions and, 7
Markolon®, 41
Massachusetts Institute of Technology patent, 128
Mastercam, 135
Material
   –blood interactions, 287
   characterization, 291
   -mediated pyrogen test, 285
   screening tests, 271
Materialise, 181, 189
Materialise NV, 138–139, 154
Matweb.com, 27
Maya®, 212
McMinn's Color Atlas of Human Anatomy, 214
MDF, *see* Medium-density fiberboard
MDR, *see* Medical device reporting
MDUFMA, *see* Medical Device User Fee Modernization Act
Medical device(s)
   biological evaluation of, 275–276
   cannibalizing of, 173
   categories, 276–277
   designer, responsibility of, 168
   manufacturer, responsibility of, 22–23
   R&D, 1
   recall authority, 249
   reporting (MDR), 227, 234, 244
   where to find, 177
Medical Device Amendments, 227, 230
Medical Device User Fee Modernization Act (MDUFMA), 227
Medical illustration, 193–216
   commercially available resources, 216
   device development, 205–206
   finding and using, 215–216
   history, 196–203
   intellectual property development, 206
   investor presentations, 209
   licensed use vs. buyout, 215
   marketing, physician training, and patient information, 209
   medical-legal, 210

medical teaching and training models, 210–211
   real structures vs., 195
   regulatory, 206
   three-dimensional animation, 212–213
   three-dimensional illustration bookshelf, 213–215
      artistic anatomy, 215
      other books, 214
   types, 203–205
      blue screen trick, 204–205
      layer technique in Photoshop, 204
      rendering from CAD programs, 204
      surgical approach planning, 203–204
      textbook illustration, 203
   value of medical illustration to medical device R&D, 194–196
Medical innovation, occurrence of, 9
Medical malpractice claims, 210
Medical photography, distinction between illustration and, 195
Medical plastics, 19–49
   biocompatibility, 21–22
   biomaterials availability, 22–23
   commodity plastics, 39–41
      ABS, 39–40
      acrylic, 40
      PC/ABS, 40
      polycarbonate, 40–41
      polyethelene, 41
      polyolefin, 41
      styrene, 41
   cross-linked thermoplastics, 25
   definition of medical-grade plastic, 25–27
   definition of polymer, 24
   elastomers, 41–44
      ethylene vinyl acetate, 44
      Kraton, 42
      K-Resin, 42
      Monoprene, 43
      Pebax, 43
      polyurethane, 42
      polyvinylchloride, 43–44
   finding plastics, 27–30
   high-performance engineering plastics for machining, 35–39
      injection molded and extruded plastics, 38–39
      polyetheretherketone, 36
      polyimide rode and sheet, 38

polysulfone and polyphenylsulfone, 37
polytetrafluoroethylene, 36–37
Ultem polyetherimide, 35–36
high-performance engineering plastics for molding, 46
materials performance, 23
plastics for machining, 30
plastics for processing by machining, 31–35
  acetal, 34
  acrylic, 31–32
  acrylonitrile–butadiene–styrene, 31
  fluorinated ethylene propylene, 35
  nylon, 34–35
  polycarbonate, 32–33
  polyethelene, 33–34
  polypropylene, 33
  polyvinylchloride, 32
processability, 23–24
sheet film and foam plastics, 47–48
  foam sheet material, 48
  PET and PETG, 47
  polyester film, 47–48
  polyimide, 48
  PVC and polyethelene film, 47
  resources, 48
  SBR foam and elastic fabric, 48
  Tyvek, 47
thermoplastic and thermosets, 24–25
thermosets, 44–46
  latex, 45–46
  nitrile, 45
  polyisoprene, 44–45
  Santoprene, 44
  silicone, 44
useful specialty plastic material forms, 46–47
  expanded PTFE, 46–47
  extruded PTFE, 46
Medical Resources, 188
Medical Sterile Products, 111
Medium-density fiberboard (MDF), 136
MedLAM™, 128
MEM elution assay, 280
Memry Corporation, 95
Menghini needle, 108
Merit Medical Systems, Inc., 87
Mersilene™/Dacron, 103
Mesh editing, 181
Metal injection molded (MIM) parts, 124

Metal tube drawing methods, 94
Microgroup, 111
Milwaukee School of Engineering, 157
Mimics®, 181
MIM parts, *see* Metal injection molded parts
MJM, *see* Multijet modeling
Model(s)
  animal, 218
  bone, 42, 188
  CAD, 167
  DNA, 145
  ergonomics studies, 118
  parametric, 181
  patient-specific computer analysis, 166
  spine, 169, 170, 172
  stereolithography, 143
  surgical planning, 143
Moisture filters, 54
Mold(s)
  balloon dip, 63
  glass dip, 64
  inserts, 137
  -making services, 137
  plaster splash, 143
  production, 61
  room-temperature vulcanate, 118
  styles of, 60
Molecular modeling, 144
Molybdenum sulfide (MoS), 38
Monofilament Nurlon™, 103
Monoprene®, 43
MoS, *see* Molybdenum sulfide
Mouse micronucleus assays, 286
MRI, *see* Magnetic resonance imaging
Multijet modeling (MJM)), 120
Mylar®, 47

N

National Institutes of Health (NIH), 5
National Library of Medicine, Visible Human Project®, 185, 202
National Sanitation Foundation, 37
NCP, *see* Nonconforming product
NDC, *see* Nitinol Devices Corporation
Nd:YAG cosmetic laser system, 131
Need finding, 10
Needle
  depth-seeking, 99
  design, 90
  grinding fixture, prototype, 98

surface-seeking, 99
types, basic, 97
vendors, 110
Needles and cannulae, introduction to, 89–112
    basic type of suture needle tips, 99
        blunt point, 99
        conventional cutting, 99
        reverse cutting, 99
        side cutting, 99
        taper point, 99
    common hypodermic tubing materials, 94–95
    glossary of needles and related terms, 105–110
    metric and English, 92
    needle gauges and sizes, 90–92
        French catheter size, 92
        gauge size, 91
    R&D needle grinding, 95
    resources, 110–112
        hypodermic tube, needle, and sharps vendors, 110–112
        sharps disposal by mail order, 112
    simple compound needle grinding fixture, 95–97
    suture attachment methods, 101
        channel, 101
        drill, 101
        nonswaged, closed eye, French eye, slit, spring, 101
        swaging sutures to needles, 101
    suture needles, 98–99
    suture sizes, 101–102
    suture types, 102–103
        natural absorbable, 102
        natural nonabsorbable, 102
        synthetic absorbable, 103
        synthetic nonabsorbable, 103
    trocars and dilators, 103–104
        blunt dilators, 103
        plastic sharps and trocars for disposables, 104
        trocars, 103
    working with hypodermic tube, 92–94
Netter, Frank, 7, 201
Netters Atlas of Human Anatomy, 213
New Atlas of Human Anatomy, 214
Nickel–titanium tubing, 94
NIH, *see* National Institutes of Health
Nitinol Devices Corporation (NDC), 95

Nitrile, 45
Nonconforming product (NCP), 259
Noncontact devices, 277
Noncontact light beam scanners, 183
Nonlinear uniform rational B-splines (NURBS), 139, 180
Northview Laboratories, 294
Not substantially equivalent (NSE) products, 238
NovaSom QSG™ system, 132
Noveon Thermedics, 42
Novofil™, 103
NSE products, *see* Not substantially equivalent products
NURBS, *see* Nonlinear uniform rational B-splines
NuSil, 44
Nylon, 34

O

OAL, *see* Overall length
Objet company
    Eden™ RP machines, 129–130
    Polyjet, 129
Obo-Werke GmbH, 137
Obturator, 108
Occupational Safety and Health Organization (OSHA), 55
OD, *see* Outside diameter
OEM, *see* Original equipment manufacturer
Office of Regulatory Affairs (ORA), 241
Olive tipped, 84
Operating system (OS), 115
ORA, *see* Office of Regulatory Affairs
Organogenesis, 148
Original equipment manufacturer (OEM), 176
OS, *see* Operating system
OSHA, *see* Occupational Safety and Health Organization
Outside diameter (OD), 91, 93
Overall length (OAL), 108
Over-the-wire technique, 83

P

Pacific Research Laboratories, 169, 188
Pacing catheter, 84
Packaging materials, 21

Paper laminating process, 128
Paragon Medical, 188
Parametric models, 181
Particle filters, 54
Passivate, 108
Pasteur, Louis, 6
Patent Office, Tesla's patent and, 14
Patents
    intellectual property and, 12
    purpose of, 12
    -specific computer analysis models, 166
    -specific prosthetics, reverse
        engineering and, 166
Pauling, Linus, 17
PC, see Polycarbonate
PC/ABS, 39
PDP, see Product development protocol
PE, see Polyethelene
Pebax®, 38, 43, 84
PEEK, see Polyetheretherketone
PEG, see Polyethylene glycol
PEI, see Polyetherimide
Pellethane®, 42
Pencil point, 108
Penn Engineering Corporation, PEM®
    inserts, 141
Perfluoroalkoxy fluorocarbon (PFA), 36
Peridot, 86
PET, see Polyethylene terephthalate
PETG, see Polyethylene terephthalate glycol
PFA, see Perfluoroalkoxy fluorocarbon
Pharmaceuticals, RP and, 152
Pharmacokinetic (PK) studies, 289
Photopolymers, stereolithography-like, 130
Photoshop, 204
Piezo inkjet, 127
Pin gauge, 94
Pitkin bevel, 108
PK studies, see Pharmacokinetic studies
Plant air, 54
Plaster splash mold, 143
Plastic(s)
    abrasion-resistance, 95
    colored, 30
    commodity, 39
    custom extrusion, 39
    elastomeric, 41
    extrusion from rigid, 38
    finding, 27
    high-performance engineering, 23, 30 35
    injection-molded, 38

    laser sintering of, 131
    medical-grade, 25
    melt temperature, 55
    prototype, 136
    radiation effects on, 49
    shapes for machining, 30
Plato, 9
Plug molding rule, 166
PLY format, 139
PMA, see Premarket approval
PMMA, see Polymethyl methacrylate
Point Technologies, 111
Polyamide, 34
Polycarbonate (PC), 32
    cost-effective alternative to, 40
    performance characteristics, 33
    radiation-stable grades, 33
    radiation sterilization and, 41
    UV cure adhesives and, 40
Polyester film, 47
Polyethelene (PE), 33, 41, 47
Polyether block amide, 84
Polyetheretherketone (PEEK), 23, 36
Polyetherimide (PEI), 23, 46
Polyethylene, 71
Polyethylene glycol (PEG), 272
Polyethylene terephthalate (PET), 47
Polyethylene terephthalate glycol (PETG), 47
Polyface mesh, 180
Polygalactin 910, 103
Polyimide, 48
Polyisoprene, 44
Polymer
    definition of, 24
    thermally stable, 36
Polymer Plastics Corporation, 30, 137
Polymethyl methacrylate (PMMA), 31
Polyolefin, 41
Polypropylene (PP), 33
Polysulfone, 46
    dimensional stability, 37
    engineering resins, 37
    FDA-recognized devices and, 37
Polytetrafluoroethylene (PTFE), 35, 36, 46, 56, 73
Polytrimethylene carbonate, 103
Polyurethane (PU), 42
Polyvinylchloride (PVC), 32, 43, 47
    most commonly used, 32
    unplasticized, 32

Polyvinylidene fluoride (PVDF), 32
PolyWorks, 186
Popper and Sons, 112
Powerpoint™, 204
PP, see Polypropylene
Practical commercialization, 8
Preclinical research, 217–221
    in vitro testing, 218–219
        animal models, 218–219
        project, 219
    in vivo study, 219–221
        data collection, 220
        good laboratory practices, 220–221
        team, 220
    overview, 217–218
Preclinical safety testing, 289
Preclinical studies, purpose of, 242
Preclinical work, most important aspect of, 218
Predicate device, 231
Premarket approval (PMA), 220, 227, 229, 232, 247
Preproduction design validation, 227
Primary skin irritation test, 284
Prodigy Plus™, 120
Product
    acceptance, 167
    development protocol (PDP), 239
    liability, 210
Pro/Engineer™, 138
Professional societies, 191
Programmable logic control, 65
Programmable RP molding, 153
Prolene™, 103
Proof-of-concept prototype, 173
Proof-of-concept work, 134
Prothrombin time assay (PT), 287
Protomed, Inc., 139, 190
Protomold, 138
Prototype
    materials, machinable, 136
    needle grinding fixture, 98
    proof-of-concept, 173
Prototype Magazine, 157
Proximal end, 108
Proximal luer fitting, 74
PT, see Prothrombin time assay
PTFE, see Polytetrafluoroethylene
PU, see Polyurethane
Pushability, 84

PVC, see Polyvinylchloride
PVDF, see Polyvinylidene fluoride

Q

QSIT, see Quality system inspection technique
QSR, see Quality System Regulation
Quality system inspection technique (QSIT), 241
Quality System Regulation (QSR), 233, 235, 240, 257
QuickCast™, 123
Quincke bevel, 108
Quintron, 145
Quosina, 75, 87

R

Radel, 37
Radiation
    cross-linking, 25
    sterilization, 41
Radio frequency (RF)
    ablation device, 173
    electrosurgery, 48
    energy, 90
    interference (RFI), 132
Rapid Prototyping, 156
Rapid prototyping (RP), 113–159, 166
    advantages of, 115
    applications in product design, 131–133
    casting patterns, 142–143
    CNC, 133–135
    cost-saving tips, 140–141
    deciding on best technology, 138
    DLP, 130–131
    FDM, 124–125
    file preparation, 138–139
    full-size VMC CNC machines, 135–136
    in-house RP vs. service bureaus, 119–121
        office-based RP machines, 120–121
        RP service bureaus, 120
    innovative applications of RP, 143–156
        analysis, 152–156
        medical products, 145–146
        pharmaceuticals, 152
        RP and RE combined into product and service, 146–148

surgical planning, 143–144
tissue engineering, 148–152
training models, 144
LOM, 127–128
machinable prototype materials, 136–137
other file formats, 139–140
overview, 114–116
panels, stereolithography, 132
parts, 133
   electroplating, 141
   machining, 141
   painting, 141
   threaded inserts, 141
Polyjet Objet printer, 129–130
rapid tooling and molding, 137–138
resolution and surface finish, 125–126
resources, 156–158
   in-print and online resources, 156–157
   professional societies and resources, 157–158
reverse engineering, 143
service bureaus, 120, 140
sintering and direct metal, 131
SLS, 123–124
Solidscape, 127
Sony SCS, 123
stereo lithography materials, 122–123
technology(ies), 116–119
   adaptation of, 148
   choice of, 119
   off-patent, 118
   strengths and limitations, 138
three-dimensional printing, 128–129
tooling, advantage to, 137
types of available RP technologies, 121
universities and organizations, 158–159
UV cure sealing to foam parts, 142
Rapid Prototyping Mailing List (RPML), 157
Rapid tooling and molding, 137
R&D needle grinding, 95
RE, *see* Reverse engineering
Reference Phantoms, 211
Regulatory affairs, 223–266
   abbreviations, 265–266
      international and national standard abbreviations, 265
      regulatory abbreviations, 265–266

basics, 228–236
   additional regulations by different states, 235–236
   device classification, 229–230
   device functional classification, 230
   device listing, 228–229
   establishment registration, 228
   exporting devices, 234–235
   510(k) premarket notification, 230–231
   importing into U.S., 234
   investigational device exemption and supporting studies, 232–233
   premarket approval submission, 232
   substantial equivalence, 231
   third-party submission review by accredited parties, 233–234
cost-effective, 225
device safety and effectiveness, 225
FDA overview and authority, 226–228
   jurisdiction acts, history, and assistance, 227
   online assistance, 227–228
good judgment, 226
good quality and procedural practices, 240–242
   good clinical practice, 241–242
   good laboratory practices, 242
   preclinical studies, 242
   quality system inspection technique, 241
   Quality System Regulation, 240–241
law enforcement, 225
special considerations, 236–240
   abbreviated 510(k), 238–239
   exemptions from 510(k) and GMP requirements, 236–237
   humanitarian use device/humanitarian device exemption, 239–240
   product development protocol, 239
   special 510(k), 237
Title 21 of CFR for medical devices, 243–265
   establishment registration, 246–248
   exemptions from federal preemption, 248
   general requirements, 243
   investigational device exemptions, 250–257

in vitro diagnostic products for
  human use, 248–249
labeling, 243–244
medical device classification
  procedures, 262–263
medical device recall authority,
  249–250
medical device reporting, 244–245
medical device tracking
  requirements, 259–261
postmarket surveillance, 261–262
procedures for performance
  standards development,
  263–264
Quality System Regulation, 257–259
reports of corrections and removals,
  246
Relay catheter, 69, 86
Repliform company, 137
Reproductive and developmental toxicity,
  288
Research, publicly funded, 5
Return on investment (ROI), 212
Reverdin's needle, 109
Reverse cutting needles, 99
Reverse engineering (RE), 114, 115,
  161–192
  abuse of, 164
  case example, 176–177
  case study, 174–176
  categories of, 168
  competitive analysis and, 187
  continuity, 181–185
    arm probe noncontact scanners, 185
    arm probe scanners, 184
    automated touch probe, 183
    light beam scanners, 183–184
    three-dimensional image
      reconstruction, 185
  destructive, 186
  inspection, 186
  methods, 169–174
    cannibalizing existing device,
      173–174
    digitizing, 169–173
    using flatbed scanner for three-
      dimensional reconstruction, 173
  resources, 187–192
    bones and bone models, 188–189
    MRI and CT reconstruction and RP
      modeling, 190

professional societies and resources,
  191–192
three-dimensional capture
  equipment, 190
three-dimensional scanning and
  manufacturing inspection, 191
three-dimensional services bureaus,
  190
three-dimensional software,
  189–190
used and reconditioned medical
  equipment vendors, 187–188
reverse modeling, radiology, and
  surgical planning, 186–187
Supreme Court and, 162
three-dimensional reconstruction,
  179–181
value of reverse engineering in patient
  care, 167–168
where to find medical devices and
  equipment, 177–179
Reverse modeling, 163
  development of in toy industry, 170
  rapid prototyping and, 116
RF, *see* Radio frequency
RFI, *see* Radio frequency interference
Rhino®, 138, 169, 171
Risk-based classification, 238
Rodin, Auguste, 3
ROI, *see* Return on investment
Roland, desktop CNC machines, 135
Room-temperature vulcanate (RTV), 44
  molds, 118, 127
  silicone rubber, 142
RP, *see* Rapid prototyping
RPML, *see* Rapid Prototyping Mailing List
RTV, *see* Room-temperature vulcanate
Ryton, 38

S

Safe Medical Devices Act, 227
SAN, *see* Styrene–acrylonitrile copolymer
SBCs, *see* Styrene–butadiene rubber
  copolymers
SBR, *see* Styrene butadiene rubber
Scanning electron microscopy (SEM), 292
SCS, *see* Solid Creation System
SE, *see* Substantial equivalence
Seldinger technique, 84, 109

Index

Selective laser sintering (SLS), 123
    advantage of, 124
    metal parts, 124
SEM, *see* Scanning electron microscopy
Sensitization assays, 284
Service bureaus, 119
Sharps
    disposal, mail order, 112
    vendors, 110
Shimadzu Biotech, Chemical Inkjet Printer, 154
Shop air, 54
Side-cutting needles, 99
Side port, 109
Sigmoidoscopes, four-way steering of, 70
Silicone, 44
Silicon Graphics, 180
Silicon Valley success story, 83
Silverman needle, 109
Simplant, 181, 185
Simpson, John, 16, 85
Simulab, 211
Sirona Dental GmbH Cerec® system, 146, 147, 166
Skived holes, 61, 62, 63, 73
SLA, *see* Stereolithography apparatus
Sleep Solutions, Inc., 132
SLS, *see* Selective laser sintering
Slug ejection, hole punching and, 61, 62
Small Parts, Inc., 86
SME, *see* Society of Manufacturing Engineers
Snow, C.P., 7
Society of Manufacturing Engineers (SME), 158, 191
Sofamor Danek, counter-torque surgical instrument, 125
Softimage®, 212
Software, three-dimensional, 189
Solid Creation System (SCS), 121, 123
Solid freeform fabrication, 158
Solidica, 131
Solidscape, 120, 127
Solidscape, Inc., ModelMaker™ RP systems, 145
SolidWorks™, 138
Solvay Advanced Polymers, 37
SOMSO Models, 210
Sones, Mason, 85
Sony Solid Creation System, 123
Special 510(k) submission, 237

Specialty plastic material forms, 46
Spine model, 169, 170, 172
SRP, *see* Subtractive rapid prototyping
Stainless steel tubing, 90
Standard for the Exchange of Product Mode Data (STEP), 140, 180
Stanford triangle format, 139
Staywell/Krames Communications, 214
Steerable catheter, 68, 70, 85
Steinmetz, Charles, 14
Stent delivery catheter, 85
STEP, *see* Standard for the Exchange of Product Mode Data
Stereolithography
    apparatus (SLA), 121
    cost of, 140
    master, production of, 132
    parts, sensitivity of, 122
    materials, 122
    models, 143
    parts, *in vitro* testing using, 123
    UV laser in, 121
.STL file, 139
Stokes, Donald E., 6
Stopcock, 85
Stop needle, 109
Stratasys corporation, 120, 124, 138
Stubs iron wire gauge, 91
Stylet, 109
Styrene, 41
    –acrylonitrile copolymer (SAN), 39
    butadiene rubber (SBR), 48
    –butadiene rubber copolymers (SBCs), 42
Subchronic toxicity, test for, 285
Substantial equivalence (SE), 230, 231
Subtractive rapid prototyping (SRP), 116, 117, 135
Surface area calculation, formulas for, 275
Surface characterization, 292
Surface-seeking needle, 99
Surfcam, 135
Surgeons, resistance of to unfamiliar, 176
Surgical planning, RP and, 143
Surgical ratchet, polycarbonate FDM and Polyjet parts in, 125, 126
SurgiGuide®, 185
Surgilon™ braided, 103
Suture
    attachment methods, 101
    European, 102

needle(s), 98, 102
    identification chart, 100
    types, basic types of, 99
    sizes, 101
    types, 102–103
Swaged needle, 109
Swaging, 109
Swan–Ganz, 85
Synbone®, 42
Synthetic rubber, 44

T

Taeus International, 187
Taper-point needle, 99
Technical Innovations, 61, 65, 73
Technology
    -driven products, appeal of, 10
    hacking of existing, 165
Tecoflex®, 42
Tecophillic®, 42
Tecothane®, 42
Teflon, 36
Teknor Apex Company, 43
Tesla, Nikolai, 13
Test turnaround time, 281–283
Tetrafluoroethylene (TFE), 35
Texas Instruments DLP technology, 130
Texloc Corporation, 41
Textbook illustration, 203
TFE, see Tetrafluoroethylene
TGA, see Thermogravimetric analysis
Therics Corporation, 152
Thermal nozzle, 56
Thermodilution catheter, 85
Thermogravimetric analysis (TGA), 292
Thermoplastic(s), 24
    cross-linked, 25
    elastomers (TPEs), 38, 41
    vulcanizate (TPV), 44
Thermosets
    examples of, 24
    shaping of, 25
Thorascopic approach planning illustration, 205
Three-dimensional animation, 212
Three-dimensional capture
    equipment, 190
    file formats
        DXF, 180
        IGES, 180
        PLY, 180
        STEP, 180
        VRML, 180
    methods of, 182
Three-dimensional image reconstruction, 185
Three-dimensional printing, 128
Three-dimensional reconstruction, 173, 179, 182
Three-dimensional scanning
    manufacturing inspection and, 191
    medical applications of, 183
Three-dimensional service bureaus, 190
Three-dimensional software, 189
Three-phase power, invention of, 14
Thrombogenicity, most common test for, 287
Time Compression Technologies, 157
Tip-forming machine, automated, 57
Tipping, 68, 71, 85
Tissue ablation, radio frequency energy for, 90
Tissue engineering, 118–119
    plotting materials, 151
    RP and, 148
Torqueability, 85
Total hip arthroplasty, 37
Touch probe scanner, 170
Toy(s)
    industry, reverse modeling in, 170
    popular material for molding, 41
TPEs, see Thermoplastic elastomers
TPV, see Thermoplastic vulcanizate
Trackability, 85
Trade secret, 164
Training models, RP and, 144
Translational Research Initiative (TRI), 5
Transseptal needle, 109
Trephine, 109
TRI, see Translational Research Initiative
Triple grind, 109
Trocars, 103, 109
Tuhoy–Borst valve, 83, 85
Tygon®, 43
Tyvek, 47

U

Udel®, 37
UDS, see Unscheduled DNA synthesis

UHMWPE, *see* Ultra-high-molecular-weight polyethelene
UL, *see* Underwriters Laboratories
Ultem, 23, 35, 46
Ultra-high-molecular-weight polyethelene (UHMWPE), 24, 33
Underwriters Laboratories (UL), 36
United Endoscopy, 187–188
Units conversion chart, 93
Unscheduled DNA synthesis (UDS), 286
Used equipment dealers, 178
Used medical equipment vendors, 187
User's Guide to Rapid Prototyping, 157
USP, *see* U.S. Pharmacoepia
U.S. patent library, online, 164
U.S. Pharmacoepia (USP), 21, 25, 101, 269
   elastomeric closures for injections, 275
   physicochemical tests, 291
   responsibility of, 26
   test methods, 26
UV cure
   adhesive, 69, 75, 86
   bonding, 32
   sealing, foam parts, 142

V

Valley of death, 10
Value Plastics, 75
Vascular closure device concept sketch, 208
Vascular highway, delivery therapies via, 67–68
Vascular system, modeling of, 186
Venture Manufacturing, 68
Venus Di Milo, 197
Veress needle, 110
Versaflex®, 42
Vertebrated catheter, 86
Vertical machining centers (VMCs), 135
Vesalius, Andreas, 7, 197–198, 199
Vespel, 38
VG Studio Max, 189
Victrex plc, 36
Video game characters, 184
Virtual reality modeling format (VRML), 139, 180
VisionTrak, 184
Vital Images, Inc., 189–190
Vita Needle Company, 112
VMCs, *see* Vertical machining centers
VRML, *see* Virtual reality modeling format

W

Westinghouse, George, 14
Westlake Plastics, 34
Wetsuit material, 48
Whittemore Enterprises, Inc., 187
Whole-body scanning, 183–184
Whole RP Family Tree, 157
Wilde, Oscar, 8
Wohler's Report, 156
Wright-Patterson Air Force Base, CNC machining and, 133

X

Xerox® copier technology, 148

Z

Z Corporation, 120
   three-dimensional printers, 128, 138, 144
   Z-cast process, 129
Zelux®, 41
Ziegler–Natta vinyl polymerization reaction, 44–45

R
856.15
.M43

2006